AF327401

OTHER MONOGRAPHS IN THE SERIES,
MAJOR PROBLEMS IN PATHOLOGY:

Published

Evans & Cruickshank: *Epithelial Tumours of the Salivary Glands*

Forthcoming

Beckwith and D'Angio: *Renal Tumors in Infants and Children* — to be published 1971.

Hartsock: *Diagnostic Histopathology of Lymph Nodes* — to be published 1973.

Melnick: *Histochemistry Applied to Pathology* — to be published 1972.

Sagebiel: *Histopathologic Diagnosis of Melanotic Lesions of Skin* — to be published 1972.

Striker and Cutler: *Use and Interpretation of Renal Biopsy* — to be published 1972.

Warner: *Gonadal Stromal Tumors of the Male and Female* — to be published 1973.

1. Ulcerative colitis. Mucosal view of furrows of ulceration (A) between edematous pseudopolypoid mucosa (B) of the descending colon. Cross section through the wall (C) reveals the superficial location of the inflammation and the absence of thickening of the wall.

2. Ulcerative colitis. Alcian blue–PAS stain of a crypt abscess revealing necrosis of the epithelium of the tip of the crypt of Lieberkühn (A) and a streamer of pus extending from the lamina propria into the gland lumen (B). Decreased mucus secretion is seen in the involved gland (C). × 100.

3. Ulcerative colitis. Reticulum stain. Adjacent section to that just shown, **2**, reveals unaltered reticulin fibers adjacent to the base of necrotic epithelium. × 100.

4. Regional enteritis. Terminal ileum is shown with thickened fibrous wall with inflammatory and proliferative changes involving all layers from the mucosa to the serosa (A). A "stony brook" appearance of the ulcerated mucosa is seen (B). The mesentery is short, thick, and retracted (C), sharply angulating the loop of intestine, and adipose tissue extends onto the wall of the intestine (D). The diameter of the ileocecal valve (E) is decreased.

5. Regional enteritis. A patch of enlarged histiocytes (A) and a giant cell (B) is surrounded by a rim of lymphocytes and plasma cells (C). Necrosis is not a feature of the lesion. × 100.

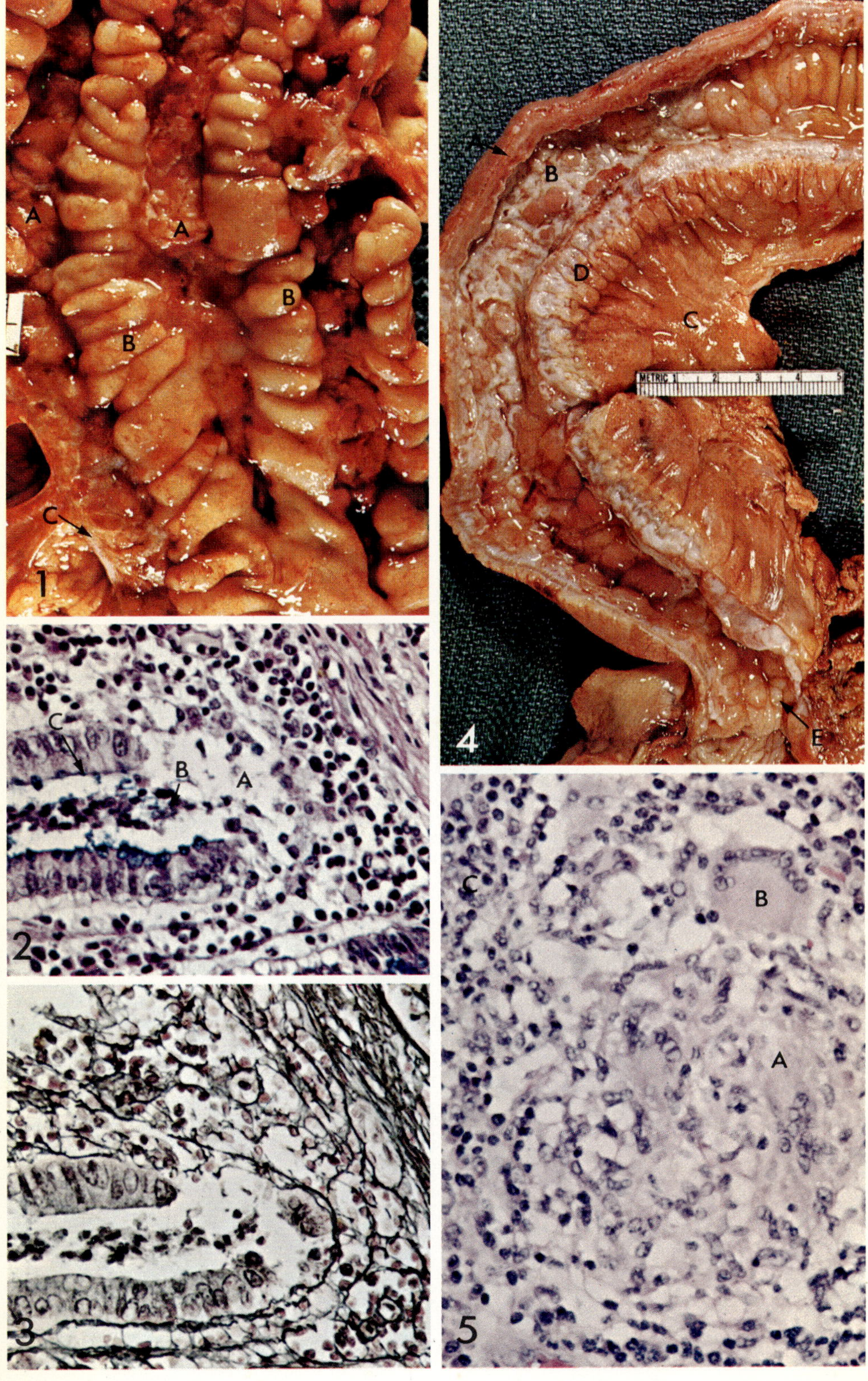

N. KARLE MOTTET, M.D.

Professor of Pathology, University of Washington
School of Medicine, and Director of Hospital Pathology,
University Hospital, University of Washington

HISTOPATHOLOGIC SPECTRUM OF REGIONAL ENTERITIS AND ULCERATIVE COLITIS

Volume II in the Series
MAJOR PROBLEMS IN PATHOLOGY
JAMES L. BENNINGTON, M.D., *Consulting Editor*
Chairman, Department of Pathology
Children's Hospital of San Francisco
San Francisco, California

W. B. Saunders Company, Philadelphia, London, Toronto, 1971

W. B. Saunders Company: West Washington Square
                         Philadelphia, Pa. 19105

                         12 Dyott Street
                         London, WC1A   1DB

                         1835 Yonge Street
                         Toronto 7, Ontario

Histopathologic Spectrum of Regional Enteritis and Ulcerative Colitis

SBN 0-7216-6570-5

Print No.:   9   8   7   6   5   4   3   2   1

To

HERBERT L. EASTLICK, Ph.D.
INSPIRING SCIENTIST AND TEACHER

who introduced me to the wonders of microscopy

EDITOR'S FOREWORD

For more than a century the diagnosis of ulcerative colitis included not only the disease now recognized by that name but also a host of other inflammatory conditions of the intestine. Among the last of the disorders to be distinguished from ulcerative colitis was regional enteritis of the small intestine. Unfortunately the idea then became firmly entrenched that regional enteritis occurred only in the small intestine while ulcerative colitis was limited to the colon.

Only in the past ten years has it been recognized that both regional enteritis and ulcerative colitis can occur on either side of the ileocecal valve; and considerable overlap often exists in the clinical as well as the pathologic features of these diseases.

Initially we failed to recognize that differences existed between regional enteritis and ulcerative colitis and in our ignorance were unable to distinguish between them. With increased knowledge we have been able to establish criteria which allow us to make a definite diagnosis in the majority of cases. The fact that it is not always possible to distinguish between ulcerative colitis and regional enteritis brings us almost full circle in our attempts to classify these two intestinal diseases.

In the absence of any known etiologic agents, efforts to differentiate between regional enteritis and ulcerative colitis have been based largely on clinical characteristics. This monograph, by a superb pathologist and long-time student of intestinal diseases, is a first attempt to approach the subject and to classify these diseases with the pathophysiologic process as the central theme.

Whether one attempts to classify these diseases by the clinical or pathologic features, it is essential that the criteria used must be clearly defined and consistently employed. Kirsner* has aptly observed that "Unless methods of study and criteria are made reasonably uniform, we may expect continuing uncertainty about the true incidence and

---

*Kirsner, J. B.: Ulcerative Colitis: "Puzzles Within Puzzles," New Eng. J. Med. *282*: 625–627, 1970.

distribution of ulcerative and granulomatous colitis, their independence and interrelationship and their clinical implications."

Dr. Mottet's exhaustive study on the morphologic findings of regional enteritis and ulcerative colitis will interest all who must deal with inflammatory diseases of the intestine and should serve admirably as a basis for case selection analysis by the clinical investigator.

JAMES L. BENNINGTON, M.D.

PREFACE

This book was written to fulfill the need for an up-to-date review of two major intestinal diseases from the vantage point of pathogenetic process. In so doing I have placed morphologic findings in principal focus and juxtaposed selected aspects of the natural history and clinical management of the diseases to make the morphologic observations more meaningful.

If I have achieved my goal, then this book should prove to be as useful a manual for the pathologist faced with the problem of diagnosing intestinal inflammatory disease as for the clinical investigator in establishing a basis for case selection and analysis. This approach demands extensive illustration; the accompanying figures have been selected to complement rather than reiterate the written word. Regional enteritis and ulcerative colitis are being diagnosed with increasing frequency throughout the world. If my efforts and approach serve to stimulate and enhance research on these problems, then I shall have been rewarded in full measure.

No previous book on the subject has utilized pathologic process as a central theme; several excellent ones have been written that have clinical features, clinical classification, and surgical or medical management as a central theme. Noteworthy among these are the clinical experiences of B. B. Crohn and H. Yarnis, who published *Regional Enteritis* (Second Edition, Grune and Stratton, New York, 1958) more than a decade ago, and a more recent book by J. C. Goligher, F. T. de Dombal, J. McK. Watts, and G. Watkinson entitled *Ulcerative Colitis* (Bailliere, Tindall & Cassell, Ltd., London, 1968). No attempt to reiterate their clinical perspective will be made here.

To break new ground in the organization of concepts entails an immense amount of work that is not apparent to the reader. There are no guidelines or time-proved organizational patterns to follow. If my approach proves to be suboptimal, but still stimulates others to pursue a more lucid analysis, then, again, I shall have been rewarded in full.

A massive literature has accumulated on the subject, especially its clinical aspects. This reflects, in part, the concern the medical profession has for the problem and the frustration it experiences in managing these protracted and debilitating illnesses. I reviewed the more than two thousand articles published in the past decade, but included only a small percentage of them in my reference lists. I am indebted to the National Library of Medicine and its MEDLARS system of information retrieval. This, plus the extensive efforts of Mr. Ralph Body, assisted by Mrs. S. P. Hammar, helped immeasurably in the preparation of my file of references and reprints. However, to keep the text readable I necessarily used references selectively based on the nature of the subject matter. Those aspects of the disease processes that are well established and on which general agreement exists have been documented with a few key references of top quality. Other aspects that are currently being explored are documented with more extensive references to the literature. It is my hope that this will ease the efforts of investigators in compiling data from the literature on selective facets of the problem. In either situation the references that are the best keys to the literature on a particular subject are included. My aim has been to evaluate and present the distilled essence of studies of the pathologic process rather than to catalog all the investigations. A risk inherent in this approach is unwittingly to insert my own particular bias. With few exceptions I have eliminated clinical studies lacking histopathologic confirmation — not intending to demean the importance of careful clinical observation, but because to have done otherwise would have contradicted the central approach of the text.

To accomplish this difficult task many people furnished invaluable assistance. Many of my professional colleagues, among them Professor John H. Yardley of the Johns Hopkins University School of Medicine, Doctor B. C. Morson of St. Mark's Hospital, London, Doctor H. Thomas Norris, of the University of Washington Medical School, and others, have provided illustrations and constructive criticism. In addition to diligently developing and double checking the bibliography, Mr. Bōdy, Chief Research Technician in my laboratory, also served as general coordinator of the efforts of the several participants. The photographic expertise of Mr. Johsel Namkung, Senior Medical Science Photographer, University of Washington, added much to the artistic quality of the illustrations. My secretaries, Mrs. K. Bishop and Mrs. J. B. Lawrence, typed the manuscript. Much credit is due the W. B. Saunders Company and its editor, Mr. Michael Jackson, who allowed me complete freedom to organize and present the subject in whatever manner I deemed best. My wife Nancy also worked diligently typing and editing drafts of the manuscript, obtaining permission for reproduction of illustrations, and doing the general secretarial work. She and my children patiently endured my at least inconvenient, often unpleasant, preoccupation with the preparation of this book over a period of three years. To all these and many others I am indeed deeply grateful.

N. KARLE MOTTET, M.D.

CONTENTS

Chapter Ten

Mixed Forms of Regional Enteritis and Ulcerative Colitis... 236

Chapter One

Natural History of Regional Enteritis

DEFINITION AND CLASSIFICATION

Regional enteritis is a granulomatous inflammatory process usually involving the terminal ileum and frequently involving other portions of the intestinal tract (Frontispiece, Fig. 1–1.). Secondary lesions are occasionally found in the lymph nodes, liver, skin, and joints. The principal and initial cellular reaction is a panhyperplasia of the perilymphatic histiocytes in all layers of the intestinal wall from the lamina propria to the serosa as well as the lymphatics and lymph nodes of the mesentery. The initial reaction in the intestinal tube is transmural regardless of its location in the tube and is frequently associated with lymphedema and infiltration with acute and chronic inflammatory cells. Later in the course of the disease the histiocytes may form giant cells and dense noncaseating granulomas resembling sarcoid. Ulceration of the mucosa usually occurs, and rarely, pus streamers may be seen in the crypts of Lieberkühn.

Implicit in this definition is its classification on the basis of pathologic process, rather than etiologic agent, of which none is known. Pathologic process is the biologic attempt of an individual to reestablish homeostasis with his environment. Quite naturally one might expect a wide variety of individual responses based on the innate variability of the individuals involved. Indeed, in some instances the response to one disease may be indistinguishable from the response to others. Some investigators of gastrointestinal disease have become overly concerned with the diversity of the process and the overlap of features between several different entities. Some have attempted to modify the definition of a disease entity to include some or all of the divergent individual responses. This has led to confusion of the identity of the disease process, and misplaced emphasis. The definition just

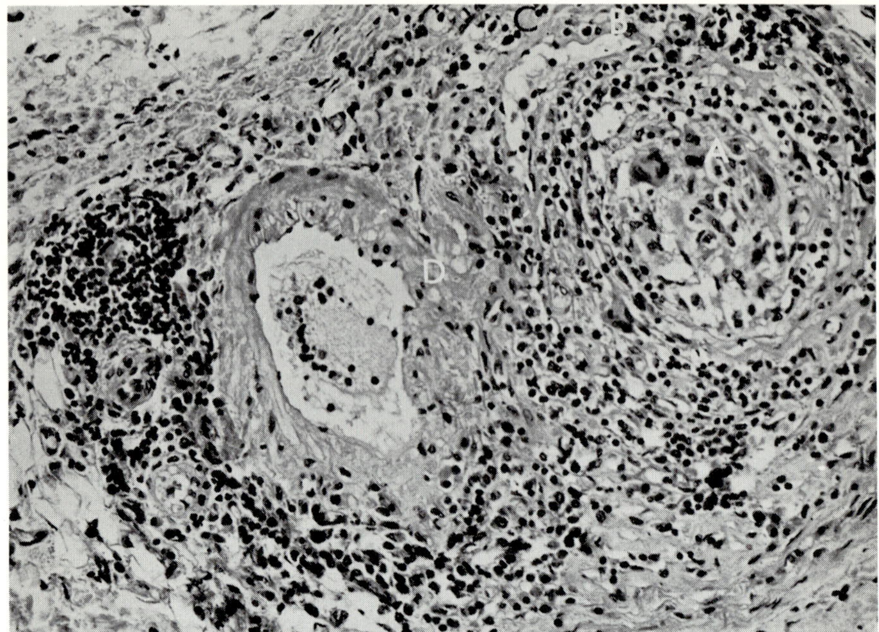

Figure 1–1   A characteristic microscopic lesion of regional enteritis consisting of a loose patch of histiocytes (A) and often including giant histiocytes surrounded by small mononuclear cells, principally lymphocytes and plasma cells (B). This lesion is located, as commonly seen, adjacent to a distended lymphatic (C) that is perivascular (D). ×64.

given is essentially a modal one and is designed to cover the vast majority of cases, recognizing that some features in individual cases vary from it. It identifies the major feature of the reaction to be proliferative and the principal cells involved to be histiocytes, particulary those adjacent to the lymphatics. Other features of the response are secondary to this one.

This classification is based on pathogenetic process rather than on etiologic, anatomic, or clinical features. The structural and functional characteristics of a pathogenetic process are the product of a dynamic interaction between an individual and his environment in an attempt to re-establish homeostasis. (Conceptually, the individual as an open system has two principal characteristics—it is inseparable from, and constantly interacts with, its external environment, and it cannot maintain a unique stationary level.) Therefore, there is an infinite variety of "normal" homeostatic patterns, all of which have in common the constancy of change. For example, in regional enteritis the characteristic features of the process in an individual may be modified by numerous factors, both intrinsic (age, sex, race, psyche, embryogenetic characteristics) and extrinsic (dietary habits, climate, bacterial flora, mechanical trauma, ionizing radiation, parasites). Because of the variability, some features may overlap with those of other intestinal diseases, and occasionally several or many features overlap, causing nosologic confusion. This should not, however, detract from the validity and utility of the pathogenetic approach. It provides both the most reliable basis for case analysis and statistics and for the development of experimental animal models.

TERMINOLOGY

In view of this variability, it is not surprising that a multiplicity of terms has been applied to regional enteritis. When Crohn and his co-workers made their seminal contribution by presenting 14 cases of the entity, they called it terminal ileitis.[1] It seemed appropriate for the initial cases reported because in each the lesion was limited to the terminal ileum. However, subsequent investigations have led to recognition that the lesion involves more than the terminal ileum in a large percentage of cases; therefore, most prefer the term regional enteritis. Others, wishing to emphasize the predominant pathologic feature of the process, have called it cicatrizing or sclerosing enteritis. Still others, wishing to indicate that it frequently involves the colon as well, have used the term regional enterocolitis. The eponym, Crohn's disease, has been applied to the process, predominantly in Great Britain. The main justification for using the eponym is that as long as the etiology remains unknown it is best to remain noncommittal. I prefer the broad anatomic term for the disease because it is easier for students to remember and to associate the pathologic process with a clinical picture; thus is less prone to confusion. Segmental enteritis and various combinations and permutations of the foregoing terms have been used by various authors; others that have been used occasionally are ileojejunitis, ileocolitis, segmental enteritis, chronic ulcerative enteritis, and terminal ileitis.

HISTORY

Because regional enteritis has such distinctive gross features, it would seem likely that an astute observer like Morgagni (1682–1771), Professor of Anatomy at Padua, having a vast experience in postmortem examination, would have clearly identified the lesion. I have carefully reviewed Book III, "Diseases of the Belly," of his monumental work *The Seats and Causes of Diseases*, translated into English in 1769 by Benjamin Alexander.[2] In his dissertation, Letter 32, on "Treats of Costiveness and of the Piles," he began with discussions of imperforate anus, intestinal atresia, and fistula. Article 5 begins as follows:

But, although this kind of disorder [obstruction] may sometimes be cured, even when there seems scarcely any hope of cure, many of them are, nevertheless, absolutely incurable, as when there is an occlusion, or adstriction, in some of the higher intestines, of which you have instances not only here in the Sepulchretum, but will also have other instances from me, at other times. And to these you will add, not only the large fleshy excrescence, said in the preceding letter to have been found within the colon by Cortesius, but also the scirrhous ring, made up of glands, which the celebrated Haaseus found in the same place, and which left a foramen scarcely sufficient to admit a slender probe; and, in like manner, the callus of the same intestine which was almost cartilagenous, and which the celebrated Christian Wenckler described, from the observation of his brother, as rendering the tube, in that part, extremely narrow.*

Though Morgagni's description here might refer to regional enteritis, he did not identify the location as the small intestine, but only as "some of the higher intestines." "Large fleshy excrescence," "scirrhous ring made up of glands," and "callus almost cartilagenous" seem more likely to describe a neoplasm producing a "napkin ring" stricture of the colon. Regional enteritis involving a segment of the colon cannot be ruled out as a possible cause of the lesion he described, but certainly he did not describe it as a distinctive entity. In Article 6 of the same letter he recounts a colleague's observations on a similar case.

Ruysch in his "Observations Anatomico-Surgical" and likewise in his "Adversaria" describes it under the name of "a scirrhous thickening and surprising coarctation of the rectum, that is to say, with its coats almost exceeding the thickness of an inch and so much indurated that he was in doubt whether to call them cartilagenous or fleshy . . . !"†

A more likely description of regional enteritis was included in Letter 34, "Treats of Pain in the Intestines." After discussing various types of hernia and diverticula (including Meckel's) he then discussed the causes of pain in the intestine in which "the cause lay entirely hid within the body," and presented descriptions of gangrene of the intestines, ruptured appendicitis, intussusception, and intestinal parasites. In Article 35 of this letter, while discussing some causes of small intestinal obstruction, Morgagni also stated, "And the obstructing causes often relate to the coats of some intestine, as, for instance that scirrhous ring spoken of in the thirty-second letter." He did not present a case description at this point; however, in Letter 35, "Concludes the Discourse upon Pains of the Intestines," Article 6 presents a case with autopsy that is rather characteristic of intestinal tuberculosis, and Article 10 more closely describes regional enteritis in "a running footman." Morgagni describes the autopsy abdominal findings as follows:

These and the other parts of the small intestines, were, in some places, extremely narrow, and, at the same time, brown, but in other places red, even

---

*Giovanni Battista Morgagni: *De Sedibus et Causis Morborum (The Seats and Causes of Diseases).* Translated by Dr. Benjamin Alexander. Facsimile of 1769 edition, New York, Hafner Publishing Company, 1960, p. 99.

†Ibid., p. 101.

the smallest vessels being so much distended from the stagnant blood, that it almost seemed as if they had been filled with an injection of red wax. And the same appearance was seen in several parts of the large intestine but especially the beginning of the colon.*

Though Morgagni had the uncanny ability to distinguish between many kinds of intestinal diseases, it is not certain from these descriptions that he actually recognized the lesions of regional enteritis as a separate entity. In 1822, William Cooke translated and edited *The Seats and Causes of Diseases*.[3] He extensively indexed, cross-referenced, and organized the autopsy findings of Morgagni on the basis of organ systems. Volume Two begins with a discussion and some editorial interpretations of Morgagni's intestinal findings (pages 45 to 165). I was unable to find any case reports that more clearly identify regional enteritis than those already cited. It seems to me that Morgagni, without the aid of a microscope, was unable to distinguish with certainty between the lesions of scirrhous carcinoma, diverticulitis, and some granulomatous inflammations of the small intestine, though it seems probable that he suspected the differences.

Dr. William Saunders informed the Royal College of Physicians, in 1813, of a case, one of a young man who had been "nervous, delicate, and troubled with costiveness and quick pulse for many years," in which the autopsy was done by Dr. Charles Combe in 1806 in the presence of Dr. Saunders.[4] In addition to the general findings of severe emaciation and unremarkable liver, spleen, kidneys, and upper gastrointestinal tract he noted the following:

The lower part of the ileum as far as the colon was contracted, for the space of three feet, to the size of a turkey's quill. The colon had three constrictions, one about three inches long at a distance of seven inches from the cecum, a second about one inch long at a distance of four inches from the former, and a third not quite half an inch long at a distance of three inches from the last. . . . Wherever the intestines were constricted, the coats were very much thickened, and exhibited an appearance of inflammation; while the blood vessels, passing through the mesentery of the intestines, were enlarged.[4]

They speculate on the mechanism as follows:

Though the lacteals were distributed to the whole of the intestines, they are most numerous about the ileum, and we believe nearly all the chyle is absorbed before the food reaches the colon. In proportion as the coats of the intestines thicken, the absorbent power of the lacteals is diminished, and in the constricted part of the ileum in this case we believe the absorbent powers of the lacteals was totally destroyed.[4]

A more recent case reported by Dr. John Abercrombie in 1828, though having some superficial features of the pathologic lesion that

---

*Ibid., p. 169.

resembles regional enteritis, more likely represents the description of bacillary dysentery or another infectious process.[5] It is interesting to note that Drs. Wilks and Moxon in their authoritative text, *Lectures on Pathological Anatomy,* published in 1875, made no reference to a regional enteritis-like lesion of the small intestine.[6] Braun described several cases of inflammatory masses of the intestine of unknown etiology.[7] Similar collections of cases were reported by Dalziel in 1913.[8] He reported six cases of regional enteritis and recorded a thorough description of the histopathology. In addition he did extensive bacteriologic studies on the specimens, ruling out tuberculosis and other enteric pathogens. He was able to isolate only *Escherichia coli.* He began his report by stating that he wished to draw attention to a new condition, which he believed had not been described and which was separate from tuberculosis of the intestine. It was Dalziel who coined the phrase, "bowel gives the consistence and smoothness of an eel in a state of rigor mortis," that has impressed medical students ever since.[8] In considering the etiology he used the analogy of Johne's disease in cattle, a chronic enteritis that is not tuberculous, but is an anatomic lesion with similar appearances. His search for a bacterial etiologic agent was unsuccessful. Tietze described several inflammatory lesions of the intestines and included some cases suggestive of regional enteritis.[9] Their delineation from other intestinal inflammatory lesions, however, is not clear. Moschcowitz and Wilensky demonstrated that many cases of granulomatous inflammation of the intestine were inappropriately diagnosed as intestinal tuberculosis.[10] They gave impetus to the evolving idea of a granulomatous disease distinct from tuberculosis and principally involving the terminal portions of the small intestine. Mock confirmed the existence of nonspecific granulomatous inflammatory lesions of the intestine.[11]

The new era in the study of regional enteritis dates to the seminal report of Crohn, Ginzburg, and Oppenheimer entitled "Regional Ileitis: a Pathologic and Clinical Entity."[1] The 14 cases they presented clearly delineated the entity that we now call regional enteritis. Most physicians of the era immediately preceding this report had the preconception that all the granulomatous disease processes of the small bowel were tuberculous in origin and nature, possibly in variant forms. Indeed, in those days, ileocecal tuberculosis was a common entity either as an end stage of pulmonary tuberculosis or as a primary intestinal involvement of bovine tuberculosis. Ileocecal tuberculosis of bovine origin was common before the establishment of tuberculosis control procedures for cattle. Doctor Crohn himself described the first clinical case of regional ileitis as follows:

. . . a young man of sixteen years of age with diarrhea, fever, a mass in the lower right abdomen accompanied by pain. X-ray of the lungs was negative for tuberculosis; the Von Pirquet test and the intradermal tuberculin test were negative. The intraperitoneal insufflation of oxygen led to no decided improvement. With scientific curiosity aroused and with the insistent urge to accomplish relief or cure, Dr. A. A. Berg was approached with the request for surgical exploration. Once again the cloud of tuberculosis preconception rose to confuse and thwart the logical demand. Dr. Berg related that at the insistence of the Saranac group he had operated upon five cases of intestinal tuberculosis in the hope of finding a cure for the local intestinal complication of phthisis. Of the five cases, three died soon after operation, two were not relieved even in their terminal hopeless state and Dr. Berg at first refused to reopen that discouraging chapter of intestinal surgery. But with argument and with presentation of the negative facts, persuasion succeeded, for Berg was an adventuresome surgeon, of great technical dexterity and well-earned self-confidence and with a mind open to the logical presentation of scientific facts.

The resection of the ileocecal and ileal segment in this case gave the opportunity for the determination of the non-specific origin of this granulomatous disease. . . . Within a year, the involved area in thirteen more cases of terminal ileitis was resected by Berg. It soon developed that the abdominal wall fistulae was the important clue to the recognition of such cases. We had in the wards many chronic cases of diarrhea with persistent abdominal fistulae, the nature of which were not discernible. They were supposedly tuberculous in nature without tubercle bacilli, or actinomycotic without actinomyces. These cases were then collected, one with eleven abdominal fistulae, and resections were performed.

. . . Dr. Leon Ginsburg and Dr. Gordon E. Oppenheimer had been collecting and studying the pathological characteristics of non-specific granulomata of the gastro-intestinal tract. Thus logically were combined the fundamental pathology of non-specific granulomas with the clinical picture of those granulomas which, because they occupied the final loop of the small bowel, led to the title of "Terminal Ileitis, A Pathological and A Clinical Entity."*

Doctor Crohn reported his findings at the American Medical Association meeting in New Orleans in 1932. Dr. J. A. Bargen, who discussed the presentation, suggested that the name of the disease be changed to regional ileitis since it was likely that the pathologic process might some day be found in involved upper segments of the ileum or even the jejunum, a conjecture that obviously has subsequently proved to be true. The existence of this entity gained rapid acceptance. It was discussed at meetings in Europe and North America, and numerous reports followed.

The 14 cases that were presented in Crohn's report, we now know in the light of further experience, had lesions that were relatively late in the course of the disease and were limited to the terminal 20 to 30 cm. of ileum. They characterized the histopathologic process as a chronic necrotizing and cicatrizing inflammation with ulceration of the mucosa and a disproportionate connective tissue reaction of the remaining wall of the involved intestine leading to stenosis of the lumen and multiple fistulas. Since this report, accumulated experience on the pathology of this disease has shown that it may occur at many sites in the intestinal tract other than the terminal ileum, with or

---

*B. B. Crohn: The early days of regional ileitis at the Mount Sinai Hospital—reminiscences. J. Mount Sinai Hosp. N.Y. *22*:143, 1955.

without terminal ileal involvement; thus, the term ileitis has been changed to enteritis or enterocolitis to account for this broader anatomic distribution. Also, it is now known that the earlier anatomic descriptions dealt almost exclusively with relatively advanced lesions and that the total spectrum of gross and microscopic features of the disease, regardless of its location in the intestinal tract, represents a continuum from early acute to late proliferative or granulomatous chronic changes. The changing morphologic patterns in this process are described in subsequent chapters.

EPIDEMIOLOGY

Analogous Lesions in Animals

The existence of regional enteritis-like disease in species other than man has recently been described. The report of Strande, Sommers, and Petrak clearly establishes the existence of a disease with the morphologic features of regional enteritis in cocker spaniel dogs.[12] In one of their cases the lesions were limited to the colon, rectum, and associated lymph nodes, whereas in the other it involved the terminal 6 cm. of ileum. Both cases had skip areas. The microscopic features of a chronic inflammation with cicatrization of the intestinal wall, producing an obliterative lymphangitis, was noted. Similar changes in the mesentery and regional lymph nodes were present, leaving little doubt as to the morphologic similarity between this disease in cocker spaniels and the human one. Van Kruiningen has collected more than 50 cases of granulomatous colitis in boxer dogs that have many of the features of regional enteritis involving the colon.[13] Here again the lymphoreticular system is the predominant tissue of involvement with eccentric thickening of the scar formation in the affected segments of colon. Kennedy and Cello have also observed this entity in boxer dogs.[14]

An extensive study of lesions found in the small intestine of swine, which has been called regional ileitis and bears many features in common with the human disease, has been reported by Emsbo from his observations of specimens obtained in meat packing houses in Denmark.[15] Similar lesions have been described by others in the United States.[16] Similar, though less convincing, reports emanating from Canada have also been recorded.[17] The existence of a terminal ileal lesion in swine has long been recognized by meat inspectors, but until Emsbo's report there was no attempt made to distinguish it from various infectious lesions of the small intestine. In his studies Emsbo obtained 58 cases from meat packing houses and carefully delineated their gross and microscopic features. Fifty-one of them were from the bacon swine, young adolescent, or young adult animals seven to eight months of age. One had acute intestinal perforation. From his study of the incidence of the lesion it appeared to occur in a very small percentage of the total swine slaughter, perhaps about 1 per cent. In one meat fodder factory in Denmark the presence of ileal lesions was found in 1.3 per cent of all animals slaughtered. In swine the lesion was strictly localized in the ileum. In 47 cases the section of the gut involved varied from 25 to 160 cm. in length with an average of about 75 cm. The greatest development of the lesion was in the terminal section of the ileum, ending suddenly at the ileocecal valve. The proximal end of the lesion gradually diminished toward the jejunum. The cecum and colon usually appeared normal although in a few cases some thickening of the mucous membrane was noted. In some cases cirrhosis of the liver, similar to that seen in the human, occurred. The external diameter of the gut varied from 1.8 to 4.5 cm. in contrast to the normal, which is about 1.5 cm. In a few cases there were no pathologic changes in the surface of the ileum; however, in over 75 per cent the mesenteric vessels were greatly dilated along the ileum, forming a dark red rim with bushy small vesssls passing from the mesentery to the subserosa. In many cases the vessels in the serosa were also markedly injected. In about half, edema of the mesentery was noted; most of these had a serosa presenting with patchy red-brown granulation tissue or fibrinous material that sometimes formed adhesions to the abdominal wall or other intestines. Emsbo was able to divide his cases into two main types: muscular and mucous. In the muscular type the main cause for the thickening of the wall was a hypertrophy of the muscular coats involving both the longitudinal and circular layers. In the mucous type the muscularis was thickened, though not as conspicuously. The ileum was usually dilated, and the mucosal changes predominated. The intestinal contents were discolored gray-brown and were fetid. It was Emsbo's opinion that the mucous type represented a further development of the muscular type, which he presumed to be an earlier stage of the disease, since he had observed transitional cases between the two. In the mucosal type of lesion the changes were very pronounced. The thickness of the mucosa was sometimes as much as 8 mm. There was a tendency to deep ulceration and necrosis, especially on the mesenteric aspect of the gut. Thus, small abscesses formed deep in the wall of the ileum. Regional lymph nodes often had a severe degree of hyperplasia. The surface of the mucous membrane had catarrhal changes with desquamation of the epithelium. The latter was often extensively detached, especially along the mesenteric aspect, so that the submucosa became denuded and appeared as a granulating wound surface. The lamina propria had cellular infiltration with plasma cells, lymphocytes, and histiocytes as well as edema and hemorrhage. The intestinal epithelium had a decreased mucous secretory activity in the involved areas and appeared somewhat dedifferentiated. Within the submucosa, accumulations of epithelioid cells and occasional giant cells were noted.

It is quite apparent from the foregoing that many features of the porcine terminal ileitis are indeed quite similar to the human disease, especially in cases of the mucous type. Perhaps its most predominant variation is the existence of a rather massive hypertrophy of the muscular coats that appears as the major feature of the muscular type of the disease and as a prominent feature of the mucous type. Other restricted reports presented only a few cases and were limited to the muscular type.[14] One from England described 20 cases of terminal ileitis in pigs.[16] Many of these derived from three litters of animals, and the possibility of familial occurrence was pointed out.

Several recent reports have described acute and chronic ileitis in the golden Syrian hamster.[18] The lesions bore very little resemblance to human regional ileitis. The lesion in the hamster was found to be acute and restricted to the ileum, which was dilated, hyperemic, and filled with watery yellow-gray fluid and blood. The ileum was enlarged to three to four times normal, markedly thickened, and had a rigid, friable wall. Foci of fibrinous peritonitis were noted, and adhesions were often present between the ileum and adjacent structures. Peyer's patches were enlarged, hyperemic, and edematous. Microscopically the principal change was hyperplasia of the ileal mucosa with infiltration of lymphocytes. Shortly thereafter a severe coagulative necrosis of the villi occurred with subsequent spread of abscesses into the submucosa and muscularis. In the advanced lesions the coagulative necrosis of the villi often extended into the submucosa and occasionally involved the entire wall of the ileum. Sinus tracts sometimes developed. Reticuloendothelial hyperplasia and microabscesses were present in the lymph nodules. The latter were frequently surrounded by whorls of connective tissue in those animals that survived. The subserosa was frequently thickened and often contained many suppurative foci as well as a marked increase in lymphocytes and plasma cells. Diffuse lymphoid hyperplasia was seen in the mesenteric lymph nodes, and reticuloendothelial hyperplasia with central necrosis was also noted. It is quite apparent that the hamster lesion is much more acute and fulminant than is regional enteritis. Second, the presence of necrosis within the hyperplastic reticuloendothelial areas and the extensive coagulative necrosis is a primary feature of the lesion. Certainly, these features are not characteristic of the human disease. Few of the animals affected with this disease recover. The 10 per cent that do recover are subsequently free from disease; it is not a chronic, relapsing lesion as is regional enteritis. There was no evidence other than its anatomic location to suggest that the lesion in hamsters represents regional enteritis.

Johne's disease (paratuberculosis) of domestic animals bears some resemblance to regional enteritis but many differences as well.[19] It is a chronic granulomatous inflammation that involves the terminal ileum principally, the proximal portion of the colon frequently, but the jejunum rarely. The lesion extends into the lymphatic channels and lymph nodes as does regional enteritis. The etiologic agent has been clearly demonstrated to be *Mycobacterium johnei,* a gram-positive, short, thick rod (1.5 by 0.5 μ), and is acid-fast with the Ziehl-Neelsen stain. The disease may attack 2 to 10 per cent of a cattle herd and also has been found in sheep, goats, deer, and llama.

The gross appearance of the lesions is one of multiple ulcers principally occurring in the lymphoid tissue of the mucosa and submucosa, similar to tuberculosis. Segments of the ileal wall may be hard and thickened though the muscularis and serosa are usually not altered. Microscopically, numerous granulomas resembling tuberculomas are seen; however, necrosis and giant cells are rarely a feature of the lesion.

The disease in rats reported by Geil does not resemble regional enteritis.[20] The process is acute with edema, dilatation of 7 to 10 cm. of ileum, coagulation necrosis of the mucosa, and hydropic degeneration of the smooth muscle. The changes more closely resemble those of vitamin B_{12} deficiency.

Geographical Distribution and Incidence

Though reports of cases of regional enteritis in humans have emanated from various parts of the world, the extent of the studies is insufficient to determine the incidence or prevalence of the disease, except for Norway, Great Britain, and North America.[21] As recently as 1966, Fone indicated that the disease appeared to be less common in Australia than in other countries, with few examples being recorded in the Australian medical literature.[22] He reported on 24 cases in the Melbourne area during the previous five years. A search of the hospital records yielded 17 more cases from earlier years.

The three major studies establishing the incidence in Northern Europe and North America are those of Evans and Acheson from Oxford, England, Gjone and co-workers from Norway, and Monk and co-workers from the Baltimore region of the United States.[23-26] The report of Evans and Acheson is the only study that has attempted to determine the incidence and prevalence in a population rather than merely the incidence or prevalence of hospital admissions.[23] Using modern statistical methods, they studied the epidemiology of ulcerative colitis and regional enteritis in the Oxford area for the decade from January 1, 1951, to December 31, 1960, the latter date being designated as prevalence day. They used multiple approaches to uncover the existence of cases in this population (which increased during the decade from 250,000 to 300,000), excluding students of Oxford University and members of the armed forces stationed in the area. The first source of information was the records of hospital admissions of the group of teaching hospitals associated with Oxford University (less than 5 per cent of the total number of hospital admissions of the population at risk occurred in hospitals outside the area). The second source of cases was responses to letters sent to all consulting physicians, surgeons, and pediatricians, asking for the identity of cases bearing certain specific diagnoses related to regional enteritis. A third avenue was a series of circular letters sent to the 219 family physicians practicing within and just outside the area of the study. The reply rate to these letters was an astounding 98 per cent. A fourth source of cases was the hospital outpatient records, and a fifth was the search of admission books of the only private nursing home that provides comprehensive service and care in the area. The Registrar General supplied a list of persons certified to have died of the disease under study while resident in the area. By culling through the lists of patients provided by these various sources, they were able to collate a final list of what appears to be virtually every case that received medical attention within the region. For regional enteritis they found an incidence rate of 0.8 case per 100,000 population per year with a standard error of 0.2. The cumulative prevalence rate on the prevalence day per 100,000 population was 9.0 cases with a standard error of 1.4.

As indicated earlier, the study of Gjone and co-workers in Norway deals primarily with hospital admissions rather than with the incidence or prevalence within a population.[24] All pediatric and medical departments of the country and a majority of small mixed hospitals gave individual information on their cases. For an eight year period from 1956 to 1963 a total of 73 patients with regional enteritis was discovered for an average annual rate of 2.6 cases per 1,000,000 population. There were no differences in different regions of the country. The study by Monk and co-workers contained information about all persons from the Baltimore area who were hospitalized for regional enteritis during a 39 month period.[25, 26] It provided a sufficiently large number of patients with well-diagnosed disease so that they could determine the hospital incidence and prevalence rates and examine various features such as sex ratio, age, race, and religion. They found an average annual incidence of 1.8 hospitalizations per 100,000 population. This incidence rate is much higher than that found in the Oxford study, though, as will be pointed out later, the mortality rates in both areas were similar. They were at a loss to explain the reason for these differences. The existence of mild forms of the disease posed a serious problem in interpreting the data where an unknown proportion of all patients are seen in private physicians' offices and never reach a hospital. It is inaccurate to relate these data to data from countries where most of the facilities for diagnosis of the disease are found in hospitals and the rates for hospitalization very closely approximate the incidence rate.

Ethnic Distribution

It is now clear that there is a much higher incidence of regional enteritis in the Jewish ethnic group than in the Gentile. The several studies referred to earlier all confirm this fact, though the extent of the preponderance varies somewhat between studies. The data supplied by Gjone in Norway is insufficient to be statistically significant on this point as there are few Jewish people in Norway and no cases of regional enteritis among them were found in his study. The report by Fone also lacks sufficient cases to have a bearing on the frequency in Jews. The study of Evans and Acheson, however, indicates that the incidence of regional enteritis among Jews was greater than among others, but the lack of data on the total number of Jews in the population under study made it impossible to calculate the ratio. The Baltimore study revealed the incidence of regional enteritis among Jews to be nine times that among non-Jews. In Israel the only reported study showed that oriental Jews, who make up about half the population, do not seem to have the disease although they have a great many other intestinal inflammatory diseases.[25] All the cases that were reported supposedly occurred in Ashkenazi Jews from Western Europe.

The hospital incidence and prevalence rates for regional enteritis are higher for whites than for non-whites. Though cases have been reported among Indians, Eskimos, and American Negroes, the data are insufficient to comment further on the incidence.[63] Social and economic factors may affect this type of data greatly because of the lesser availability of hospital admissions to these groups. Whether the incidence of this disease in these various non-white groups is equal to that of the whites remains to be determined.

Age and Sex Distribution

The several reports are in close agreement regarding the age distribution of onset of regional enteritis. A case has been reported by Koop and co-workers having the histologic features of regional enteritis in a newborn.[28] During the first decade of life the onset of regional enteritis is extremely rare. From ages 10 to 19 approximately one fourth as many cases occur as occur in each decade between 20 and 60 years of age. Van Patter and co-workers found 85 (14 per cent) of their series of 600 cases of regional enteritis to have had an onset of symptoms prior to the age of 15.[29] Mosley reviewed the cases admitted to Mount Sinai Hospital and those from the personal files of Dr. Crohn and found 28 cases of childhood regional enteritis in an eight to nine year period at that hospital.[30] Figure 1-2, from Acheson's study, shows the age of onset during the various decades of life.

The sex distribution of regional enteritis is approximately equal

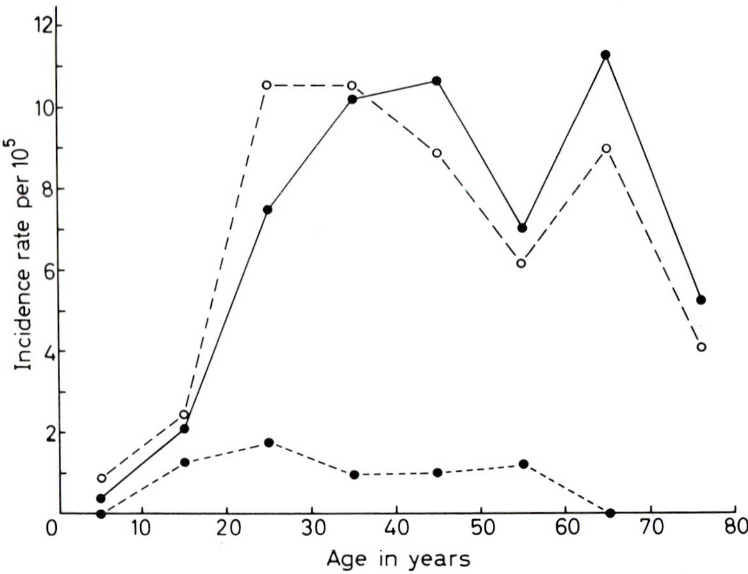

Figure 1-2   Average annual age-specific incidence rates (1951-60) for ulcerative colitis and regional enteritis in the Oxford area. Continuous line = U.C. (age at first diagnosis); interrupted line = U.C. (age at onset of first symptoms); dotted line = R.E. (age at first diagnosis). (Courtesy of E. D. Acheson, *in* Recent Advances in Gastroenterology, Chapter 2, 1965, and J. and A. Churchill, Ltd., London.)

though the larger studies show a small male preponderance. For example, in Monk's study in Baltimore, white males outnumbered white females with 6.77 cases per year per 100,000 population to 5.73 for females. Similarly, the study of Gjone in Norway revealed an annual rate of 2.6 male cases per million and 2.5 female. Fone's study in Australia revealed 22 females and 19 males in their series of 41 cases.[22] A massive review of the literature revealed a 57 per cent male preponderance.[31] Crohn and Yarnis reported a 56 per cent male preponderance in 542 cases, and Van Patter found it to be 57 per cent in 600 cases at the Mayo Clinic.[21, 29] The Oxford study by Evans and Acheson revealed an equal male to female ratio of 0.8 case per 100,000 population per year, whereas the cumulative prevalence rate showed a slight female preponderance of 9.8 to 8.2. This suggests that though the number of cases occurring in men and women is comparable, the women tend to remain ill longer.

Pregnancy and Regional Enteritis

Because about half the regional enteritis patients are women and most of them are in the child-bearing age group, the question of the effect of pregnancy on their illness arises. This question must be divided into two parts: What is the effect of pregnancy on a patient who has pre-existing regional enteritis? This is the situation most likely to be faced by a physician. The second aspect of the question is: Does pregnancy or the postpartum period precipitate the onset of regional enteritis? Crohn and his co-workers reported on their own personal experience in the study of 84 pregnancies in 53 patients who had or had had regional enteritis. They divided their patients into four groups: those with enteritis quiescent at conception, enteritis active at conception, onset during pregnancy, and onset during the postpartum period. Of the first group, those who had a previous history of regional enteritis, there were 45 pregnancies in 34 patients. Of these, 62 per cent had uneventful and favorable pregnancies, whereas 38 per cent (17) had recurrences of their enteritis during pregnancy or postpartum. Of those who had had regional enteritis treated with prior surgery, 81 per cent had uneventful pregnancies and 19 per cent had recurrence during pregnancy or postpartum. In contrast, of those who had had a previous history of regional enteritis that was not treated with prior surgery, only 27 per cent had uneventful pregnancies and 73 per cent had recurrences during pregnancy or postpartum. In the second group, 30 patients in whom enteritis was active at the inception of pregnancy, the majority had moderately severe cases of enteritis. Pregnancy did not appear to alter the course of the disease in 12 of these, and in 14 there was subsidence of the inflammatory process during pregnancy. In only four was the enteritis aggravated during pregnancy or the postpartum period. The authors concluded that pregnancy exerted an unfavorable effect on enteritis, particularly in those in whom the enteritis was active at the time of conception.

A markedly different picture occurs when enteritis begins during pregnancy. This is an extremely rare occurrence, fortunately. In Doctor Crohn's large study only three patients had the onset of enteritis during pregnancy; two of these were primigravida and all three went on to premature delivery. The course of the disease was severe in all three cases and represented a serious threat to both fetus and mother. Blair and Allen reviewed the literature on the problem and presented a case of their own.[33] They also summarized the experiences of others.[34, 35, 36] A complete review of the literature confirms the extreme rarity of this complication of pregnancy and its poor prognosis for both the mother and the fetus. Of the total of seven cases in the literature, all went to premature labor and only four infants survived. There was one maternal death, and one mother died four years later from the regional enteritis.

Familial Incidence

Numerous case reports of the familial occurrence of regional enteritis have been written. Rather than review these here, I refer the

TABLE 1–1   Familial Occurrences of Regional Enteritis*

Authors	No. Families
Lewisohn (1938)	1 (2 sisters)
Brown, Scheiffly (1939)	1 (2 sisters, brother)
Bockus (1946)	1 (2 cousins)
Kirsner, Owens, Humphreys (1948)	1 (father, son)
Reich (1948)	1 (2 sisters, first cousin)
Armitage, Wilson (1950)	1 (brother, sister)
Edwards (1954)	2 (2 brothers; female identical twins)
Felsen, Wolarsky (1955)	21 (mixed)
Eudel, Viguié (1955)	1 (2 sisters)
Heard, John (1956)	1 (mother, son)
Metzger, Frobese (1956)	1 (mother, son)
Houghton, Naish (1958)	1 (brother, sister) (7 families, ulcerative colitis, regional enteritis)
Freysz, Haemmerli, Kartagener (1958)	1 (female twins, ages 59, 63)
Steigmann, Shapiro (1961)	2 (father, son, father's brother; father, daughter, father's sister)
Cornes, Stecher (1961)	2 (1/86 patients — 1/45 patients "Reg. Ent. Colon")
Niederle (1961)	1 (female identical twins)
Sherlock, Bell, Steinberg, Almy (1962)	1 (4 siblings, sibling child, first cousin)
Crohn (1962)	16 (860 patients)
Kirsner, Spencer (1963)	20 (185 patients, 22 family members) 5 (70 ileocolitis patients, 5 family members)

*Literature listed in yearly sequence. (Courtesy of J. B. Kirsner and J. A. Spencer: Ann. Intern. Med. *59*:133–144, 1963, and the American College of Physicians.)

reader to the study by Kirsner and Spencer, in which these case reports are listed and discussed (Table 1-1).[37] In the same report a series of 185 cases of familial regional enteritis is presented. This represented about 10 per cent of all the cases of regional enteritis seen in the University of Chicago Clinic. The second large series of 21 cases of familial occurrence was reported by Felsen and Wolarsky.[38] In Crohn's own experience of 860 patients with regional enteritis, 16 cases occurred within families.[17] These three large series suggest an over-all frequency of familial occurrence of at least 1 to 2 per cent. In addition, there are several reports in the literature that show 3, 4, or more individuals within a kindred who had the disease. Almy and Sherlock reviewed the genetic aspects of regional enteritis and, on the best available evidence of the prevalence of the disease, postulated the likelihood of a chance or a coincidental occurrence within a family.[39] Based on an over-all incidence of 10 or more cases per 100,000 population, the probability of a familial occurrence due to chance alone is about one in 25 million cases; thus it seems clear that regional enteritis at least in some instances tends to occur on a familial basis.

MORTALITY

The reports of Acheson and of Mendeloff and co-workers provide accurate data on the mortality ascribed to regional enteritis.[25-27, 40] Figure 1-3 compares the average death rate per 100,000 population in the United States and in England and Wales for regional enteritis on an age-specific basis. It also compares the death rate with that of ulcerative colitis. The average age-adjusted death rates ascribed to regional enteritis in the United States, Canada, and England and Wales are 0.08, 0.09 and 0.11 death per hundred thousand, respectively (Table 1-2). The death rate for ulcerative colitis is about five to seven times greater. Although the death rate in the United States is slightly higher for males than females, in England and Wales it is about equal. As can be seen from the graph, the death rate increases somewhat with age. Why it should be higher in England and Wales than it is in Canada and the United States remains unexplained.

From the various reports the most common cause of death is intestinal perforation and peritonitis. Less frequently death is caused

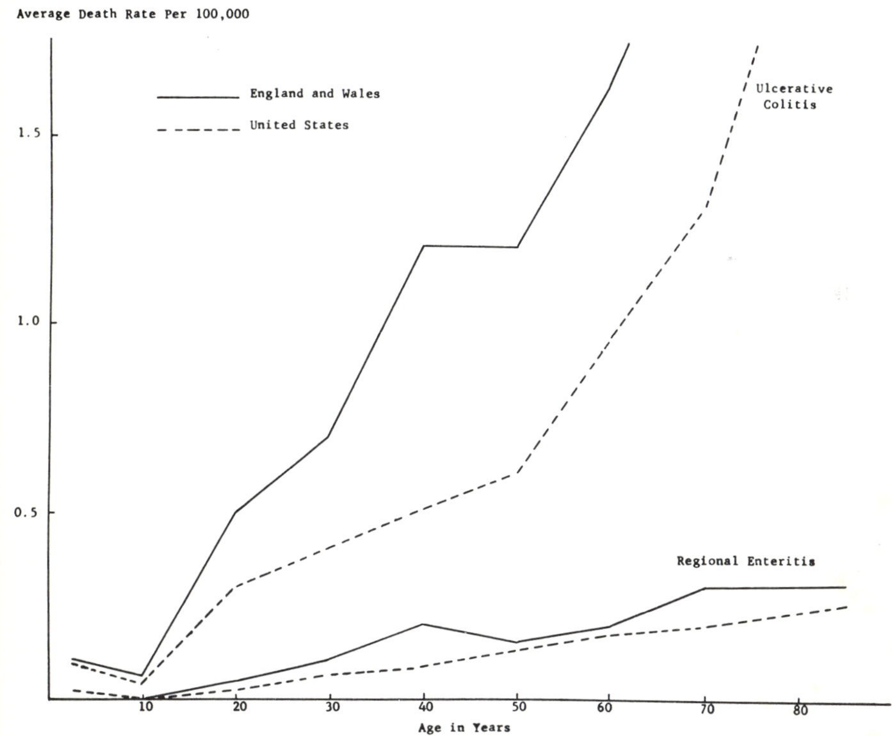

Figure 1-3 Average age-specific death rates per 100,000 for ulcerative colitis and regional enteritis U.S.A. (all races) and England and Wales. (Courtesy of E. D. Acheson, J. Chron. Dis. *10*:481–487, 1959, and Pergamon Press Ltd., Oxford.)

TABLE 1–2   Regional Enteritis Annual Death Rate per 100,000*

England and Wales (1952–1956)	0.11
United States (1950; 1952–1956)	
White races	0.08
Colored races	0.06
Canada (1952–1957)	0.09
New Zealand (1954–1958)	0.07

*Modified from E. D. Acheson, in *Recent Advances in Gastroenterology,* London, J. and A. Churchill Ltd., 1965.

by intestinal obstruction and its consequences, renal failure, malnutrition, liver abscess, or complications associated with surgery. Recent reports have confirmed these findings.[41]

ETIOLOGY

My original intention in preparing this monograph was to devote a chapter or more to considerations of etiology. However, as I critically reviewed the many articles and suggestions on etiology, it became apparent that the amount of factual information was so limited that the question arose in my mind whether etiology should be mentioned at all. Not only is the etiology of regional enteritis completely unknown, but there seems to be a dearth of controlled research. Perhaps this is true because of the relatively low incidence of this disease in comparison to other diseases, which tends to limit the opportunity for investigation. There has been a surprising lack of effort to construct an animal model for the disease. Recognizing these limitations, it would be inappropriate to analyze extensively the various suggestions as to etiology because there is so little factual information and controlled investigation. Suffice it to say that as with other chronic diseases of unknown etiology characterized by relapses and remissions, affecting as broad an age group as regional enteritis, the stimulus for many theories of etiology exists.

Infectious Agents

Virtually every category of agent has been suggested at one time or another. Infectious agents, either bacterial or viral, were among the first etiologic agents considered. However, extensive investigation on the bacterial flora of the intestine does not reveal any unique organism or unique pattern of flora. Viral agents have been less extensively studied; however, those investigations that have been carried out have been essentially negative. Attempts have been made to identify antibody for the adenovirus or group B Coxsackie viruses, using neutralization tests on sera from patients with active disease and after variable periods thereafter. There are no significant differences recorded between antibody titers of patients with active disease and those encountered in the general population. Similar results were obtained when portions of intestinal wall or lymph nodes were cultured for viruses. An interesting possible viral mechanism was suggested by the investigations of Sneierson and co-workers.[42] They investigated an epidemic of viral etiology in Green, New York, which involved between 250 and 300 school children and a few adults. The physical signs and symptoms mimicked Coxsackie virus infection of the abdominal type. Stool and blood cultures were negative for virus; 11 of the children were hospitalized with signs and symptoms of acute appendicitis. Surgical exploration in eight revealed that all had enlarged mesenteric lymph nodes in the ileocecal region. Four of these chiildren had the gross pathologic picture of acute regional enteritis. No corrective surgery was done and follow-up studies three months later showed completely negative physical findings. This investigation, though it does not establish a viral factor in the etiology of regional enteritis, does suggest an interesting possibility that viral or similar agents may set up an inflammatory process that becomes self-perpetuating. Therefore, in the usual sequence of events, by the time a patient with regional enteritis presents himself to the physician the evidence of the viral infection may have been muted.

Whether mesenteric lymphadenitis, as suggested by Erskine, represents a primary etiologic factor for both appendicitis and regional enteritis or whether these are separate morphologic and clinical entities is interesting but unproved speculation.[43] Other surgeons have focused attention on severe fibrosis of the appendix and have stressed its similarity to the appendiceal fibrosis that frequently accompanies regional enteritis.[44]

Defective Immunologic Responses

Defective immunologic responses are another suggested mechanism of the onset of regional enteritis. Both autoimmune phenomena and allergic responses to common foodstuffs have been suggested. Allergists point to the fact that the localization, its spreading tendency, the remissions and recurrences, and the occasional inherited predisposition support the allergic concept. Frequently when patients are placed on special diets to eliminate allergens their illness will enter remission. Whether there is a causal relationship, however, remains to be proved because many patients, perhaps an equal number, who are not put on elimination diets will enter remission as well. Others have suggested that regional enteritis may be a variant of sarcoidosis because of the similarity of the granulomas to those of sarcoid. Careful study of these relationships have been carried out by Williams, who found no evidence to support the relationship between regional enteritis, tuberculosis, sarcoidosis, or hypersensitivity reactions in general.[45] Using the Kveim, Mantoux, and precipitin tests, he studied 50 patients with regional enteritis and was unable to demonstrate the presence of immunologic relationships.

Absorption of Toxic Substances

Absorption of toxic substances from either the food ingested or the product of bacterial action within the intestine has also been suggested as an etiologic mechanism.[46] However, objective evidence of a relationship is lacking.

Inherited Metabolic Defect

Inherited metabolic defect is another etiologic mechanism suggested by those who have been interested principally in the existence of the familial occurrence of regional enteritis and in some instances ulcerative colitis. Chalfin and Holt have demonstrated a lactase enzyme deficiency in five patients with regional enteritis.[47] Three of these five patients had abnormal oral lactose tolerance tests and a history of milk intolerance that antedated the onset of their intestinal complaints. A glucose-6-phosphate dehydrogenase enzyme deficiency in regional enteritis was reported.[48, 49] Four out of five patients with regional enteritis were deficient in this enzyme in their erythrocytes. The limitations of interpretation imposed by the low percentage of patients with the deficiency ruled out the suggestion of a causal relationship.[50]

Psychosomatic Mechanisms

Psychosomatic mechanisms have also been incriminated. Proof of the relationship remains doubtful. The occurrence of certain personality types and personality features in many patients with regional enteritis has given impetus to this concept. However, whether the personality traits are a cause or a result of the disease remains unproved. The fact that regional enteritis does occur in dogs and pigs would suggest either that these animals have psyches similar to those of humans with the disease, or that the human psychologic factor is not primary.

Developmental Mechanisms

Developmental mechanisms have also been suggested. Some regional enteritis patients have an anomalous blood supply to the small intestine or malrotation. Pope and O'Neal reported a case of intestinal vascular insufficiency and the development of a regional enteritis-like cicatrizing lesion.[51] Whether the frequency of these anomalies in such patients exceeds that in the general population is not known. Importance of the vascular lesions has been added to by the frequently observed occurrence of an episode of acute trauma to the abdomen shortly before the onset of symptoms. Indeed, Crohn, in one of his early investigations, had noted this point.[21] The problem has been reviewed by Huff and co-workers.[52]

The presence of metaplastic epithelium in the small intestine in many cases of regional enteritis has led some pathologists to speculate on this as an etiologic factor. Brunner's glands were found in the distal small intestine in 16 of 34 cases by Kawel and Tesluk.[53] They believed this metaplasia a consequence of the inflammatory process. Lee studied a series of 92 pathologic specimens from the small intestine with a variety of inflammatory and neoplastic lesions as well as normal ones.[54] He concluded that the metaplasia was not specifically related to chronic inflammation or ulceration and was not a congenital heterotopia. He noted that it was particularly common in regional enteritis.

SYMPTOMS AND SIGNS

In the adult the presenting complaint varies, depending on the acuteness and severity of the process. The majority of patients present a history suggestive of a chronic disease process characterized principally by gradually increasing diarrhea of perhaps six to eight stools per day, mostly at night or in the morning, and a gradual weight loss of up to 10 pounds. Not infrequently patients will present with the symptoms of acute abdominal inflammation with a sudden development of right lower quadrant pain, tenderness with fever, guarding, diarrhea, and constipation. Occasionally a patient will present with a fever of unknown origin without localizing features. The history and physical examination, in all major studies thus far completed, indicate that virtually all patients have some degree of abdominal pain, and the various reports indicate that one quarter to one half of the patients have a palpable abdominal mass in the right lower quadrant. Frequently these patients have abdominal scars, especially an appendectomy scar. The mass in the right lower quadrant is usually moderately tender, fixed posteriorly, and firm and probably represents the inflammatory reaction in the terminal ileum. Various reports indicate anorectal fistulas are present in 20 to 50 per cent of the cases. Diarrhea is present in one third to two thirds, whereas fever or weight loss are present in less than half. Bloody stools are quite common, and whereas diarrhea is present in many of the patients, constipation is also seen in some, approximately 10 per cent. Nausea and vomiting are found in about a third of the patients. Laboratory examinations reveal anemia in approximately 20 per cent. Usually the history and physical findings are sufficient to make the diagnosis, confirmation being derived by x-ray examination. The "string sign" first described by Kantor is characteristic of the disease, but is rarely seen (Fig. 1-4).[55] The clinical differential diagnosis usually includes bacillary dysentery, intestinal parasites, sarcoid, tuberculosis, appendicitis, or intestinal neoplastic diseases such as malignant lipoma of the ileum. Other clinical features may be present

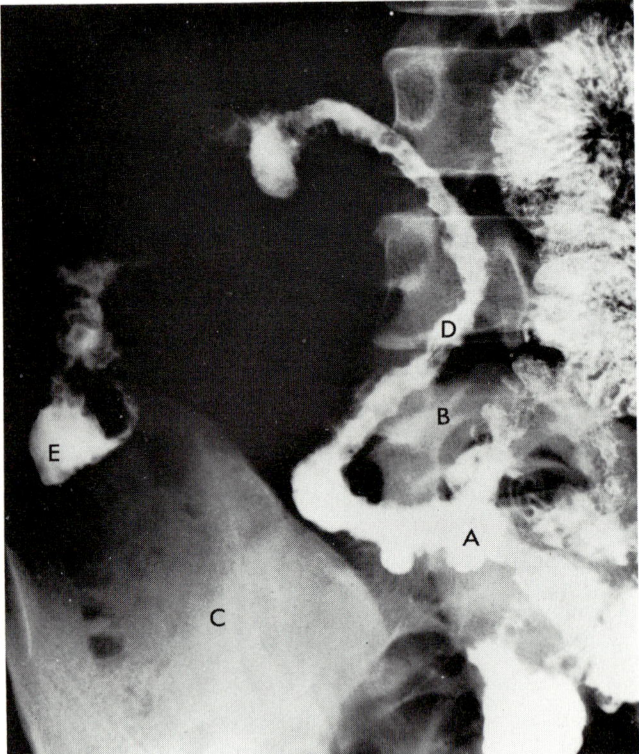

Figure 1-4   Regional enteritis involving the terminal ileum as revealed by barium study radiographs. Uninvolved intestine (A) is seen overlying the vertebral column (B) and near the pelvis (C). The diseased segment of ileum (D) curves upward medially, then downward to a partially filled cecum (E). The involved segment has a narrowed lumen and a markedly irregular surface. The prominent shadow at the upper extent of the loop represents an ulcer surrounded by induration that separated the involved segment of intestine from the cecum and other segments of bowel. This radiographic appearance of regional enteritis is much more commonly seen than the "string sign." Compare this view of the lesion with that seen grossly in Figures 4-1, 4-2, and 4-3. (Courtesy of M. M. Figley, M.D., Professor and Chairman, Department of Radiology, University of Washington School of Medicine.)

occasionally such as steatorrhea, arthritis, erythema nodosum of the skin, perineal abscesses, malnutrition, or personality changes.

Childhood regional enteritis presents with clinical findings somewhat at variance to those just described. Frequently the disease in children begins with extraintestinal findings such as fever, arthralgias, anemia, or retarded growth and development. Diarrhea is frequently absent at the onset, and the presenting complaint is usually a vague abdominal pain in the right lower quadrant. In about one fourth of the children the abdominal pain may be sufficiently intense to provoke laparotomy. In about one of eight children anorectal fistulas may develop early in the course of the disease. The sudden onset of fever, leukocytosis, and pain in the right lower quadrant frequently make the condition indistinguishable from acute appendicitis. Many of these children are operated upon and the surgeon finds a terminal ileum that is congested, thickened, relatively rigid, with an associated mesenteric adenitis. Approximately half of the children so identified with acute regional enteritis subsequently undergo spontaneous remission, while the remainder develop the chronic disease. Whether this represents, as Erskine suggested, mesenteric lymphadenitis as a primary etiologic factor for both appendicitis and regional enteritis or whether these are separate morphologic and clinical entities is an interesting but unproved speculation.[43]

Winkelman studied 61 cases of regional enteritis in adolescents (10 to 19 years of age) and noted that the incidence of pain and diarrhea and their severity were comparable to those of regional enteritis in the adult.[56] Diarrhea was a presenting complaint in one third of his patients and it was often intermittent and described variously as watery, semisolid, loose, and rarely foul or bloody. The number of stools per 24 hour period varied from 2 to 5 usually, though occasionally it ranged as high as 10. Intermittent low-grade fever was present in about half his adolescent patients.

It is not the purpose of this monograph to present in detail or to analyze the clinical features of this disease. Readers seeking more information should refer to the clinical reports.[22, 57, 58, 59, 60, 61]

References

1. Crohn, B. B., Ginzburg, L., and Oppenheimer, G. D.: Regional ileitis: A pathologic and clinical entity. J.A.M.A. *99:*1323-1328, 1932.
2. Morgagni, Giovanni Battista: De Sedibus et Causis Morborum (The Seats and Causes of Diseases). Translated by Dr. Benjamin Alexander. London, A. Millar and T. Cadwell, Publishers, 1769. Facsimile of the 1769 edition, New York, Hafner Publishing Company, 1960.
3. Cooke, William: Morgagni's The Seats and Causes of Disease. London, J. and A. Churchill Ltd. 1822.
4. Combe, C., and Saunders, W.: A singular case of stricture and thickening of the ileum. Med. Trans. Roy. Coll. Phys. *4:*16-21, 1813.

5. Abercrombie, J.: Pathological and Practical Researches on Diseases of the Stomach, the Intestinal Canal, the Liver, and Other Viscera of the Abdomen. 4th American from last London edition (1828). Philadelphia, Lea and Blanchard, 1845.

6. Wilks, S., and Moxon, W.: Lectures on Pathological Anatomy. 2nd Ed. London, J. and A. Churchill Ltd., 1875.

7. Braun, H.: Ueber entzündliche geschwülste am Darm. Deutsch. Z. Chir. *100:*1–12, 1909.

8. Dalziel, T. K.: Chronic interstitial enteritis. Brit. Med. J. *2:*1068-1070, 1913.

9. Tietze, A.: Über entzündliche dickdarmgeschwülste. Ergebn. Chir. Orthop. *12:*211-273, 1920.

10. Moschcowitz, E., and Wilensky, A. O.: Non-specific granulomata of the intestine. Amer. J. Med. Sci. *166:*48-66, 1923.

11. Mock, H. E.: Infective granuloma: Nonspecific chronic tumor-like productive inflammations of the gastro-intestinal tract. Surg. Gynec. Obstet. *52:*672-689, 1931.

12. Strande, A., Sommers, S. C., and Petrak, M.: Regional enterocolitis in cocker spaniel dogs. Arch. Path. *57:*357-362, 1954.

13. Van Kruiningen, H. J.: Granulomatous colitis of boxer dogs: Comparative aspects. Gastroenterology *53:*114-122, 1967.

14. Kennedy, P. C., and Cello, R. M.: Colitis of boxer dogs. Gastroenterology *51:*926-931, 1966.

15. Emsbo, P.: Terminal or regional iletis in swine. Nord. Vet. Med. *3:*1-28, 1951.

16. Field, H. I., Buntain, D. I., and Jennings, A. R.: Terminal or regional ileitis in pigs. J. Comp. Path. *63:*153-158, 1953.

17. Nielsen, S. W.: Muscular hypertrophy of the ileum in relation to "terminal ileitis" in pigs—a preliminary report. J. Amer. Vet. Med. Ass. *127:*437–441, 1955.

18. Boothe, A. D., and Cheville, N. F.: The pathology of proliferative ileitis of the golden Syrian hamster. Path. Vet. (Basel) *4:*31-44, 1967.

19. Control of Johne's disease. Report of the Organization for European Economic Cooperation; Project 207. Paris, 1967.

20. Geil, R. G., Davis, C. L., and Thompson, S. W.: Spontaneous ileitis in rats—a report of 64 cases. Amer. J. Vet. Res. *22:*932-936, 1961.

21. Crohn, B. B., and Yarnis, H.: Regional ileitis. 2nd Ed. New York, Grune and Stratton, 1958.

22. Fone, D. J.: Regional enteritis (Crohn's Disease). Med. J. Aust. *1:*865-873, 1966.

23. Evans, J. G., and Acheson, E. D.: An epidemiological study of ulcerative colitis and regional enteritis in the Oxford area. Gut *6:*311-324, 1965.

24. Gjone, E., Orning, O. M., and Myren, J.: Crohn's disease in Norway 1956-63. Gut *7:*372-374, 1966.

25. Mendeloff, A. I., Monk, M., Siegel, C. I., and Lilienfeld, A.: Some epidemiological features of ulcerative colitis and regional enteritis. Gastroenterology, *51:*748-756, 1966.

26. Monk, M., Mendeloff, A. I., Siegel, C. I., and Lilienfeld, A.: An epidemiological study of ulcerative colitis and regional enteritis among adults in Baltimore. I. Hospital incidence and prevalence, 1960 to 1963. Gastroenterology *53:*198-210, 1967.

27. Acheson, E. D.: On the mortality ascribed to regional enteritis. J. Chronic Dis. *10:*481-487, 1959.

28. Koop, C. E., Perlingiero, J. G., and Weiss, W.: Cicatrizing enterocolitis in a newborn infant. Amer. J. Med. Sci. *214:*27-32, 1947.

29. Van Patter, W. N., Bargen, J. A., Dockerty, M. B., Feldman, W. H., Mayo, C. W., and Waugh, J. M.: Regional enteritis. Gastroenterology *26:*347-450, 1954.

30. Moseley, J. E., Marshak, R. H., and Wolf, B. S.: Regional enteritis in children. Amer. J. Roentgen. *84:*532-539, 1960.

31. Ravdin, I. S., and Johnson, C. G.: Regional ileitis. A summary of the literature. Amer. J. Med. Sci. *198:*269-292, 1939.

32. Crohn, B. B., Yarnis, H., and Korelitz, B. I.: Regional ileitis complicating pregnancy. Gastroenterology *31:*615-628, 1956.

33. Blair, J. S. G., and Allen, N.: Crohn's disease presenting acutely in pregnancy. J. Obstet. Gynaec. Brit. Comm. *69:*648–651, 1962.

34. Babson, W. W.: Terminal ileitis with obstruction and abscess complicating pregnancy. New Eng. J. Med. *235:*544-547, 1946.

35. Williams, D. L., and Davis, D. R.: Regional enteritis; report of case complicating pregnancy with review of literature. South. Surg. *12*:342-351, 1946.
36. Jones, R. L., and Soltau, D. H. K.: Pregnancy in association with Crohn's disease. J. Obstet. Gynaec. Brit. Emp. *65*:811-816, 1958.
37. Kirsner, J. B., and Spencer, J. A.: Family occurrences of ulcerative colitis, regional enteritis, and ileocolitis. Ann. Intern. Med. *59*:133-144, 1963.
38. Felsen, J., and Wolarsky, W.: Familial incidence of ulcerative colitis and ileitis. Gastroenterology *28*:412-417, 1955.
39. Almy, T. P., and Sherlock, P.: Genetic aspects of ulcerative colitis and regional enteritis. Gastroenterology *51*:757-763, 1966.
40. Acheson, E. D.: On the mortality ascribed to ulcerative colitis. J. Chronic Dis. *10*:469-480, 1959.
41. Banks, B. M., Zetzel, L., and Richter, H. S.: Morbidity and mortality in regional enteritis. Report of 168 cases. Amer. J. Dig. Dis. *14*:369-379, 1969.
42. Sneierson, H., Cunningham, J. R., and Artuso, D.: Epidemic virus infection (not identified); acute mesenteric lymphadenitis and acute regional ileitis. Amer. J. Gastroent. *40*:293-301, 1963.
43. Erskine, E. B.: The pathologic relationship of mesenteric adenitis, ileitis and appendicitis. Amer. J. Clin. Path. *11*:706-712, 1941.
44. Ravdin, I. S., and Rhoads, J. E.: Regional ileitis and fibroplastic appendicitis. Ann. Surg. *106*:394-406, 1937.
45. Williams, W. J.: A study of Crohn's syndrome using tissue extracts and the Kveim and Mantoux tests. Gut *6*:503-505, 1965.
46. Dotevall, G., and Kock, N. G.: Absorption studies in regional enterocolitis (Mb. Crohn). Scand. J. Gastroent. *3*:293-298, 1968.
47. Chalfin, D., and Holt, P. R.: Lactase deficiency in ulcerative colitis, regional enteritis, and viral hepatitis. Amer. J. Dig. Dis. *12*:81-87, 1967.
48. Sheehan, R. G., Necheles, T. F., Lindeman, R. J., Meyer, H. J., and Patterson, J. F.: Regional enteritis and granulomatous colitis associated with erythrocyte glucose-6-phosphate-dehydrogenase deficiency. New Eng. J. Med. *277*:1124-1126, 1967.
49. Katsaros, D., and Truelove, S. C.: Regional enteritis and glucose-6-phosphate-dehydrogenase deficiency. New Eng. J. Med. *281*:295-296, 1968.
50. Motulsky, A. G.: Crohn's disease and G-6-PD deficiency. New Eng. J. Med. *278*:281-282, 1968.
51. Pope, C. H., and O'Neal, R. M.: Incomplete infarction of ileum simulating regional enteritis. J.A.M.A. *161*:963-964, 1956.
52. Huff, J. F., Black, B. M., and Bartholomew, L. G.: Regional enteritis following acute trauma to the abdomen. J.A.M.A. *180*:491-492, 1962.
53. Kawel, C. A., Jr., and Tesluk, H.: Brunner-type glands in regional enteritis. Gastroenterology *28*:810-820, 1955.
54. Lee, F. D.: Pyloric metaplasia in the small intestine. J. Path. Bact. *87*:267-277, 1964.
55. Kantor, J. L.: Regional (terminal) ileitis: Its roentgen diagnosis. J.A.M.A. *103*:2016-2020, 1934.
56. Winkelman, E. I.: Regional enteritis in adolescence. Pediat. Clin. N. Amer. *14*:141-158, 1967.
57. Crohn, B. B.: Regional ileitis. Med. Clin. N. Amer. *40*:513-518, 1956.
58. Rappaport, H., Burgoyne, F. H., and Smetana, H. F.: Pathology of regional enteritis. Milit. Surg. *109*:463-502, 1951.
59. Gilbert, J. A., and Sartor, V. E.: Regional enteritis: Disease patterns and medical management. Canad. Med. Ass. J. *91*:23-27, 1964.
60. Neeley, J. C., and Goldman, L.: Regional enteritis. Surg. Clin. N. Amer. *42*:1257-1266, 1962.
61. Hunt, T., Morson, B. C., and Lockhart-Mummery, H. E.: Crohn's disease. Trans. Med. Soc. London *81*:87-95, 1965.
62. Crohn, B. B.: The early days of regional ileitis at the Mount Sinai Hospital—reminiscences. J. Mount Sinai Hosp. N.Y. *22*:143-146, 1955.
63. Ratzlaff, N., and Jacobs, W. H.: Regional enteritis in the American Negro. Amer. J. Gastroent. *53*:252-258, 1970.

Chapter Two

Natural History of Ulcerative Colitis

DEFINITION AND CLASSIFICATION

Ulcerative colitis is a recurrent, predominantly mucosal, acute inflammatory process of all or any part of the large intestine (including the rectum) of unknown etiology. The earliest identified morphologic lesion is the simultaneous occurrence of regressive changes in the epithelium deep in the crypts of Lieberkühn and the transmigration of polymorphs from the adjacent lamina propria through the altered epithelium to the lumen of the crypts (Frontispiece, Fig. 2–1). Necrosis of the crypt epithelium and adjacent lamina propria produces the crypt abscess, a characteristic feature of the disease. Extension and coalescence of the crypt abscesses produce a shaggy mucosal ulceration. Intense hyperemia of the mucosa occurs. Later in the course of the disease intense lymphocytic and plasma cell infiltration surrounds the abscesses and ulcers, producing a chronic inflammatory response that is situated in the mucosa and the superficial aspect of the submucosa. However, in spite of the extensive necrosis and mucosal inflammation, fibroblastic proliferation and collagen fiber formation, usual features of inflammatory repair, occur minimally and late in the process, if at all. Very uncommonly, the deeper layers of the bowel wall may be involved. A bloody mucopurulent discharge into the lumen of the intestine with varying proportions of blood, mucus, and pus is seen. Occasionally the lesion may extend to the vermiform appendix or terminal ileum. Extraintestinal lesions are occasionally found in the skin, liver, or joints, and in rare cases the existence of the secondary lesion may precede or overshadow the severity of the intestinal process.

The etiology of ulcerative colitis is unknown. As with regional enteritis and other diseases, in the absence of an etiologic classification the most fruitful approach is to characterize the disease process on the

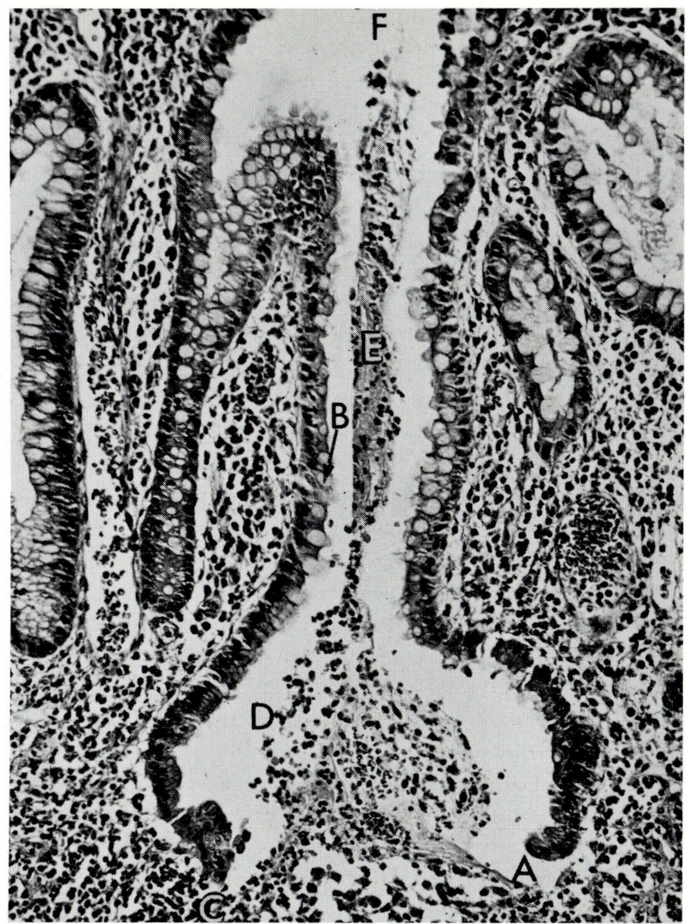

Figure 2–1   A crypt abscess, the characteristic and commonly observed microscopic lesion of ulcerative colitis. Epithelial necrosis has occurred at the base of a crypt of Lieberkühn (A) of a gland with decreased mucous secretion (B). Polymorphs and necrotic debris extend from the lamina propria (C) into the lumen of the distended gland (D) and form a streamer of pus (E) extending to the lumen of the bowel (F). ×40.

basis of its histopathologic process. This enables the clinician and researcher alike to group cases of comparable pathologic process together in order to analyze and deal with them more successfully. By defining the pathologic process and delineating its boundaries with similar entities one can group like responses for constructive study. The central purpose of this book is to characterize the pathologic processes of two distinctive intestinal inflammations and to compare them with similar inflammatory intestinal processes. The observer must constantly bear in mind that the characteristic features of the process in an individual may be modified by numerous intrinsic and extrinsic factors that cause variability in the morphologic change. Because of this variability, there is usually some overlapping with the features of other intestinal diseases, which occasionally is a source of nosologic confusion.

TERMINOLOGY

In their second edition of *Lectures on Pathological Anatomy,* published in 1875, Wilks and Moxon not only clearly delineated ulcerative colitis as an entity distinct from dysentery, but firmly implanted the term ulcerative colitis, which has been generally accepted since that time.[1] Because it is clearly appropriate to the nature of the process, there has been little attempt to change or modify the name. Variations that have occurred include the insertion of the word "idiopathic" or "nonspecific" in an attempt to emphasize the fact that as yet the cause is unknown, and that clinically the diagnosis is often reached by exclusion of other diseases of the colon of known etiology by demonstration of the etiologic agent. Occasionally the colitis portion of the term has been changed to proctocolitis to emphasize the fact that the disease frequently involves the rectum, a feature that is commonly accepted as understood by the users of the term ulcerative colitis. Others have tended to use the terms primary, suppurative, or chronic, a practice that has little to recommend it. Though the disease may follow a prolonged or chronic clinical course, throughout much of it the inflammatory infiltrate is clearly an acute rather than a chronic type of cellular exudate. Rarely the terms colitis ulcerosa or colitis gravis have been used to denote this process, especially on the European continent. More recently the term thromboulcerative colitis has been used, principally by those who emphasize the possibility that the disease entity may have a vascular occlusive origin. This usage also seems to be premature until conclusive evidence of the etiologic and pathogenetic mechanisms has been found.

HISTORY

Recognition of the existence of a noncontagious type of diarrhea associated with colonic inflammations probably evolved during the early Christian era in Europe. According to Goligher and co-workers,

One fascinating and detailed early description of ulcerative colitis-like disease is attributed to Aretaeus of Cappadocia (*c.* A.D. 300). He described a large number of different types of diarrhea including one which consisted of chronic noncontagious diarrhea of a foul type found chiefly in adults, more common in women than in men, occasionally seen in elderly persons and in older children but never found in infants! It is arguable that some cases of Crohn's disease or idiopathic steatorrhea might have been included under this heading but Aretaeus' account is one which many present day clinicians would accept as descriptive of ulcerative colitis. Certainly he has reproduced the age specific incidence of this latter disease with uncanny precision! Similar, though less precise, descriptions of a condition like ulcerative colitis were recorded by a number of other physicians in Roman times including one from Epheus (*c.* A.D. 117), whose name "Soranus" seems curiously apt.[2]

Much credit for the delineation of ulcerative colitis as a separate clinical and pathologic entity should be given to the Union Army Medical Corps during the American Civil War. In the Surgeon General's publication, *Medical and Surgical History of the Rebellion, U.S.A.,* published in 1865, the pathologic and clinical features of ulcerative colitis and its distinction from other forms of dysentery were described as follows:

The series illustrative of diarrhoea and dysentery consists of over 200 specimens, grouped as follows:

The first group embraces the examples of follicular ulceration of the colon. The specimens present all the transition forms of simple enlargement of the solitary follicles of the colon, the rupture of the same, and the formation of punched-out ulcers of moderate size. The colon is usually more or less thickened, the thickening, in some cases, amounting to a quarter of an inch. The ulcers are usually rounded or oval, extending nearly or quite to the muscular coat, and looking much as if they had been cut out with a punch; when received fresh at the Museum, the appearances varied with the stage of the process. In the few cases in which the solitary follicles were simply enlarged, without ulceration, the intestine was seldom thickened. It was often normal in color; sometimes, however, slate or ash colored; sometimes it presented patches of congestion. The enlarged solitary follicles were often the seat of pigment deposits; sometimes also an areola of pigment, deposited in and among the glands of Lieberkühn, surrounded the enlarged and blackened solitary follicles. These patients had generally died of some other disease, as of camp fever supervening upon the diarrhoea, with lesions of the small intestine—of gunshot wounds, etc. In the more serious cases of diarrhoea, the colon was more or less thickened, and presented punched-out ulcers which had originated in the solitary follicles. The colon was then seldom normal in its color. Sometimes it was red, reddish brown, or reddish black; at other times greenish, slate, or ash colored; at others, again, unnaturally pale. Its texture, when cut into, was sometimes tough and lardaceous; sometimes it was softened. The ulcers usually presented a grayish or yellowish-gray base. They were sometimes filled with mucus, at other times contained pus. In the majority of the cases of this class, the small intestine was not involved, unless camp fever had existed as a complication.

In the second group of cases, the follicular ulcers have extended until, in extreme instances, the greater part of the mucous membrane of the colon is destroyed by the vast erosions thus produced. The follicular ulcers usually extend by burrowing in the submucous connective tissue; in this way, in some of the specimens, several of these ulcers communicate with each other in the submucous tissue, though still retaining distinct orifices. The mucous layer containing the glands of Lieberkühn, undermined by the extension of the ulcer, not unfrequently hangs in shreds like a fringe from its edge; the undermined portion being occasionally destroyed by ulceration, but more frequently perishing by sloughing. In such specimens, when received fresh at the Museum, the mucous membrane was generally of a dark-red, brownish, greenish-brown, or slate color. The ulcers presented yellowish-brown or yellowish bases, often with blackish or brown sloughs adhering to their surface or edges. It would appear that this second group of cases represents simply a more advanced stage of the disease shown in the first group; and that the conditions determining the degree of ulceration are the duration of the disorder on the one hand, on the other, the constitutional condition of the patients; those who labored under the scorbutic taint, or who were otherwise brought to an extremely adynamic condition, presenting the most extensive ulcers.

In the third group, the cases present more or less ulceration of the bowel, similar to that seen in the first and second group; but, in addition, the surface of the gut is more or less coated with a yellowish or greenish-yellow pseudo-membranous layer, like that observed in the air-passages in diphtheria. This condition is generally the result of an acute dysenteric process supervening upon a previous diarrhoea of long standing. The appearances of the gut, when fresh, are masked by the plastered layer of greenish-yellow or yellowish pseudo-membrane which coats its surface.[3]

Their series of specimens on diarrhea and dysentery was preceded by others with typhoid and paratyphoid lesions and was followed by groups of lesions involving the small and large intestine, principally tuberculous. Their description of the first and second groups of the diarrhea and dysentery series is consistent with ulcerative colitis, but does not, however, rule out amebic dysentery. Their emphasis on the changes in the crypts suggests that, for the most part, they had separated ulcerative colitis from other colonic inflammations. Their report includes a photograph of one of the cases described and documents their recognition of a type of colitis separate from dysentery (Fig. 2-2). In their discussion of the lesions they note that "two forms of ulceration have been observed in the colon in these cases of chronic diarrhoea." The authors then describe what is obviously lymph follicle hyperplasia with secondary ulceration and the "glandular" type of lesion shown in the photograph. The former most assuredly represents a dysentery or paratyphoid type of lesion (see Chapter Six). They conclude the circular with the following paragraph:

The second form of ulceration begins by an abrasion or denudation of epithelium at some point which does not correspond to the position of a solitary follicle. The follicles of Lieberkühn are next destroyed, and the ulcer spreads in the connective tissue by the process which has just been described. The central ulcer of the plate is of this variety. Such ulcers are much rarer than those of the first kind and probably are always secondary to them. It is not possible to go further into details in this direction at present, but it is hoped that a careful and fully illustrated account of the minute anatomy of these diseases will be presented to the medical profession in the Medical History of the War.[3]

The evidence indicates that they recognized the existence of what we call ulcerative colitis, though they did not name it or pursue its significance. It is a striking testimonial to their medical acumen, espe-

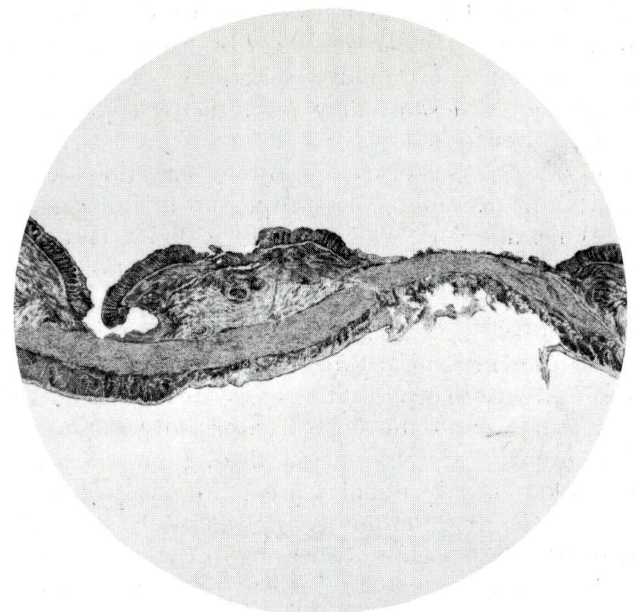

A

Outline of the accompanying plate. A A A A. Follicles of Lieberkühn. B B. Muscle of Brücke. C C C C. Submucous connective tissue. D D D D. Circular muscle of the colon. E E E. Longitudinal muscle, cut transversely; At H H, two of the longitudinal bands of this layer. F F F. Peritoneal layer. G G G G. Points of very active cell multiplication. I I. An artery and vein cut through transversely. 1. A deep follicular ulcer, extending to the muscular layer. 2. A small superficial ulcer, which has penetrated to the submucous connective tissue. 3. An ulcer of greater size, penetrating nearly to the muscular layer, which is covered with granulations.

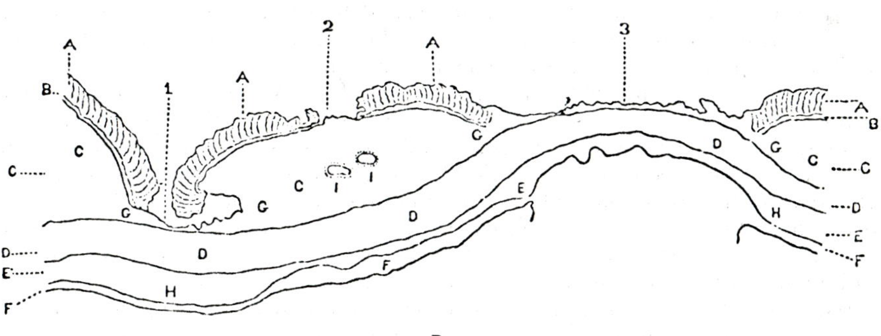

B

Figure 2–2   *A*, Reproduction of a lithographic photomicrograph made in 1865 of a case of "chronic diarrhoea" observed by medical officers of the Union Army during the American Civil War. The anatomic features portrayed are consistent with what we now call ulcerative colitis. It appeared in Circular No. 6 of the Surgeon General's Office, November 1, 1865. It was accompanied by a woodcut outline, *B*, identifying the specific anatomic features of the photolithograph.

The author is indebted to Mr. James B. Rhoads, Archivist of the United States, and Mr. Elmer O. Parker of the Old Military Records Division, who conducted an extensive search to find this report.

cially when one considers that it was accomplished only seven years after the publication of *Cellular Pathology* by Rudolf Virchow, in 1858, and before the era of determinative bacteriology. In their discussion of the microscopy of the lesions they refer to the concepts "argued by Virchow and the Berlin School."

Following on the heels of these astute observations, a rapid succession of reports on ulcerative colitis appeared in Europe. In England, Sir Samuel Wilks and Dr. W. Moxon provided a careful study and description of ulcerative colitis in the second edition of their book, *Lectures on Pathological Anatomy*, published in 1875.[1] (In a letter to the *Medical Times and Gazette*, Sir Samuel Wilks had described "The Morbid Appearance of the Intestine of Miss Banks," which was a report of an autopsy presenting the typical findings that we now know to be ulcerative colitis of the severe acute type of "toxic megacolon" in 1859. He described an erosion of the mucosa throughout all regions of the rectum and colon and terminal ileum with massive sloughing and hemorrhage.) In the first edition of the book by Dr. Wilks there was no description of ulcerative colitis. However, in the preface to the second edition Dr. Moxon indicated the need to revise and extend the concepts based on the extension of our knowledge of cellular pathology by Virchow. The second edition, published in 1875, has a section on "Inflammations of the Large Intestine" in which ulcerative colitis was clearly defined and named:

> The term colitis is sometimes used as though synonymous with dysentery. Our usual language has indeed been too indefinite, nay, incorrect, in speaking of all affections of the large intestine as dysenteric; for the true dysenteric process, although in many features like simple ulcerative colitis, yet it is a disease having certain definite characters.
>
> There is quite as much reason to regard febrile epidemic dysentery as a disease distinct from simple ulcerative colitis as there is to regard febrile epidemic dyptheria as a disease distinct from croup. . . .
>
> Cases of idiopathic colitis are rare, and stand, as we have said, in the same relation to true dysentery as croup does to dyptheria, from the absence of those peculiar features which give dysentery the characters of a specific fever. For example, we have seen a case attended by discharge of mucus and blood where, after death, the whole internal surface of the colon presented a highly vascular, soft, red surface, covered with tenacious mucus or adherent lymph, and here and there showing a few points of ulceration; the coats, also, were much swollen by exudation into the mucous and submucous tissues. In other examples there has been extensive ulceration, commencing in the follicles, and spreading from them to destroy the tissue around, thus producing a ragged ulcerated surface. . . .[1]

Following this Doctor Moxon proceeds to describe "pellicular or dyptheritic colitis" and describes the pseudomembrane of a case of Bright's disease. Within a decade following the publication of the textbook by Wilks and Moxon, several reports relating to the entity were published.[4, 5, 6]

EPIDEMIOLOGY

Analogous Lesions in Animals

The existence of a naturally occurring ulcerative colitis-like disease in domestic or laboratory animals has not been conclusively demonstrated. Many types of inflammatory lesions of the colon have been described; however, none of them have the characteristic histopathology of ulcerative colitis. Reports such as that of Stewart and Jones clearly are not the human type of pathologic process.[7] In their study of a spontaneous disease occurring in the cecum of rats the inflammation was predominantly perivascular in location with a periarteritis and endarteritis obliterans. Prominent lymphangitis and lymphostasis were also noted. When the animals recovered, intensive scarification of the sides of the ulcers occurred, in some instances producing a stricture.

A lesion strikingly similar to ulcerative colitis was produced in laboratory rats and rabbits by means of radiation by Sommers and Warren (Figs. 2–3, 2–4, 2–5, and 2–6).[8, 42] They irradiated 346 parabiotic rat pairs plus 72 additional pairs in which one partner had been adrenalectomized prior to irradiation. Total body irradiation was administered always to the right-hand partner in single doses of 400, 800, 1200, or 1600 r. Eighteen single control rats were similarly irradiated at each of these dose levels. After irradiation the animals were killed at intervals from one hour to 29 days, and complete autopsies were performed. Crypt abscess lesions were found in 9 per cent of the parabiotic rats. The crypt abscesses have a striking similarity to the characteristic lesions of ulcerative colitis. No lesions of this type were found in the protected (nonirradiated) parabiont or in the nonirradiated controls. It must be appreciated that while the colonic lesion was developing, other changes characteristic of radiation disease were developing in other organs of the body. The time when crypt abscesses occurred was not that of the maximal radiation damage, but tended to precede it. Infections seemed an unlikely explanation because the inflammatory change was limited to the crypts and did not involve the surface aspects of the epithelium. Studies of human and animal gastrointestinal tissues after ionizing radiation have not revealed crypt abscesses. However, these studies have not been extensive, and measurements of dosage level and distribution have not been carefully controlled.

Recently Watt and Marcus produced lesions strikingly similar to those of ulcerative colitis in rabbits and guinea pigs by including carrageenins in their feed.[43, 44] The carrageenins were derived from red seaweed, *Eucheuma spinosum.* After undegraded or degraded carrageenins were included in the diet of guinea pigs, ulcerations (includ-

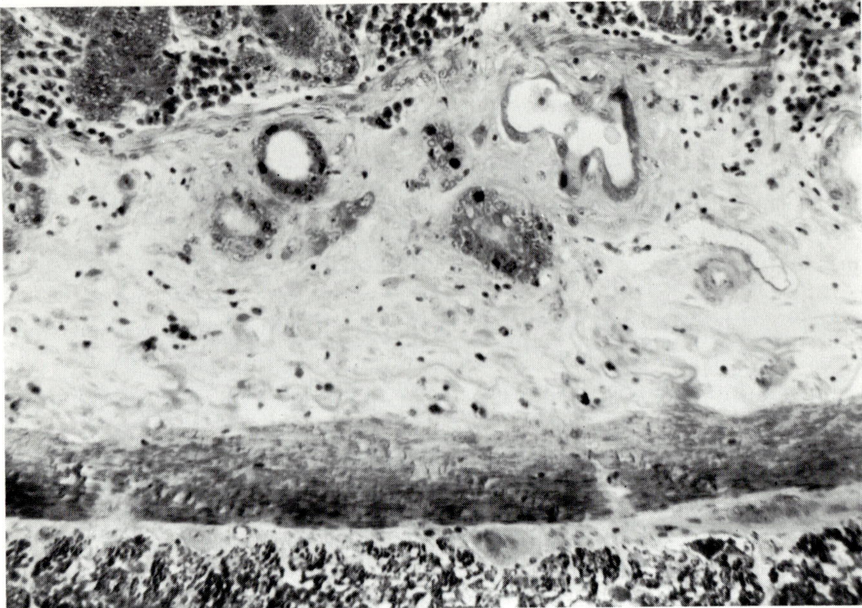

Figure 2-3   Radiation changes in the intestine of a rabbit. Note edematous submucosa, abnormal epithelial cells in the glands, extensive edema, and the beginning of inflammatory change. ×300. (Courtesy of S. Warren, M.D., of the Cancer Research Institute, New England Deaconess Hospital, Boston.)

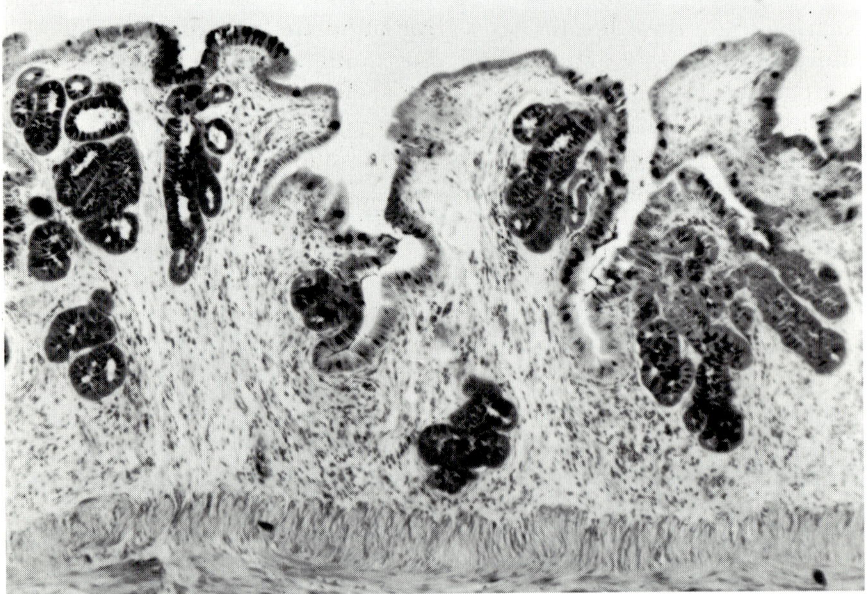

Figure 2-4   Rabbit colon during the first month after irradiation (8 to 10 doses of 400 to 500 r daily) showing atrophic mucosa interspersed with hyperplastic regenerating glands. Diffuse inflammatory infiltrate is seen in the lamina propria. ×100. (Courtesy of N. B. Friedman and S. Warren, Arch. Path. *33*:326-333, 1942, and the American Medical Association.)

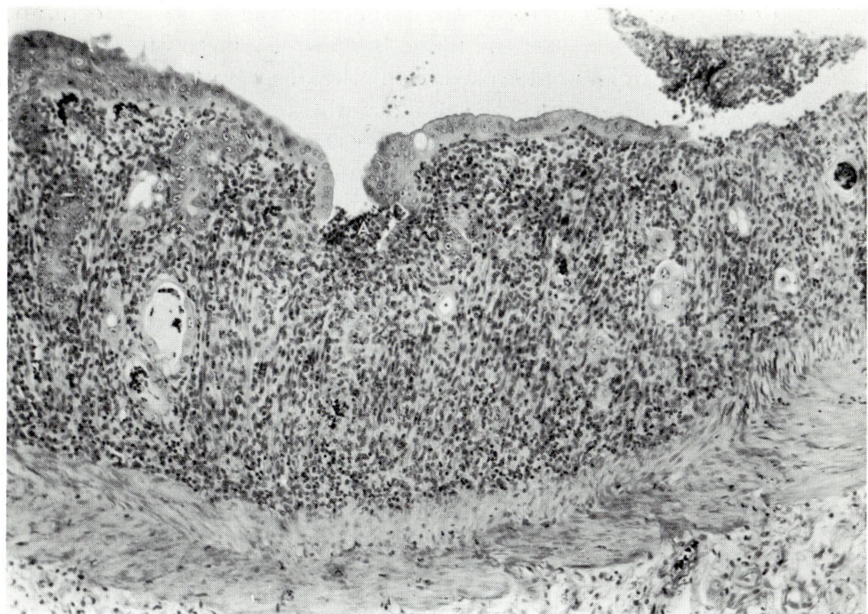

Figure 2–5 Rabbit colon during the first month after irradiation showing atrophic mucosa with early ulceration (A) and diffuse inflammatory infiltrate of the lamina propria of polymorphs, lymphocytes and eosinophiles. Changes are confined to the superficial layers. ×150. (Courtesy of N. B. Friedman and S. Warren, Arch. Path. *33*:326-333, 1942, and the American Medical Association.)

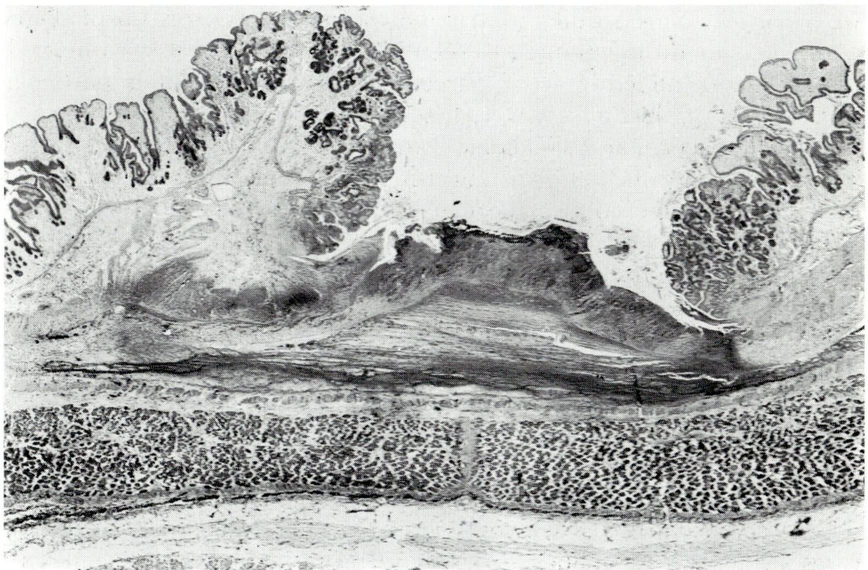

Figure 2–6 Rabbit colon during the third month after irradiation showing a large ulcer in an abnormal mucosa. The colonic lesion produced by irradiation has many similarities to the lesions of human ulcerative colitis (see Chapter Five). Crypt abscesses have been reported in about 10 per cent of the experimental lesions. ×100. (Courtesy of N. B. Friedman and S. Warren, Arch. Path. *33*:326-333, 1942, and the American Medical Association.)

ing crypt abscesses) occurred in the large intestine in 80 per cent and 100 per cent respectively of the animals within 30 days. Similar results were obtained in rabbits. Microscopically the ulcers involved mainly the mucosa with the characteristic cellular infiltrate, vascular congestion, and crypt abscesses. Though additional research is necessary to further elucidate the phenomenon, it appears significant for at least two reasons: It may provide a convenient experimental model for study of the etiology and pathogenesis of ulcerative colitis in humans; and caution should be exercised in utilizing foods or medicinals containing carrageenins until more is known of their biologic effects.

Geographical Distribution and Incidence

That ulcerative colitis in the human has a worldwide distribution is unquestionable. Of doubtful validity are many of the reports of varying incidence in different regions. The *incidence* of a disease is the number of individuals in whom that disease is diagnosed in any given year, divided by the population at risk. The *prevalence* of a disease is the number of individals suffering from the disease at any given date, divided by the number of people at risk at that specific time. Thus, a disease that persists on the average of 10 years before death or cure will have a prevalence rate about 10 times the incidence rate. It is quite apparent that the gathering of data for the denominator of this ratio is usually much easier than gathering the data for the numerator. The weakness of many studies is that the data are based on hospital first admissions or numbers of cases seen in a hospital. There are obviously many factors affecting what percentage of all cases of a particular disease will present at a hospital, such as type of hospital, pattern of physician practice, and sociologic characteristics of the populace. When a disease is as difficult to distinguish from other intestinal inflammations as ulcerative colitis, one can appreciate the unreliability of the data. To compare the reports from one country to another is quite unreliable. Goligher and co-workers in Chapter IV of their book, *Ulcerative Colitis,* have collected reports from various countries of the world.[2] It is apparent from the literature that ulcerative colitis has been diagnosed on every continent in the world and that it exists in virtually all major subdivisions of the human race.

For many years the fiction persisted that ulcerative colitis did not occur in the tropics. An increasing number of case reports from tropical countries, as the diagnostic procedures for distinguishing the dysenteries from ulcerative colitis improved, revealed more and more cases of ulcerative colitis. For example, Chuttani and colleagues reviewed the existence of ulcerative colitis in the tropical zone of India by gathering the admission rate of cases of ulcerative colitis to various hospitals.[9] Diagnoses based on modern clinical methods revealed that the disease was not rare on the Indian subcontinent. Their observation that the admission rate in different hospitals varied tenfold further confirms the unreliability of hospital admission rates as a guide to the incidence of a disease unless a detailed study of the population at risk and the hospital under study clearly shows that they account for approximately the total medical care for colonic diseases in the region. Reports of the existence of ulcerative colitis have also emanated from Mexico, Iran, Israel, Egypt, Brazil, and Greece.[10] The tropical and subtropical distribution of ulcerative colitis is broad.[45] For these reasons I do not place any credence in the actual incidence as given in these many case reports beyond the generalization that the disease exists in these countries. The reader who wishes to pursue these reports further may refer to the aforementioned chapter. I shall confine my discussion to the thorough and statistically valid studies in defined populations.

As with regional enteritis, there are three studies using modern statistical methods and pursued with great care that present the closest approximation to the actual incidence of the disease in Northern Europe and North America. Paramount among these are the several reports of Acheson, who studied the incidence, prevalence, and mortality of ulcerative colitis in the Oxford area of England and the mortality of the disease in the United States Army. He has reviewed and summarized his various studies on the epidemiology of ulcerative colitis.[1] Monk and co-workers studied the epidemiology of ulcerative colitis and regional enteritis in the adult population of the Baltimore area.[12, 13] Their method of finding cases was based on hospital admissions to the 17 general hospitals in the city of Baltimore plus two Federal hospitals, which serve virtually all the population of the metropolitan area. Therefore the study of hospital admissions in this instance provides a reasonably good estimation of the total incidence of the disease in the population defined in the study. However, it must be appreciated that some cases of ulcerative colitis in this region may have been treated in private physicians' offices and not referred to the major hospitals so that the incidence may have been shown as somewhat less than its actuality. The third major study of ulcerative colitis was conducted by Gjone and Myren in Norway, where by virtue of the National Health program virtually all cases that occur within the country are recorded.[14] Prior to these major studies on the epidemiology of ulcerative colitis, Houghton and Naish used the records of a group of hospitals in Bristol, England, which together, like the Baltimore study, represent a definable population.[15] Their results are quite similar to the more recent and extensive studies in the Oxford area. Acheson and co-workers, by laboriously pursuing several sources of cases (described in Chapter One under Epidemiology), were able to uncover virtually every case in a definable population of Oxford, England, and its surrounding countryside.[11] They examined the in-patient records of the hospitals of the region, they queried the general practitioners and consultants in the area, and they found that the average annual in-

TABLE 2–1   Average Annual Incidence of Ulcerative Colitis Per 100,000 White Population

	Male	Female	Total
England (Oxford area)	5.8	7.3	6.5
United States (Baltimore area)	3.9	5.2	4.6
New Zealand			5
Norway	2.0	2.1	2.1

cidence of ulcerative colitis was 6.5 cases per 100,000. The prevalence rate was 79.9 cases per 100,000 (Table 2–1). The study of Gjone and Myren in Norway, using first hospitalization rates, revealed an incidence rate of 2.1 cases per year per 100,000 population, which is considerably lower than that of the Oxford area.[14] Wigley and McLaurin, in a similar relatively thorough study of the first hospitalization rate in the white population of New Zealand, found the rate to be 5 to 6 per 100,000, which is quite similar to that found by Acheson in Oxford.[16] The already noted study of Monk and co-workers established the average annual incidence of first hospitalization rate for ulcerative colitis per 100,000 white population in the Baltimore area to be 4.6. Thus, the data from Oxford, New Zealand, and Baltimore are quite similar; however, Norway records a much lower incidence. Whether the low incidence in Norway is an artifact of the case finding or reporting methods or is in actuality an ethnic difference remains to be proved.

Ethnic Distribution

Whether the foregoing incidence deciphered for predominantly Caucasian populations is comparable with other races and ethnic groups in general remains to be demonstrated. Within certain subdivisions of the human race the observation of cases of ulcerative colitis is extremely rare and worthy of note. For example, Wigley and McLaurin were able to find only two cases in New Zealand that involved the Maori population.[16] Though this could be attributed to a low diagnostic rate due to the stoic personality and rural habitat, which would tend to diminish the use of medical care, it seems quite unlikely. As the authors point out, the Maoris do avail themselves of the National Health program. For example, there was no difference in the admission rate between Maori and European males for coronary disease. Unless one assumes that coronary heart disease was much more common in the Maoris than in whites (which has not been substantiated), their utilization of the hospitals was about equal to that of the white population. Wigley and McLaurin concluded that the paucity of cases of ulcerative colitis among the Maoris was a genuine racial difference. Bebchuck and co-workers have shown that cases of ulcerative colitis are also extremely rare among some Indian tribes of North America.[17]

Reichenbach conducted an autopsy study of 328 American Indian deaths from the tribes of the Southwestern region of the United States.[18] This represented about one in five deaths occurring over a five year period. He found that the incidence of several disorders (e.g., cholelithiasis, diabetes mellitus, congenital anomalies, tuberculosis) varied greatly from tribe to tribe. In a personal communication he stated that in his experience no cases of regional enteritis or ulcerative colitis were diagnosed though bacillary dysentery was quite common, especially among the young.

Undoubtedly the best-documented ethnic variance in the incidence of ulcerative colitis has been shown for the Jewish ethnic group. Paulley was among the first to demonstrate that the incidence of ulcerative colitis among the Jewish patients in two London hospitals was far in excess of that of the Gentiles.[19] Subsequent studies by Acheson on the well-defined group of young males of the United States Army veterans found a fourfold excess of ulcerative colitis among Jews when compared to Gentiles.[20] Acheson and Nefzger pursued these investigations further and found that the higher risk in Jews was present regardless of the region within the United States in which they were born or whether they were residents of large cities or rural areas.[21] Acheson also noted a greater number of Jews in the Oxford survey. Further confirmatory evidence was provided by Birnbaum, Groen, and Kallner, who studied the occurrence of ulcerative colitis amongst the various ethnic subgroups in Israel.[22] The results suggest that the disease was more frequent among the Occidental than the Oriental Jews. Also, Monk and co-workers in the Baltimore study, using detailed methods to eliminate sampling bias, concluded that Jews have a rate that is two to four times higher than non-Jews. The ratio of Jewish to non-Jewish women hospitalized for the first time is over four to one; it was unchanged for each decade of life except among women over 60 years of age.

Whether the incidence of ulcerative colitis in the American Negro is the same or different from the Caucasian remains unproved. In Acheson and Nefzger's study of the U.S. Army population there was no significant difference between the American Negro and the white enlisted man. It has long been the clinical impression that fewer American Negroes have ulcerative colitis than whites; however, this type of observation is subject to extensive error. The Baltimore area study, which included the largest American Negro population yet studied for the disease, revealed the incidence of ulcerative colitis to be much lower in the non-white population than in the white. Whereas the Baltimore white population had 3.5 first hospitalization cases per 100,000 population per year, the non-white population had 0.45. Therefore, from the fragmentary evidence that exists, the incidence of ulcerative colitis probably is lower in the American Negro than in his Caucasian countryman.

Age and Sex Distribution

Coll and Stevenson reported a case of ulcerative colitis with onset of symptoms at an age of three weeks that eventually necessitated colectomy.[23] Bargen and Kennedy and Hughes reviewed the problem of infantile ulcerative colitis and reported a series of cases.[24, 25] The age incidence and bimodal pattern of ulcerative colitis was revealed by the Oxford study as shown in Figure 2-7. From this graph one observes that the incidence was extremely low during the first decade of life, but at about the age of puberty it began to rise sharply and reached a peak in the 20 to 40 age groups. There followed a decline in the incidence of new cases in the subsequent decade, but it again increased at the age of 60. This is in sharp contrast to the age distribution of regional enteritis, also shown in the figure. It represents one of the strong evidences against the unity of the two diseases. Reasons for the bimodal shape of the ulcerative colitis curve remain obscure. Whether this reflects a variation in the exposure to extrinsic etiologic agents or biologic

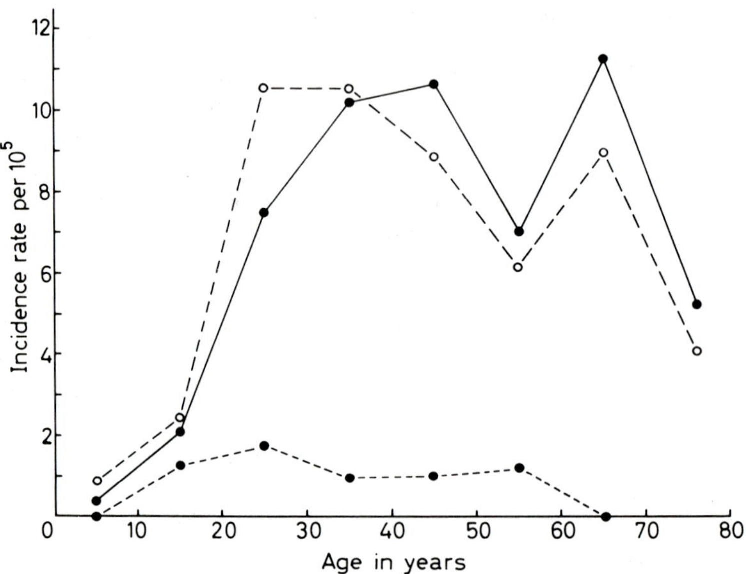

Figure 2-7 Average annual age-specific incidence rates (1951–60) for ulcerative colitis and regional enteritis in the Oxford area. Continuous line = U.C. (age at first diagnosis); interrupted line = U.C. (age at onset of first symptoms); dotted line = R.E. (age at first diagnosis). (Courtesy of E. D. Acheson, in Recent Advances in Gastroenterology, Chapter 2, and J. and A. Churchill, Ltd. London.)

changes within the host is completely unknown. Whether the bimodal distribution holds true for the disease in other countries is also not known.

Several major epidemiologic studies reveal that there is a very slight female preponderance of cases of ulcerative colitis. The ratio of female to male as given by Acheson is 1.3 to 1. The excess risk in women was found to be present in every age group except for the adolescent. Monk and co-workers gave the female to male ratio in the Baltimore study as 1.5 to 1. Thus, the careful statistical studies support the long-standing clinical impression that women are more often liable to ulcerative colitis than men.

Pregnancy and Ulcerative Colitis

The relationship between ulcerative colitis and pregnancy has been extensively studied by Maddix and by Krawitt.[26, 27] A review of the literature uncovered 605 cases that have been reported. Of the 605 pregnancies, 10 per cent resulted in spontaneous abortions and 5 per cent in therapeutic abortions, and only 2 per cent in premature birth and 1 per cent in cesarian section. Ulcerative colitis had its onset during pregnancy in 17 per cent of the women, and aggravation of the disease process occurred in 44 per cent, with an uneventful gestation in 38 per cent. Of the 183 cases in which ulcerative colitis was quiescent at the time of onset of pregnancy, aggravation occurred in 37 per cent. Of the 154 cases in which the disease was active at the time of the onset of pregnancy, in 51 per cent the disease was aggravated, whereas 23 per cent improved, while 27 per cent were unchanged. Therefore it appears that about one of three cases of quiescent ulcerative colitis will be activated by pregnancy, and that about half the active ulcerative colitis patients will be worse with pregnancy. The existence of ulcerative colitis had no effect on the rate of abortion, prematurity, or cesarean section. Krawitt attributes great importance to the attitude of a patient toward her pregnancy as a determinant in the course of ulcerative colitis and emphasizes the importance of the doctor-patient relationship in managing these pregnant women.

Familial Incidence

Major reviews of the familial incidence of ulcerative colitis have been made by Felsen and Wolarsky, by Houghton and Naish, by Kirsner and Spencer, and by Almy and Sherlock.[15, 28, 29, 30] One of the features of epidemiologic studies has been the overlap in the occurrence of ulcerative colitis, regional enteritis, and spondylitis in the same families. Sloan, Bargen, and Gage reviewed more than 2,000 cases of ulcerative colitis and found 26 (1.3 per cent) to have a family history of the disease.[31] In a similar study of more than 1,000 patients Kirsner and Spencer found 66 cases (5.2 per cent). In addition, in the same study, the latter authors found a 10.8 per cent incidence of regional enteritis. Almy and Sherlock calculated that the chance occurrence of these various diseases in the same family would be one in a million for ulcerative colitis and one in 25 million for regional enteritis. Thus, the foregoing demonstration of a family occurrence of at least 1 to 2 per cent indicates that the overlap is significant. Felsen and Wolarsky found positive family histories in 3.1 per cent of 1,204 patients studied, and Houghton and Naish obtained similar results in Bristol. Therefore an increased familial occurrence of these diseases is unquestionable.

MORTALITY

Table 2-2 presents the annual death rate for ulcerative colitis compiled from the several studies just noted. For unexplained reasons the death rate for ulcerative colitis is almost twice as high in England and Wales as in North America. This may be an artifact of diagnostic procedures or death certificate terminology, or a more fatal type of disease may occur in these countries. The death rate for regional enteritis in these countries is similar. The mortality data from a wide variety of countries and several continents all show a lower mortality rate than that shown for England and Wales. However, these reports are subject to error as already described.

TABLE 2–2   Annual Death Rates from Ulcerative Colitis and Regional Enteritis Taken from Various Periods in the Decade 1951–60 per 100,000*

	AVERAGE ANNUAL DEATH RATES	
	Ulcerative colitis (572.2)	*Regional enteritis* (572.1)
England and Wales (1952–56)	0.9†	0.11†
U.S.A. (1950; 1952–56)		
White races	0.5†	0.08†
Coloured races	0.3†	0.06†
Canada (1952–57)	0.5†	0.09†
New Zealand (1954–58)		
White races	0.9	0.07
Maoris	0.0	—
Denmark	0.6	—
Israel	0.5	—

*Courtesy of E. D. Acheson, in *Recent Advances in Gastroententerology* (Chapter 2). London, J. and A. Churchill Ltd., 1965.
†Age-adjusted to U.S. population, 1950.

ETIOLOGY

The cause of ulcerative colitis is completely unknown despite many years of research effort. Innumerable suspected causative factors have been suggested,[46] often with minimal objective evidence in their support. Because the disease does not occur spontaneously in animals the development of an experimental model has been tardy. Investigation has been largely confined to human clinical situations, which are cumbersome and often inexact. Its unpredictable course characterized by spontaneous remissions and exacerbations complicates the accurate evaluation of cases. Because the disease is not a common one it is difficult for any one physician to accumulate a large series of patients and to carry out personally carefully controlled studies except in a few centers. Indeed, confusion has been sufficiently extensive to lead many to suggest that ulcerative colitis is not a single disease but a constellation of related diseases. Some believe it is a "final common pathway" of pathologic process due to a variety of causes. Others have suggested that regional enteritis and ulcerative colitis are merely variations of the same process, presumably having the same cause.

Infectious Agents

For many years clinical investigators have attempted to link ulcerative colitis with specific infections of the colon. Even though ulcerative colitis was identified as a morphologic and clinical entity distinct from dysentery more than a hundred years ago, physicians have repeatedly attempted to link the process with infection. The clinical course of a patient who is febrile and toxic with bloody stools and with rapid onset of the problem has led many physicians to attempt to show a relationship between ulcerative colitis and specific colonic infectious processes. All these attempts have failed thus far. None of the colonic organisms studied, whether bacterial, protozoal, viral, or fungal, have been demonstrated as a causative agent. Study of the intestinal flora in cases of ulcerative colitis has revealed no clearly pathogenic bacteria or parasites. Fecal bacterial growths from ulcerative colitis patients generally yield the same organisms, i.e., streptococci, staphylococci, and coliform bacilli. Some studies have revealed the total bacterial count of the stools of ulcerative colitis patients to be much in excess of controls. The significance of this overgrowth is doubtful because the preponderance of evidence indicates that the contents of the colon of patients with ulcerative colitis is a good culture medium and bacterial overgrowth is to be expected. Decreasing the bacterial count by means of antibiotics does not alter the course or the pathologic features of the disease.

Felsen and Wolarsky have been recent proponents of a relationship between *Shigella* infection and ulcerative colitis.[28] Their conclusions rely heavily on positive agglutination tests, which are, at best, of doubtful significance. Occasionally the onset of ulcerative colitis closely coincides with an attack of dysentery. Investigators have been unable to demonstrate the presence of *Shigella* in the stools of ulcerative colitis patients or in samples taken from the ulcers. More recently a 20 year follow-up on the incidence of ulcerative colitis in World War II veterans who had bacterially proved bouts of *Shigella* dysentery has been reported. These individuals did not have an abnormal amount of ulcerative colitis during the period of follow-up. An abnormal bacterial profile in the colon resulting from the use of some antibiotics produces an acute pseudomembranous enterocolitis that is pathologically distinct from ulcerative colitis (see Chapter Three). The preponderance of evidence to date does not support bacteria as a direct primary causative agent.

Viral agents have been suggested, but again, cultures of feces and biopsy tissue and animal inoculation procedures have not uncovered an etiologic agent. Lymphopathia venereum virus has been suggested; however, the Frei test is virtually always negative in ulcerative colitis patients, and neutralizing serum antibodies for the virus are absent. A generation ago protozoal infection with *Entamoeba histolytica* was suggested as an etiologic agent even though the appearance of the ulcerated lesions is quite dissimilar. Since the development of effective amebacides and their trial in ulcerative colitis patients, it has generally been shown that there is no significant effect on the course of the disease and that the ameba seems to be an unlikely agent.

Though infectious agents have not been shown to be a primary etiologic factor in ulcerative colitis, the likelihood of their having a part in the morphologic appearance and perpetuation of the lesion as secondary invaders seems much more plausible. Unfortunately the precise role of secondary invasion of bacteria in the pathogenesis of ulcerative colitis has not been elucidated. One can only state that bacteria appear to contribute to the severity and chronicity of the lesion and to some of the features of its histopathology, which is discussed in a subsequent chapter.

Psychologic Factors

Since the early work of C. D. Murray and of Sullivan and Chandler, the possibility of a psychosomatic mechanism producing ulcerative colitis has been considered.[33, 34] Psychiatrists generally characterize the personality structure of patients with ulcerative colitis as being one of immaturity with a dependent attitude toward others and a diminished ability to tolerate frustration or to assume responsibility. These individuals have difficulty in facing up to life situations demanding decisive or aggressive action. They are often intelligent and ambitious, but have great difficulty in carrying out successful patterns of activity. Many show obsessive, compulsive traits as a means of compensating for this difficulty. They are often oversensitive and withdrawn, submissive, and display placating attitudes and conforming behavior. Groen and Bastiaans reported their results with 29 patients who were treated exclusively with psychotherapy, which consisted of sympathetic listening, attentiveness, kindess, protection, and the opportunity for the patient to discharge aggressive feelings.[35] Of the 29 patients treated with this type of supportive psychotherapy, 14 remained well for a year after treatment, 7 improved, and 8 either had recurrence of the disease or became much worse. Certainly this psychotherapy is as effective in treating ulcerative colitis as are the current chemical agents. Grace, Pinsky, and Wolff also did a very carefully controlled study of 34 patients with ulcerative colitis.[36] Their controls consisted of a matched pairing of patients, 34 in number, with regard to age, sex, severity of illness, and duration of illness prior to treatment. Therapy was aimed at alleviating stress in the patients. Considerable improvement was noted in those treated by psychotherapy, in both the roentgen appearance of the colon and the over-all clinical result.

Though patients with ulcerative colitis appear to represent a more definable psychologic type than those with regional enteritis, little evidence has been provided in terms of the psychosomatic mechanism involved. Physiologists have long known that vascular reactions such as vasodilatation or vasoconstriction occur in the intestinal tract as a result of fright, rage, or pain. These observations have been made not only on experimental animals, but in the human with various kinds of intestinal stoma or fistula. Evocation of resentment, hostility, or rage produces not only a hypermotile bowel, but hyperemia, edema, and a friable mucosa with petechial hemorrhages. The experience of fright can produce a rapid and extensive pallor or vasoconstriction in a patch of the colon that may last for half a minute or more. Painful stimuli similarly produce a temporary blanching. Just as the skin color changes from pallor with fear to hyperemia with rage as a consequence of vascular changes mediated through the autonomic system, comparable changes occur in the bowel mucosa. Though one may perceive the physiologic mechanism whereby the emotional state of the individual may produce or predispose to ulcerative colitis, there is no evidence that this actually does happen as a cause of ulcerative colitis.

Vascular Abnormalities

Vascular phenomena have been invoked by others seeking organic explanations for ulcerative colitis. The diminution of the vascularization of the bowel or parts of it, owing to endarteritis or vasoconstriction, has been seen in some pathologic specimens of ulcerative colitis. The pathologic features of ischemic colitis have been well defined and these changes do not resemble them (see Chapter Six). In our own observations on newborn infants with ischemic colitis, the gross and microscopic appearances of the lesions are distinct from those described for ulcerative colitis. It seems quite unlikely that interference with the vascular supply alone can produce the lesion characteristic of ulcerative colitis, though it may be an additive factor.

Lunderquist and Lunderquist studied the vascular supply of the colon in 10 patients with ulcerative colitis and 3 normal controls by angiography.[37] Two of their ulcerative colitis patients were symptom free at the time of examination and revealed a normal vascularization of the colon. Each of the 8 remaining patients had an inferior mesenteric artery that was diminished in diameter to 4.5 to 6.5 mm. The vasa recta did not taper in the usual manner and often terminated bluntly as if occluded. The mucosa of the intestine was supplied only by very narrow, irregularly distributed arteries. The veins were markedly dilated, had an irregular course, and filled with the contrast media more quickly than normal. Warren and Sommers first reported the existence of vasculitis lesions in some cases of ulcerative colitis and classified them as a separate subtype.[38] Many, however, lack morphologically demonstrable vascular lesions. Whether the vascular lesions are a cause or a consequence of the colitis remains to be proved.

Motility

Others seeking a physiologic mechanism in the genesis of ulcerative colitis have noted that intestinal motility is altered in patients with the disease. The motor phenomena in ulcerative colitis have been objectively studied using physiologic methods. In contrast to normal patients, those with ulcerative colitis have an over-all reduction in bowel motility, particularly in those motions that are associated with the to-and-fro mixing of the bowel contents. In contrast to this, the powerful major propulsive waves of contractility spread over the entire colon, in large part replacing the mixing and absorption-inducing motility, and these major propulsive excretory mass movements are increased. Patients with inactive ulcerative colitis, however, who do not have diarrhea, exhibit normal motility patterns in the colon. It has been impossible to determine whether altered motility patterns are a cause or a consequence of the disease, because there is, as yet, no way of identifying and delineating the motor function of the colon of pre-ulcerative colitis individuals.

Mucolysis

Several research groups have advanced the hypothesis that, under normal circumstances, the mucus produced in the colon protects the wall from other injurious agents, and perhaps ulcerative colitis patients have either an insufficiency or an inappropriate type of mucus with properties inadequate to protect the wall. The corollary of this line of reasoning would be that a noxious agent within the contents of the bowel might inhibit the production of the appropriate mucus or alter it in such a way as to render it ineffective in protecting the mucosa. Attempts to identify alterations in the character of the mucopolysaccharides of ulcerative colitis patients have been unsuccessful. There is no consistent difference between these mucins and those of normal patients. Also attempts to identify enzymes and other agents that might lyse the mucin and set up the conditions for the inflammation have not yielded convincing results. Attempts to identify enzyme constituents of bile and of pancreatic, gastric, or intestinal juices, which may leak into the colon through the intestinal lumen and produce unusually irritating contents, have been unsuccessful. Similarly, attempts to isolate nutritional factors that might alter the relationship between bowel contents and bowel wall resistance have been inconclusive.[39]

Immunologic Mechanisms

A variety of immunologic mechanisms have been suggested as the cause of ulcerative colitis. Some investigators propose that allergies to certain foods, such as wheat, eggs, potatoes, oranges, tomatoes, or milk, represent the etiologic factor. Indeed, a very small percentage of patients will show improvement when milk or one of the other foods is removed from the diet. However, a causal relationship remains to be demonstrated. That dietary alterations may be associated with improvement in the clinical state of the individual does not prove an etiologic relationship. Dietary manipulation has profound psychologic effect on the individual; in addition, dietary manipulations may alter the bacterial flora of the colon. The incidence of allergic disease in ulcerative colitis patients and their families is not significantly different from that in control series.

The Shwartzman reaction as a cause for ulcerative colitis has its proponents. This reaction produces severe capillary damage, thrombosis, and hemorrhage. The lesions of ulcerative colitis involve the mucosa and upper submucosa and are associated with vascular and histologic changes similar to those seen in the Shwartzman reaction. It would also explain the general pattern of exacerbations and remissions. The hypothesis proposes a vascular reaction following the intravenous absorption of a bacterial endotoxin. The reaction would appear only at the site where the endotoxin had been injected or absorbed, in this case the colon. With repeated exposures and reactions, the exacerbations and remissions could be explained. Toxins from antigenically unrelated organisms could induce the response in a previously sensitized mucosa. Though this concept fits attractively with the appearance and behavior of the pathologic process, there is as yet no proof that it actually is involved. It certainly is worthy of further investigation.

Autoimmunity has attracted the attention of several investigators searching for a cause of ulcerative colitis.[40, 41, 47] With the demonstration of autoimmune diseases in other organs, such as the thyroid, the possibility of an autoimmune mechanism in ulcerative colitis exists. Proponents of this mechanism hypothesize that the absorption of antigen from the epithelial or related cells of the mucosa of the colon results in the production of antibodies specific to those cells, which in turn destroy them and produce the necrosis of crypt abscesses that initiates the inflammation. This further produces antigen, which accelerates the cycle. The morphology of the mucosal lesion, the appearance of the lymph nodes, and the demonstration of intestinal mucosal antibodies in the serum of patients with ulcerative colitis produce presumptive evidence in support of the mechanism. However, whether this autoimmunity is a cause or a result of the process also remains to be demonstrated.

Whereas with many disease entities there seems to be little to suggest an etiologic agent, with ulcerative colitis the numerous possibilities have presumptive positive evidence in their support; however, proof is lacking.

SYMPTOMS AND SIGNS

Diarrhea, with or without the passage of blood and mucus in the stools, represents the initial symptom in virtually all cases of ulcerative colitis. Crampy abdominal pain, tenesmus, weight loss, or vomiting occur in about two thirds of the patients shortly after the initial symptoms and may be of varying severity. Quite uncommonly, the patient may present with a fever of unknown origin, joint pains, skin lesions, or symptoms related to liver disease. The onset may be insidious; however, most frequently the onset of bloody diarrhea is abrupt. The past history of other intestinal problems such as spastic colitis is virtually never antecedent. Abdominal pain, when it occurs, is usually associated with defecation. Though in many patients with ulcerative colitis the physical examination may be unrewarding, in others it may provide useful confirmatory evidence. The patient may appear emaciated, and with skin pallor, and there may be evidence of anemia or dehydration as a consequence of the diarrhea. Abdominal examination may reveal point tenderness to pressure and rebound tenderness with guarding and rigidity. In cases in which the bowel is acutely distended (toxic megacolon) the abdomen may appear distended and tympanitic.

Further confirmation of the existence of the disease may be obtained by sigmoidoscopic and radiologic examination. The findings on sigmoidoscopic examination are essentially a part of the gross features of the lesion and are described in Chapter Five.

Following the onset of the disease, the clinical course is extremely variable and any individual case may be placed on a different point of a continuous spectrum, ranging from a very mild disease with occasional attacks to a very severe, acute, fulminating one. As a result, clinicians have established many systems of classification on the basis of clinical behavior. The most characteristic feature of ulcerative colitis is the unpredictability of its clinical course. In some, the illness is relatively mild, being limited to the rectum and rectosigmoid, and on radiologic examination the bowel appears normal. In others whose symptoms are severe, sigmoidoscopic changes are pronounced, and in still others with minimal symptoms, there may be very extensive involvement of the bowel. Usually there is a tendency for progression, though in rare circumstances there has been complete disappearance of evidence of the disease. Generally, those who are very young at the time of onset of the disease will have a more severe course. Also the prognosis appears to be related to the initial severity of the disease. A very mild onset, in about three of four cases, will be followed by a mild course, with improvement or recovery, whereas of those who have a severe, fulminating onset, three of four will have a severe course with probable early death. Mortality during the first year of the disease is quite variable in different reports, ranging from about 25 to 50 per cent. The patient's response to treatment when based on signs and symptoms is difficult to evaluate. Those patients whose colitis is characterized by vasculitis have a higher mortality than those characterized by crypt abscesses. There is a rough correlation between the anatomic extent of the disease and the clinical course. Limited to the left side of the colon, principally the rectum and sigmoid, it has a more favorable prognosis than that involving the entire colon or another segment of it. Patients with right-sided colitis may develop extension of the disease to the descending colon, sigmoid, and rectum, and the prognosis then is that of generalized colitis. Also, the right-sided colitis tends to follow a rapid course with a poor prognosis and to involve the terminal ileum.

References

1. Wilks, S., and Moxon, W.: Lectures on Pathological Anatomy. 2nd Ed. London, J. and A. Churchill Ltd., 1875.
2. Goligher, J. C., de Dombal, F. T., Wattis, J. McK., and Watkinson, G.: Ulcerative Colitis. London, Baillière, Tindall and Cassell, Publishers, 1968.

3. Medical and Surgical History of the Rebellion, U.S.A., Nov. 1, 1865. Circular No. 6, pp. 139-151, Reports on the extent and nature of the material available for the preparation of a medical and surgical history of the rebellion.

4. Allchin, W. H.: Acute extensive ulceration of the colon. Trans. Path. Soc. London *36:*199-202, 1885.

5. White, W. H.: On simple ulcerative colitis and other rare intestinal ulcers. Guy's Hosp. Rep. *30:*131-141, 1888.

6. White, W. H.: Colitis. Lancet *1:*537-538, 1895.

7. Stewart, H. L., and Jones, B. F.: Pathologic anatomy of chronic ulcerative cecitis: A spontaneous disease of the rat. Arch. Path. *31:*37-54, 1941.

8. Sommers, S. C., and Warren, S.: Ulcerative colitis lesions in irradiated rats. Amer. J. Dig. Dis. *22:*109-111, 1955.

9. Chuttani, H. K., Nigam, S. P., Sama, S. K., Dhanda, P. C., and Gupta, P. S.: Ulcerative colitis in the tropics. Brit. Med. J. *4:*204-207, 1967.

10. Zevgolatis, C., Economopoulos, P., and Sakellaropoulos, N.: Ulcerative colitis in Greece: A study of 181 cases. Proc. Roy. Soc. Med. *62:*261-262, 1969.

11. Acheson, E. D.: The epidemiology of ulcerative colitis and regional enteritis. In Recent Advances in Gastroenterology. Chapter 2. Pages 202-226, 1965.

12. Monk, M., Mendeloff, A. I., Siegel, C. I., and Lilienfeld, A.: An epidemiological study of ulcerative colitis and regional enteritis among adults in Baltimore. I. Hospital incidence and prevalence, 1960 to 1963. Gastroenterology *53:*198-210, 1967.

13. Monk, M., Mendeloff, A. I., Siegel, C. I., and Lilienfeld, A.: An epidemiological study of ulcerative colitis and regional enteritis among adults in Baltimore. II. Social and demographic factors. Gastroenterology *56:*847-857, 1969.

14. Gjone, E., and Myren, J.: Colitis ulcerosai Norge. Nord. Med. *71:*143-145, 1964.

15. Houghton, E. A. W., and Naish, J. M.: Familial ulcerative colitis and regional ileitis. Gastroenterologia (Basel) *89:*65-74, 1958.

16. Wigley, R. D., and Mclaurin, B. P.: A study of ulcerative colitis in New Zealand showing a low incidence in Maoris. Brit. Med. J. *2:*228-231, 1962.

17. Bebchuck, W., Rogers, A. G., and Downey, J. L.: Chronic ulcerative colitis in a North American Indian. Gastroenterology *40:*138-140, 1961.

18. Reichenbach, D. D.: Autopsy incidence of diseases among southwestern American Indians. Arch. Path. *84:*81-86, 1967.

19. Paulley, J. W.: Ulcerative colitis; A study of 173 cases. Gastroenterology *16:*566-576, 1950.

20. Acheson, E. D.: The distribution of ulcerative colitis and regional enteritis in United States veterans with particular reference to the Jewish religion. Gut *1:*291-293, 1960.

21. Acheson, E. D., and Nefzger, M. D.: Ulcerative colitis in the United States Army in 1944. Epidemiology: Comparisons between patients and controls. Gastroenterology *44:*7-19, 1963.

22. Birnbaum, D., Groen, J. J., and Kallner, G.: Ulcerative colitis among the ethnic groups in Israel. Arch. Intern. Med. *105:*843-848, 1960.

23. Coll, I., and Stevenson, D. L.: Case of infantile ulcerative colitis. Brit. Med. J. *4:*952-954, 1958.

24. Bargen, J. A., and Kennedy, R. L.: Chronic ulcerative colitis in children. Postgrad. Med. *17:*127-131, 1955.

25. Hughes, E. S.: Course and prognosis of ulcerative colitis developing in childhood. Med. J. Aust. *1:*443-444, 1969.

26. Maddix, B. L.: Ulcerative colitis and pregnancy. Minnesota Med. *45:*1097-1102, 1962.

27. Krawitt, E. L.: Ulcerative colitis in pregnancy. Obstet. Gynec. *14:*354-361, 1959.

28. Felsen, J., and Wolarsky, W.: Familial incidence of ulcerative colitis and ileitis. Gastroenterology *28:*412-417, 1955.

29. Kirsner, J. B., and Spencer, J. A.: Family occurrences of ulcerative colitis, regional enteritis, and ileocolitis. Ann. Intern. Med. *59:*133-144, 1963.

30. Almy, T. P., and Sherlock, P.: Genetic aspects of ulcerative colitis and regional enteritis. Gastroenterology *51:*757-763, 1966.

31. Sloan, W. P., Jr., Bargen, J. A., and Gage, R. P.: Symposium on diseases of the colon; life histories of patients with chronic ulcerative colitis; a review of 2000 cases. Gastroenterology *16:*25-38, 1950.

32. de Dombal, F. T., Burch, P. R. J., and Watkinson, G.: Aetiology of ulcerative colitis. Gut *10*:270-277, 1969.
33. Murray, C. D.: Psychogenic factors in the etiology of ulcerative colitis and bloody diarrhea. Amer. J. Med. Sci. *180*:239-248, 1930.
34. Sullivan, A. J., and Chandler, C. A.: Ulcerative colitis of psychogenic origin: A report of six cases. Yale J. Biol. Med. *4*:779-796, 1932.
35. Groen, J., and Bastiaans, J.: Psychotherapy of ulcerative colitis. Gastroenterology *17*:344-352, 1951.
36. Grace, W. J., Pinsky, R. H., and Wolff, H. G.: The treatment of ulcerative colitis. Gastroenterology *26*:462-468, 1954.
37. Lunderquist, A., and Lunderquist, A.: Angiography in ulcerative colitis. Amer. J. Roentgen. *99*:18-23, 1967.
38. Warren, S., and Sommers, S. C.: Pathogenesis of ulcerative colitis. Amer. J. Path. *25*:657-674, 1949.
39. Montgomery, R. D., Frazer, A. C., Hood, C., Goodhart, J. M., Holland, M. R., and Schneider, R.: Studies of intestinal fermentation in ulcerative colitis. Gut *9*:521-526, 1968.
40. Lagercrantz, R., Hammarstrom, S., Perlmann, P., and Gustafsson, B. E.: Immunological studies in ulcerative colitis. IV. Origin of autoantibodies. J. Exp. Med. *128*:1339-1352, 1958.
41. Deodhar, S. D., Michener, W. M., and Farmer, R. G.: A study of the immunologic aspects of chronic ulcerative colitis and transmural colitis. Amer. J. Clin. Path. *51*:591-597, 1969.
42. Friedman, N. B., and Warren, S.: Evolution of experimental radiation ulcers of the intestine. Arch. Path. *33*:326-333, 1942.
43. Watt, J., and Marcus, R.: Ulcerative colitis in the guinea-pig caused by seaweed extract. J. Pharm. Pharmacol. *21*:Suppl., 1875–1885, 1969.
44. Watt, J., and Marcus, R.: Ulcerative colitis in rabbits fed degraded carrageenan. J. Pharm. Pharmacol. *22*:130–131, 1970.
45. Aktan, H., Paykoc, Z., and Ertan, A.: Ulcerative colitis in Turkey: Clinical review of sixty cases. Dis. Colon Rectum *13*:62–65, 1970.
46. de Dombal, F. T., Burch, P. R. J., Watkinson, G.: Aetiology of ulcerative colitis. Gut *10*:270–284, 1969.
47. Bardana, E. J., and Pirofsky, B.: Autoimmune hemolytic anemia and ulcerative colitis: A multisystem immunodeficiency disease? Int. Arch. Allerg. *37*:325–336, 1970.

Chapter Three

Examination Procedure for Intestinal Specimens

The importance of a thorough pathologic work-up of inflammatory lesions of the intestinal tube cannot be overemphasized. Monk and co-workers, in their extensive statistical analysis of intestinal inflammations in the Baltimore area, found that 79 per cent of the diagnoses were established by histopathologic examination.[1]

Pathologists in general have been well indoctrinated in the importance of careful assessment of the size, location, and extension of neoplastic disease as a basis for their selection of samples for microscopy. The resultant detailed descriptions of morphologic types, stages, and relationships have provided clinicians with a factual basis to correlate clinical findings. The accurate identification of inflammatory lesions of the small and large intestine, delineation of their size and extent, and characteristics of the particular disease process are equally important in the management of patients so afflicted. Regional enteritis, ulcerative colitis, and many of the other intestinal inflammatory diseases involved in the differential diagnosis are chronic and recurring with periods of remission and exacerbation. In our current state of medical knowledge this commits the patient, then, to a protracted period of medical management. Because of the prolonged and debilitating nature of these diseases, it behooves the pathologist to work diligently in diagnosing and establishing an accurate record for these patients. Almost certainly, the initial pathology report will be reviewed many times as the patient repeatedly returns for medical care. Not only because of its value to the individual patient under therapy, but also because of our need for histogenetic classification, owing to the limitations of our knowledge of their etiology, it is imperative that precise description and diagnosis of the processes be rendered if clinical investigation is to improve the management or provide the cure for these diseases.

Throughout my experience, both as a pathologist and director of laboratories in a community hospital and as pathologist for a large University referral center, I have seen two types of error frequently recur in the work-up of intestinal specimens. Unquestionably the principal source of error is the inadequate gathering of objective data owing to insufficient sampling or the failure to have obtained slides from previously resected specimens from the patient (another form of insufficient sampling). In view of their clinical chronicity and the repeated operations that patients with these intestinal diseases are frequently subjected to, a particular specimen may be only a small fragment of the disease process in the patient at a specific point in time. One cannot reliably describe and identify the pathologic process from such a limited sample. One must review all previous specimens and study their gross description to update the diagnosis.

The second major source of error is the production of artifacts by inappropriate handling of the specimen. First among these is the failure to examine immediately and fix the specimen at the time of excision. Autolysis and bacterial putrefaction begin immediately with the interruption of blood supply by the surgeon. Unless the specimen is appropriately prepared at once the microscopic appearance will be greatly distorted. Descriptions in the existing manuals on methods of surgical pathologic investigation are inadequate for the proper work-up of intestinal inflammatory disease specimens. Therefore it is necessary to present a detailed account of an adequate work-up. The procedures for examination of the surgically resected bowel, the intestinal biopsy, and the autopsy in intestinal disease are presented in order. The latter two are discussed with reference to additional features not presented in the portion on the surgically resected bowel.

SURGICALLY RESECTED SPECIMENS

The pathologist is usually confronted with a bowel examination either by a call from the operating room or the presentation of a pan full of intestines. By far the preferable procedure is for the pathologist to appear in the operating room at the time the specimen is removed and immediately perform an initial examination to demonstrate the lesion to the surgeon. In all events, the specimen should not be left until the end of the operating room day when an attendant routinely delivers specimens to the pathology laboratory. The size of the specimen and its fecal contents indicates that, even under refrigeration in the operating suite, autolysis and putrefaction will ensue with consequent changes in texture and coloration. It is appropriate that the pathologist carefully open the bowel and demonstrate the nature and extent of the gross lesion to the surgeon. Neither the surgeon or gastroenterologist nor any unqualified individual should open the specimen unless a trained pathologist is not available.

The initial examination of the specimen immediately upon removal, whether in the operating suite or at the surgical pathology cutting table, consists of identification and measurement of the entire specimen. This not only establishes what has been excised for medical purposes, but also has a major medicolegal value. It is surprising how frequently measurements are not made and how frequently the surgeon and pathologist, on a subsequent recurrence of the disease, are faced with uncertainty as to exactly what and how much was resected at the first operation. In addition to the over-all identification and measurements, needed data about the specimen are: What is the total length of small intestine removed (whether in one piece or multiple segments)? Was the appendix removed? What is its size and position? Was the large intestine totally removed? What is its length and diameter? Is the anal canal included? How much mesentery, lymphoid tissue, and other structures were excised?

Normal Dimensions

It is essential to measure intestinal specimens as soon after removal as possible and prior to fixation. Variations in muscle tone will alter the dimensions greatly. Adding to this, the shrinkage of fixation will result in erroneous measurements. In considering whether the dimensions of a specimen are within the normal range or not, one must appreciate the fact that both the small and the large intestines average 8 per cent smaller in women than in men. The length also decreases with age.

Small intestine	
Length (total)	7.0 M.
Diameter	
duodenal	4.0 cm.
ileal	2.5 cm.
Mesentery (bowel to base width)	18–20 ± 4 cm.
Large intestine	
Length (cecal tip to distal sigmoid)	
male	140.0 cm.
female	130.0 cm.
Diameter	
cecal	7.5 cm.
rectal	4.0 cm.

Preparation of Specimen

Once the initial external examination is accomplished, including the recording of the color, over-all diameter, consistency, and any unusual surface features of the specimen such as adhesions, one may then with a sharp knife (not scissors) incise the intestinal tube along its long axis on the antimesenteric side. To remove the contents of the bowel, gentle washing with 10 per cent neutral formalin is preferred. Blunt scraping instruments, sponges, anything solid, must not be used as it will abrade the surface of the mucosa. Instead one should wash the lumen by gently directing a stream of formalin over the mucosa to remove the contents. Once this is done the specimen is ready for photography, which is an ideal method of recording the appearance of the bowel for future reference.

When the specimen cannot be examined in the operating suite but must be transported to the surgical pathology laboratory, it should neither be transported "dry" nor be immersed in fixing solution undissected. Transport should be accomplished by covering the specimen with a towel soaked in a balanced salt solution (such as Tyrode's or Ringer's solution) to keep the surface moist. In either instance the specimen must be examined, incised, and cleaned for fixation as soon after resection as possible.

The least expensive and most versatile all-purpose fixative available is 10 per cent formalin, and it should be used in liberal quantities. It should be neutral in pH to prevent deposition of formalin pigments in the tissues.

An alternative method for fixation and preservation of the specimen that gives better results but requires more attention is the application of the principle employed in many butcher shops to keep stale meat brightly colored. Addition of ascorbic acid to keep the hemoglobin oxidized is an effective way to retain color. The specimen, however, must then be kept in a sealed container. We prepare this fixative in the following manner: To 5 gals. 10 per cent neutral formalin add 17 gm. Prague powder and 34 gm. ascorbic acid. Immediately upon addition of the Prague powder and ascorbic acid to the formalin the solution must be placed in a sealed container or stoppered bottle so that the oxidizing capacity of the ascorbic acid is not dissipated. Specimens immersed in this solution, fixed, sectioned, and stained are microscopically indistinguishable from those in formalin.

The specimens are now ready for detailed gross examination, selection of samples, and preparation for fixation for 24 hours. Clamps, pins, and other metallic devices are not recommended for positioning the specimen for fixation; pinning it on a board produces undesirable distortions. If it is necessary to hold it open or to separate part from part, it is preferable to break a wooden tongue blade to the desired length and use it as a truss between the various folds of the bowel. The specimen is fixed in at least 20 times its volume of fixative. The detailed gross examination can be carried out either concomitant with the initial dissection and photography or at the end of the fixation period. Photography must be done before the specimen has been in fixative for more than 15 minutes; otherwise the appearance of colors will be altered. I find that gross observations are enhanced if a slight amount of fixation precedes the detailed examination. Brief fixation slightly hardens the tissues and enhances the delineation between anatomic structures.

Gross Examination

The complete gross examination should be carried out in an orderly and systematic manner so that review of the report is facilitated and a visual image of the lesion is more easily reconstructed. This is most easily done by recording observations in a proximodistal and a mucosa-to-serosa sequence with ancillary structures described thereafter. Thus, the description of the small intestine precedes the description of the colon, appendix, and rectum, and is followed by that of mesenteric lymph nodes and blood vessels. A description of the mucosa is followed by a description of the submucosa, muscularis, and serosa.

QUESTIONS TO BE ANSWERED IN THE GROSS DESCRIPTION

1. What organs are received; what are the length, diameter, and thickness of the walls of each? What ancillary structures are received?

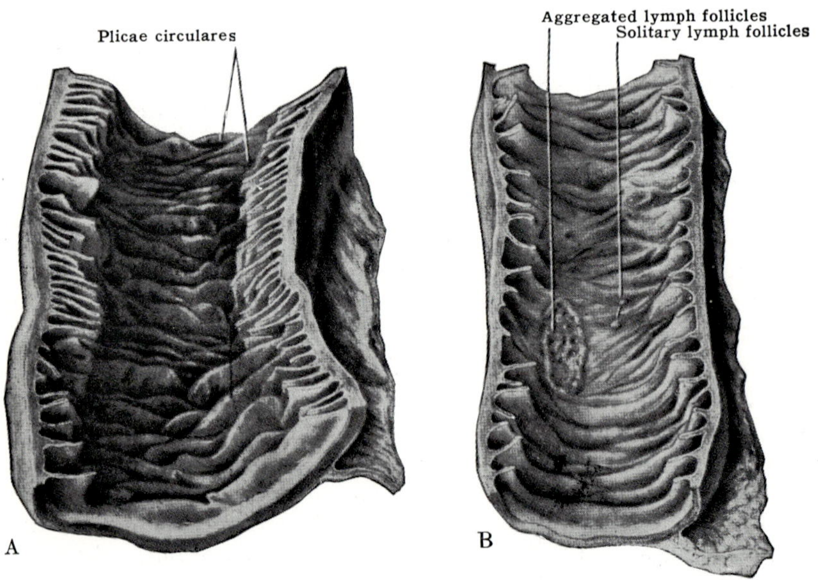

Figure 3–1   Surface view of the mucosa of small intestine. Four-fifths actual size. *A*. Jejunum, numerous high plicae circulares. *B*. Ileum, low plicae circulares, and an aggregated lymph nodule and solitary lymph nodules. (From *Morris' Human Anatomy*, 12th Edition, by B. J. Anson. Copyright © 1966, the Blakiston Division. Used with permission of McGraw-Hill Book Co.)

(If an organ or structure is not clearly recognizable, one may use the term "resembling.")

2. What are the color, consistency, and unusual external features of each organ or structure in sequence?

3. What are the size and distance of such lesions as ulcers or polyps from well-known landmarks such as the ileocecal valve, the anal ring, or the edge of the surgical dissection; what are the diameters of ulcerated or polypoid lesions; what are the size, color, contour, and consistency of the lesions?

4. What is the distribution of the localized lesions? Are they mesenteric, antimesenteric, or circumferential? Are Peyer's patches involved (Fig. 3-1)? How deep is the base of the ulcer? Does it extend through the muscularis? Are there adhesions between loops of bowel?

5. What is the thickness of the wall in each segment of the bowel? What is the diameter of the lumen of uninvolved portions versus

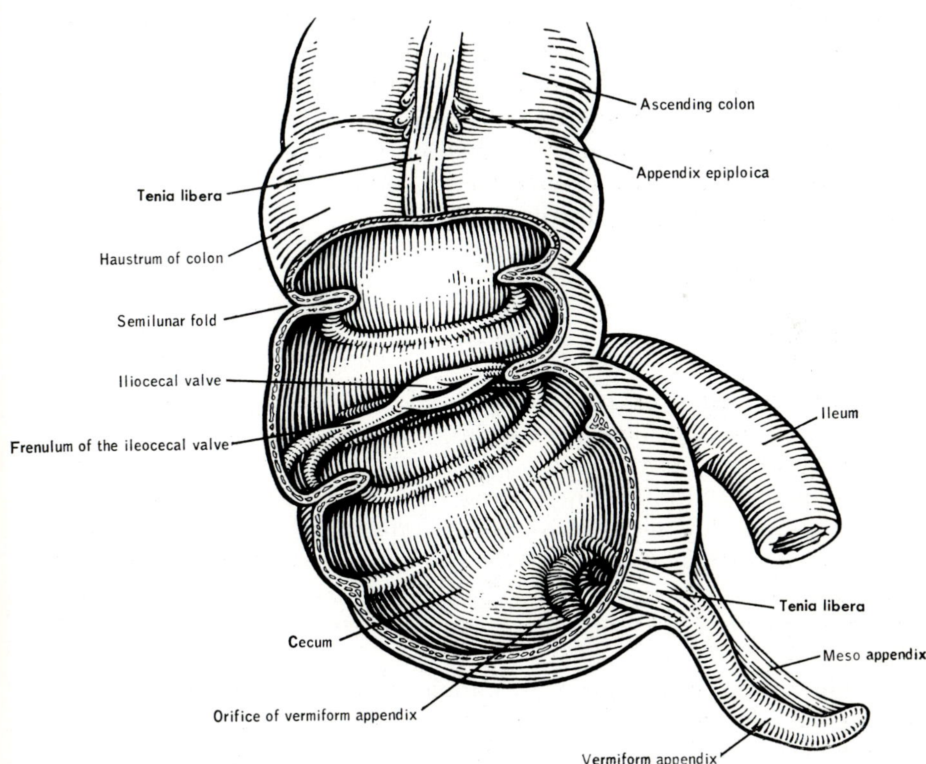

Figure 3-2 Cecum and ascending colon, partly opened, showing ileocecal valve, ventral view. Note the tenia libera leading to the veriform appendix. (From *Morris' Human Anatomy*, 12th Edition, by B. J. Anson. © 1966, the Blakiston Division. Used with permission of McGraw-Hill Book Co.)

involved portions? Is the mesentery thick or short? What are the diameters of the mesenteric lymph nodes? Do the mesenteric lymphatics appear prominent? What is the consistency of the mesenteric fat? Are abscesses seen within it?

6. Does the ileocecal valve appear competent or loose and patulous (Fig. 3-2)?

7. Is the mucosa covered with a pseudomembrane? What is its thickness in involved versus uninvolved portions? Are diffuse or focal lesions present? Are there skip areas of inflammation? What is the relative thickness of the mucosa and submucosa? Is the muscularis thickened by hypertrophy or inflammatory infiltrate or fibrosis?

8. Is the appendix involved in an inflammatory process?

9. What is the thickness of the serosa? Is it fibrous? Is it covered with a fibrinous exudate or fibrous adhesions between loops of bowel or other structures? Are there healed suture lines present? Are fistulous tracts identifiable? Are white punctate nodules scattered on the serosa?

10. What is the distance of the surgical margin from the nearest lesion?

11. Are there mucosal cysts? What are their size and location and the color of their contents? Are the contents clear or creamy?

12. What does transection of the blood vessels reveal? Are there any occlusions, narrowing, or inflammatory zones in their walls?

13. Is there any localized dilatation or constriction of the bowel?

14. Are there any diverticula or fistulas? If so, what are their lengths, diameters, and distribution?

Sampling

Once careful gross observations and measurements are completed, one is then in a position to make an intelligent selection of specimens for microscopy. Slabs of tissue, 1 to 2 mm. thick and up to 5 to 6 mm. in length and width, may be removed and identified as to location. To excise samples for microscopy, scissors must never be used, as they will produce a crush artifact. Similarly, forceps must be used with extreme care for the same reason. Ideally, a sharp instrument such as a scalpel or razor blade is the only instrument that should be used to cut the tissues.

One common mistake is to sample only the lesions. In differentiating between the various inflammatory diseases of the intestinal tract it is important not only to sample the edges of the major gross lesions that one can see, but also it is equally important to sample the minimal early lesions. Microscopically they often reveal the primary disease process without the confusing aspects of secondary inflammatory response to nonspecific bacterial action. Third, one must sample liberally the grossly uninvolved portions of the intestine. This is especially true in the differential diagnosis of ulcerating lesions of the colon, as frequently the early crypt abscesses will not be recognized grossly. Sampling of lymph nodes is as important in intestinal inflammatory diseases as it is in neoplastic diseases. As is pointed out elsewhere in this text, thorough sampling of the lymph nodes in regional enteritis will reveal the presence of the characteristic granulomas in most cases. Typhoid and paratyphoid dysenteries also produce characteristic changes in lymphoid tissue.

Another important point in removing the samples is that the instruments and dissecting board must be carefully cleaned between surgical specimens. Tissue samples from one specimen may be contaminated by scraps from another. The tissue blocks should rarely if ever be cut thicker than 4 mm., and generally, multiple small samples are preferable to a few large ones. Samples should also be taken from the surgical resection margins and identified so that the presence or absence of inflammatory changes at the site of the resection can be evaluated. To evaluate the inflammatory disease process adequately in a major resection specimen, at least 10 or 20 samples are necessary. Only in this way can one assess the true nature and extent of the disease process.

Staining

The staining procedures recommended are those described in *Manual of Histologic Staining Methods of the Armed Forces Institute of Pathology* edited by L. G. Luna.[2] Hematoxylin and eosin remain the basic morphologic tissue stain, though the more recent celestin blue–alcian green–saffron staining procedure for examining lung tumors has excellent applicability to the intestine. This combined stain provides a measure of the amount of mucous secretion, shows the presence of mast cells, and differentially stains collagen and smooth muscle. Therefore, one can evaluate the fibrosis, reactiveness of the epithelium, and muscular hypertrophy in the same specimen. Because of the alteration in mucous secretion in regions of incipient inflammatory change, often the alcian blue–PAS stain may be useful. To stain microorganisms the Ziehl-Neelsen stain may be used to demonstrate acid-fast bacilli. Ulcerating lesions of the colon that may contain amebas should have a special ameba stain. We prefer the naphthol green B and aniline acid eosin method.[2] Amebas stain blue-green, whereas the connective tissue components are dark green. Ingested erythrocytes within the cytoplasm of the ameba stain a deep rose color.

Microscopy

Thorough examination of all microscopic specimens is also done systematically. By appropriately identifying the site of the sample, one can relate the microscopic observation to the specific lesion seen grossly. Microscopic observations are to be recorded in the same sequence as that used for the gross examination: proceeding with a proximodistal sequence and describing changes from the mucosa through the serosa. These are followed by descriptions of mesenteric fat, lymph nodes, appendix, rectum, and so on. In addition to the usual description, one should carefully identify the presence or absence of metaplastic changes in the epithelium of the small intestine and the general proportion of various cell types in the inflammatory exudate.

BIOPSY SPECIMENS

Open or closed biopsies of the small intestine are not practical for the diagnosis of inflammatory diseases, therefore need not be discussed further. In contrast, biopsies of the large intestine during sigmoidoscopy are of immense value in the diagnosis of inflammatory diseases. They also have value in distinguishing regional enteritis involving the large intestine from other granulomatous inflammations such as tuberculosis. Recently Anderson and co-workers studied the use of large bowel biopsies in cases of regional enteritis of the small intestine.[4] They found mild nonspecific inflammatory changes in about half their cases, which were of no help in identifying regional enteritis involving the small intestine. However, the validity of rectal and anal biopsies in identifying regional enteritis involving the colon and its distinction from ulcerative colitis has been well established by Morson and by Lockhart-Mummery.[5, 6] Biopsies were immensely valuable in distinguishing between these lesions involving the large intestine.

Of even greater value is the use of the large bowel biopsy in the diagnosis of ulcerative colitis. Matts did an extensive study of the procedure and clearly established its validity.[7] He analyzed the results of more than 500 sigmoidoscopies, personally performed, of ulcerative colitis patients and found that in active cases of the disease biopsy revealed the lesion in virtually 100 per cent, whereas in the quiescent phase of disease 79 per cent of the biopsies were positive. The value of the biopsy will, of course, vary somewhat with the expertise of the sigmoidoscopist in selecting the site for sampling. Because ulcerative colitis is predominantly a superficial mucosal lesion and has the crypt abscess as a characteristic if not pathognomonic feature of the minimal and early lesion, it provides a fortuitous combination of circumstances, and the procedure yields excellent results in expert hands. Careful sigmoidoscopic examination is necessary to assess the distribution of grossly visible changes within the colon. Then, under direct vision, a suitable area is selected for biopsy, and the specimen is removed and immediately placed in fixative.

The second potential use for the rectal biopsy in ulcerative colitis is to serially sample the colon in chronic or long-standing cases so that precancerous changes can be identified. This would enable the surgeon to remove the bowel prior to the development of malignancy yet permit the patient to retain a functional colon as long as possible. The precancerous changes associated with ulcerative colitis have been described by Dawson and Pryse-Davies and are presented in a subsequent chapter.[8] Essentially, the precancerous lesions resemble villous and sessile adenomatous polyps and epithelial atypism of varying severity on the flat mucosa. Morson and Pang recently completed an evaluation of the rectal biopsy as an aid to the diagnosis of precancerous lesions and further elaborated their histologic features.[9] Precancerous changes were recognized on rectal biopsy in nine patients with ulcerative colitis. One or more foci of invasive carcinoma along with extensive precancerous changes were found in the resected specimens of five. These investigators recommend that rectal biopsy be used in conjunction with clinical and radiologic methods to determine when an ulcerative colitis patient enters a precancerous phase.

For the pathologist, the preparation of the specimen is of prime importance. With the sampling and gross observations completely under the control of the clinician, it remains for the pathologist to orient the specimen carefully so that right-angle sections through the mucosa will be achieved. Many laboratories find Carnoy's, Bouin's, or Zenker's fixatives preferable to formalin for biopsy specimens. These impart slightly firmer consistency to the specimen and under these controlled conditions of fixation give mucosal epithelial cells a more attractive appearance. Serial or step sections should be prepared on all biopsies to enable one to identify the mucosal lesion in a greater pcercentage of cases than is possible with the mere random specimen.

Microscopic findings in biopsy specimens of the colon reveal many of the mucosal changes described in Chapter Five. Lacking these findings, occasionally biopsies from the colon in diseases other than ulcerative colitis may yield nonspecific inflammatory changes. These are in sharp contrast to the granulomatous type of inflammation seen with other diseases previously mentioned.

AUTOPSY PROCEDURES

The principal intestinal lesions will have been previously removed in most autopsies of patients who suffered from intestinal inflammations. It is imperative that the prosector obtain the microscope slides and pathology reports of these specimens in order to render a complete autopsy analysis. Second, it is important that a careful examination be done of the liver, biliary tract, skin, and joints (particularly the vertebral column) for evidence of the lesions described in Chapters Six and Seven. A careful search for amyloidosis should also be carried out as well as for sarcoidosis and pulmonary mycosis or tuberculosis.

References

1. Monk, M., Mendelhoff, A. I., Siegel, C. I., and Lilienfeld, A.: An epidemiological study of ulcerative colitis and regional enteritis among adults in Baltimore. I. Hospital incidence and prevalence, 1960 to 1963. Gastroenterology *53:*198–210, 1967.
2. Luna, L. G. (ed.): A Manual of Histology Staining Methods of the Armed Forces Institute of Pathology. 3rd Ed. New York, McGraw-Hill Book Co., 1968.
3. Histological Typing of Lung Tumors. World Health Organization, 1967, pp. 27–28.
4. Anderson, F. H., and Bogoch, A.: Biopsies of large bowel and regional enteritis. Canad. Med. Ass. J. *98:*150–153, 1968.
5. Morson, B. C., and Lockhart-Mummery, H. E.: Anal lesions in Crohn's disease. Lancet *2:*1122–1123, 1959.
6. Lockhart-Mummery, H. E., and Morson, B. C.: Crohn's disease of the large intestine. Gut *5:*493–504, 1964.
7. Matts, S. G.: The value of rectal biopsy in the diagnosis of ulcerative colitis. Quart. J. Med. *30:*393–407, 1961.
8. Dawson, I. M. P., and Pryse-Davies, J.: The development of carcinoma of the large intestine in ulcerative colitis. Brit. J. Surg. *47:*113–138, 1959.
9. Morson, B. C., and Pang, S. C.: Rectal biopsy as an aid to cancer control in ulcerative colitis. Gut *8:*423–434, 1967.

Chapter Four

Intestinal Histopathology of Regional Enteritis

EARLY ACUTE LESIONS

As emphasized in Chapter One, the presenting signs and symptoms of regional enteritis are often those of acute abdominal crisis and may be clinically indistinguishable from acute appendicitis. Surgeons operating on suspected acute appendicitis occasionally find a normal appendix but a terminal ileum involved in an acute inflammatory process.[1-16] Indeed, this has led some to consider the possibility of a common etiologic factor in these processes. Understandably, surgeons are usually reluctant to perform a biopsy of the intestine or to excise the inflamed segment. However, some of these procedures have been done and provide the basis for the documentation of the appearance of the early lesion.

One of the difficulties in being certain that one is observing an acute phase of the disease is that at the time of operation one cannot rule out the possibility of a chronic subclinical process with acute exacerbation. Since symptoms are likely to become more severe during an acute exacerbation, laparotomies are more likely to be done at that time. Therefore, one cannot state with certainty how early in the course of the disease the lesion we call "early acute" actually is in the reports just cited. Many cases are included in which the patient describes a history of abdominal symptoms of a few hours' to several days' duration. Anticipating acute appendicitis the surgeon does a laparotomy only to find a normal appendix, but on exploration discovers the characteristic gross lesion of regional enteritis. Appendectomy is usually done and appears to have no deleterious effects.[88] Symptom-free patients with the histopathologic lesion of regional enteritis at autopsy following death due to trauma have been recorded.[17]

Gump and co-workers reviewed reported cases of acute regional enteritis; from their findings Table 4-1 was prepared.[18] The reader

**TABLE 4–1   Fate of Patients Following Operation for
Acute Regional Enteritis***

First Author	Acute Cases	Progress to Chronic Disease	No Further Difficulty	Inadequate Follow-Up
Koster	6	0	2	4
Myer	4	1	2	1
Eliason	14	1	5	8
Eckel	11	2	8	1
Sneierson	8	0	8	0
Holloway	5	0	4	1
Smithy	3	0	2	1
Pugh	3	0	1	2
Rose	3	0	2	1
Homb	33	0	28	5
Crohn	16	10	4	2
Armitage	10	0	10	0
O'Callaghan	8	0	3	5
Storrs	8	0	7	1
Siegel	42	9	28	5
Bolton-Carter	12	7	5	0
Austin	33	0	24	9
Crohn	15	5	10	0
Gump	34	0	0	—
Totals	368	35	153	46

*Modified from F. E. Gump, M. Lepore, and H. G. Barker: Ann. Surg. *166*:942–946, 1967. Philadelphia, J. B. Lippincott Co.

may quickly calculate that about 13 per cent of the cases of acute ileal inflammation progress to chronic regional enteritis. One should recognize that the chances for error in this figure are overwhelmingly on the low side because of the likelihood that other acute intestinal inflammations are included inadvertently. Certainly, all the acute inflammations of the terminal ileum are not regional enteritis, and what proportion of those reported actually have the histopathologic features of regional enteritis cannot be discerned without biopsy. Most types of inflammation of the small intestine of known etiology tend to be more prevalent in the terminal ileum than in any segment anterior to it. The lymphoid system, a principal reacting tissue in inflammations, is concentrated largely in the terminal ileum. Though solitary follicles of 0.6 to 3 mm. diameter are scattered throughout the small intestine in the lamina propria, they are more numerous and larger in the distal ileum. Peyer's patches, as a rule, occur only in the ileum though they occasionally are found proximally, even in the duodenum. They usually number about 30 to 40, but are highly variable depending on age. In some elderly people they may be absent. They occur opposite the mesentery, are oval, have a maximum diameter of 20 mm. with the long axis aligned with the long axis of the intestine. The significant points to be derived from the collection of cases are: (1) Some acute lesions have been observed to progress to regional enteritis. (2) Whether the granulomatous disease evolves from the group of acute inflammations of various causes or whether regional enteritis has a separate cause that happens to be lumped with other acute inflammations remains moot. (3) Biopsies and resections have provided a sufficient number of specimens to establish the histopathology of the early lesion. The similarity between the early lesions and the minimal lesions found in advanced cases is described later in this chapter.

Warren and Sommers, in their monumental study of the pathology of regional enteritis, described the gross appearance of the early lesion when observed in the operating room.[19] Meadows and Batsakis also reported observations on 35 surgical specimens derived from 29 patients with regional enteritis and provided a systematic description of the histopathologic evolution of the disease from its earliest recognizable form to the late changes.[20] In their three cases of early regional enteritis the lesion was entirely limited to the ileum. In the intermediate or transitional phase of their nine cases, five had lesions both in the ileum and colon, three in the ileum alone, and one in the jejunum alone. Late lesions represented approximately two thirds of their specimens (23 of 35), of which 5 involved the ileum and colon, 16 were limited to the ileum, and 2 were found in the jejunum alone. In Austin's series the preoperative diagnoses were acute appendicitis, small bowel obstruction, and ruptured ectopic pregnancy.[21]

On laparotomy the characteristic findings macroscopically are edema, vascular congestion, slight serosal fibrinous exudate, enlarged mesenteric lymph nodes, and thickened mesentery involving the terminal 5 to 6 cm. of the ileum. In 14 cases reported by Austin, subsequent laparotomies for other reasons revealed the terminal ileum to be entirely unremarkable. Ficarra observed the acute lesions following epidemic mesenteric lymphadenitis, and Crohn reported two cases of acute regional enteritis unexpectedly discovered at operation.[22, 23] Williams described a series of 61 surgical specimens in which he attempted to divide the cases into three types: early nonspecific, diffuse granulomatous, and focal granulomatous.[24] Erb and Farmer reported an autopsy on a two and one half year old girl who died after eight days of illness characteristic of regional enteritis.[17] There was marked edema of the terminal ileum, cecum, and proximal colon with closure of the ileocecal valve, membrane covered ulcers on the mucosal surfaces of Peyer's patches, and enlarged regional lymph nodes. Microscopically the edema was most prominent in the submucosa but involved the subserosa as well. The inflammatory exudate consisted mostly of large leukocytes with pale vesicular nuclei. There were also some polymorphonuclear cells and a striking necrosis of lymph follicles. Some small veins were thrombosed and lymphatics were distended with granular pink material. Sinusoids of the lymph nodes were widely dilated and at times filled with large mononuclear cells. The case of regional enteritis in a newborn reported by Koop and co-workers had comparable pathologic features.[25] Warren and Sommers reported three acute cases in young women.[19] The gross and microscopic changes were similar to those described by Erb and Farmer. The acute inflammatory changes were accompanied by numerous large round monocytic cells lying free or clumped in lymphatic spaces and in interstitial tissue. Ulceration was present in two of the cases, and in one the acute reaction extended into the colon and ileum.

In the early acute lesions, characteristically, the segment of inflamed bowel is red-purple or maroon in color with a sharp distal margin at the ileocecal valve and often an equally abrupt transition to normal appearing intestine at the proximal boundary (Figs. 4-1, 4-2, 4-3, and 4-4). It grossly consists of a segmental thickening of the terminal 4 to 50 cm. of the small intestine with some narrowing of the lumen (Fig. 4-5). This is the result of severe edema of the entire wall, especially marked in the submucosa. On palpation it has an indurated consistency, and the serosal surface reveals increased prominence of

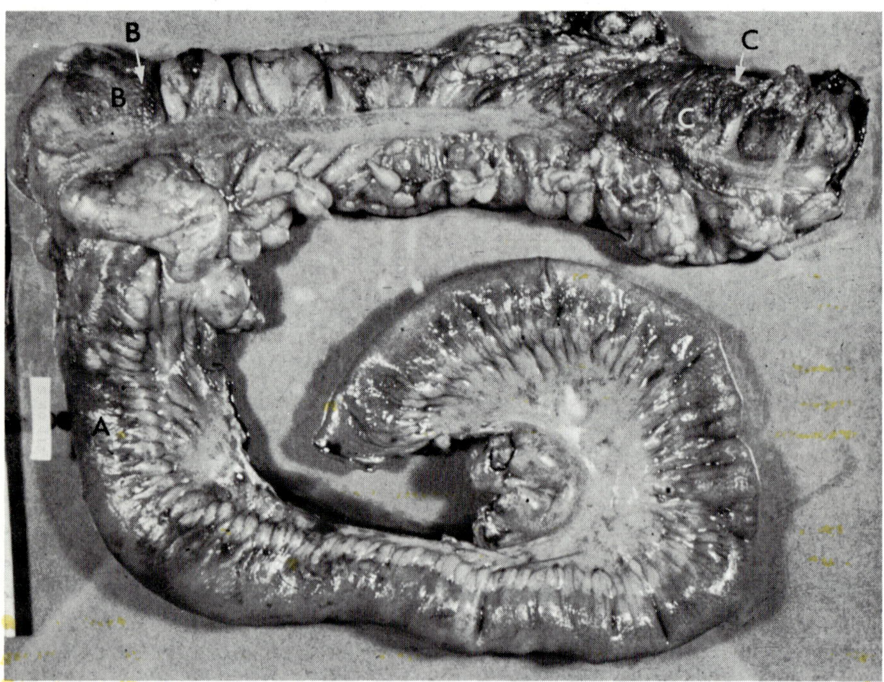

Figure 4-1 Terminal ileum, cecum, and ascending colon revealing the external appearance. Even at this relatively early phase of the disease one can see changes on the serosal aspect at the terminal 10 to 15 cm. of ileum (A), cecum opposite the ileocecal valve (B), and ascending colon (C). The color is dull red-maroon, and the consistency is firm. The mesentery is retracted and thick, producing sharply angular loops of intestine, and the mesenteric fat extends onto the lateral wall of the intestinal tube.

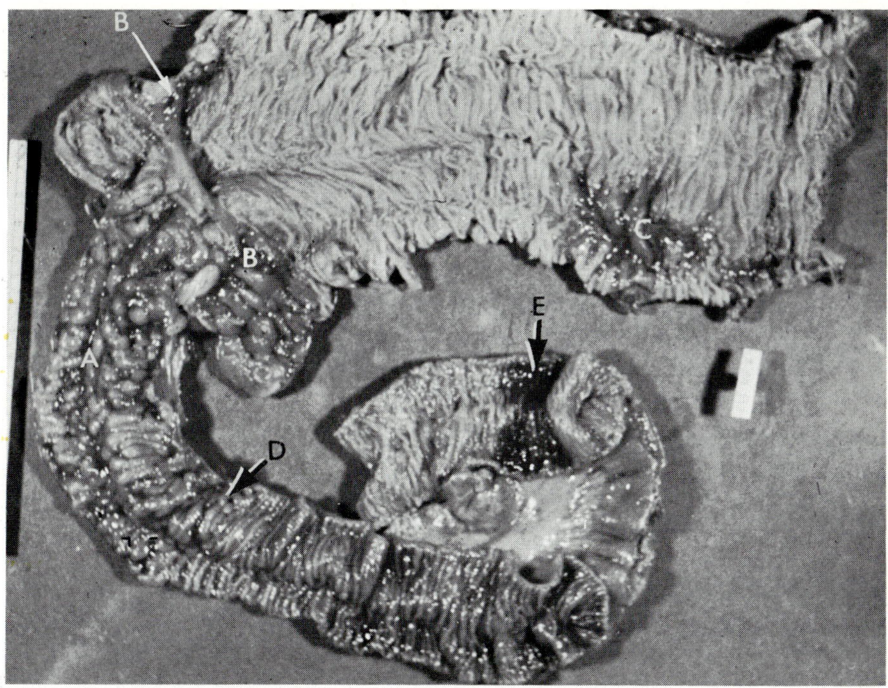

Figure 4–2　Same specimen longitudinally incised and opened. Note the "stony brook" appearance of the ulcerations and remaining patches of mucosa corresponding to the area of serosal change shown at A, B, and C in Figure 4-1. Thickening and flattening of mucosal folds adjacent to the lesions are visible (D). An early skip lesion is also shown (E).

distended blood vessels (hyperemia) and may have some fibrinous exudate with loose fibrinous adhesions to adjacent loops of intestine. A small amount of cloudy fluid is usually seen in the peritoneal cavity. On the mucosal surface, ulceration is sometimes absent and the mucosa appears to have a fine cobblestone texture; the cut surface reveals a thickening of the mucosa and submucosa to about 2 to 3 mm. In other cases the mucosal surface may have some foci of ulceration covered with a loose purulent exudate. The duration of the early acute phase is unknown and may be quite variable in different cases. Skip areas have been occasionally seen even in the early lesions (Fig. 4-4). The muscularis is only slightly thickened, if at all, and the serosa and subserosa may be slightly thickened owing to congestion and edema. At this stage the mesentery and mesenteric lymph nodes in the involved segment are also thickened and very soft and edematous, but no evidence of fat crowding around the lateral walls toward the antimesenteric surface is seen. Crohn described oval mucosal ulcerations about 1 cm. in diameter with axial polarity located especially beneath the attachment of the mesentery.[23]

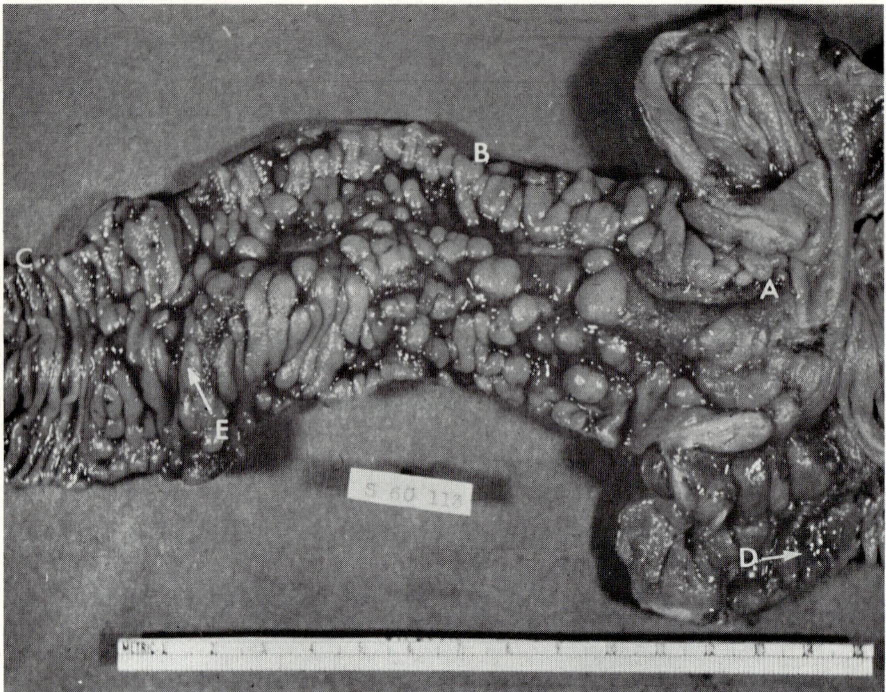

Figure 4–3 An enlarged view of the ileal lesion of regional enteritis shown in Figures 4-1 and 4-2 emphasizing the absence both of pseudomembrane and of increase in the diameter of the orifice of the ileocecal valve (A). The proliferative response of histiocytes and fibroblasts is not yet sufficiently extensive to produce an impressively thickened intestinal wall in this relatively early phase of the disease, though minimal thickening is recognizable (compare the thickness at B with C). The gross features of early regional enteritis in the cecum (D) are comparable to those of the ileum. One can also discern that the ulcers begin at the base between mucosal folds (E).

Microscopically the changes are most prominent in the mucosa and submucosa, and there is a tendency toward a patchy rather than a diffuse distribution of cellular and fluid exudate (Figs. 4-6 to 4-15). Lymphangiectasia with surrounding lymphedema is a prominent feature throughout all layers of the intestinal wall extending to the mesentery and adjacent lymph nodes, though the extent of this change is variable in different regions of the involved bowel. The goblet cell population of the mucosa and mucous secretion appear generally increased, though a decrease is noted in the immediate vicinity of the lesions (Figs. 4-8 and 4-10). The characteristic evidences of chronicity such as fibrosis, chronic inflammatory cells, and muscular hypertrophy are absent. Villous blunting occurs early and is associated with a thickening of the lamina propria owing to cellular infiltrate and edema fluid (Figs. 4-12 and 4-13). The cellular exudate is not specific in the early lesion and consists principally of mononuclears (lymphocytes and

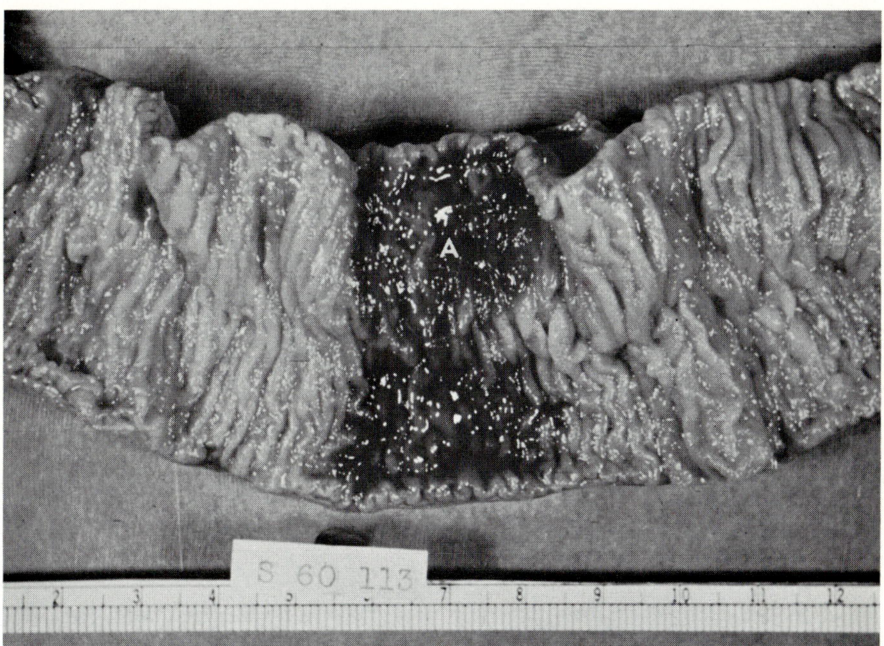

Figure 4-4 Ileal skip lesion (A) proximal to the terminal ileal lesion shown in Figure 4-3. The skip lesion also has the gross features of an early stage of development.

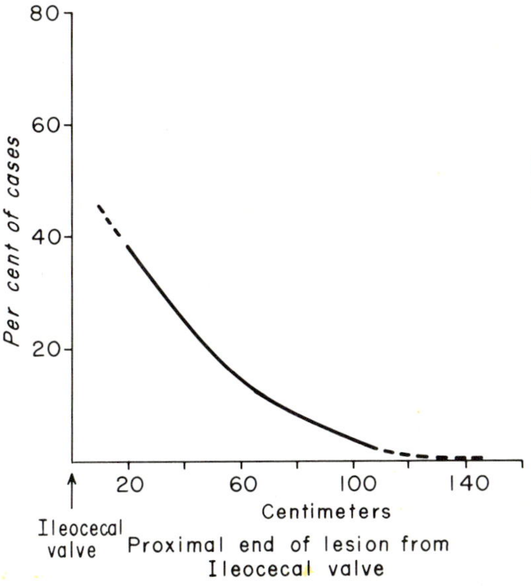

Figure 4-5 Length of terminal ileal lesion.

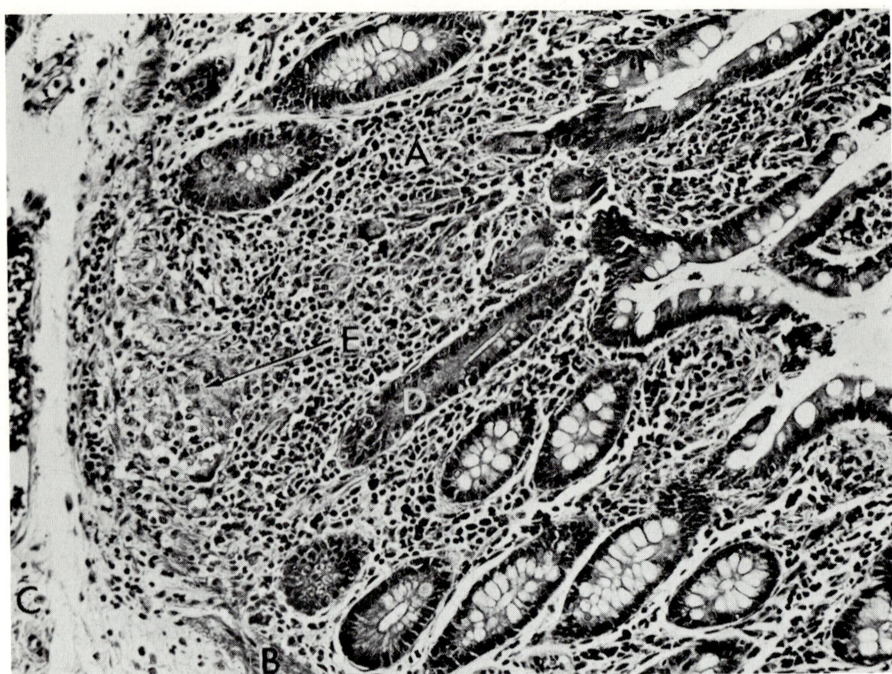

Figure 4–6   Microscopic view of an early or minimal lesion of regional enteritis located in the lamina propria (A) near the muscularis mucosae (B). The superficial part of the submucosa is also shown (C). The mucosal glands (D) are splayed apart by an ill-defined focus of histiocytes (E). Serial sections revealed this to be the center of the lesion. ×40.

monocytes and, less commonly, some plasma cells) and polymorphs and eosinophils. The polymorph infiltrate is predominant in these instances and is seen in the region of mucosal ulceration and at the base of clefts in the mucosa.

Histiocytic proliferation is scanty at this stage, and giant cells are not frequently found. Thus, the cellular response is largely limited to the mucosa and submucosa at this stage. Peyer's patches may be massively enlarged and edematous with germinal follicles less distinct than normally. The germinal centers contain a moderately increased number of histiocytes rather loosely arranged, accentuating the cobblestone appearance seen grossly. In about one of four early lesions small cleft-like ulcerations may be seen that have overhanging edges of mucosa, producing a slit-like ulcer. The ulceration often overlies Peyer's patches and usually superficially involves the mucosa only, but may lead subsequently to deeper microabscesses. At this stage fibroblast proliferation and collagen formation are present but scanty; the general thickening of the wall is largely due to the inflammatory infiltrate and edema rather than to a proliferative response. The cellular exudate tends to be aggregated around lymphatic channels and capillaries (Fig. 4–14).

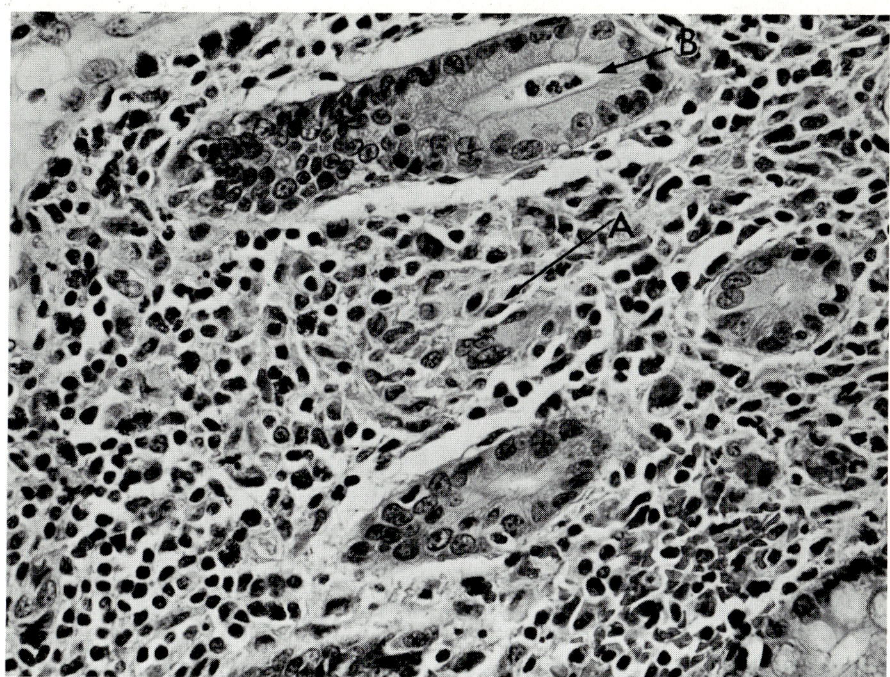

Figure 4–7　Microscopic view of another early or minimal lesion situated somewhat higher in the lamina propria than the one shown in Figure 4-6. Note the loose and ill-defined aggregation of histiocytes and the giant cell between the glands (A). Ulceration of the mucosa has not occurred. Polymorphs are also shown in a gland lumen (B). This occurs rarely in regional enteritis for unexplained reasons. ×100.

The absence of fibrosis coupled with the deep penetration of ulcerative clefts and microabscesses may account for the occasional perforation of the bowel and the fistula tracts that are seen, rarely, even in the early phases of the disease. No vasculitis has been reported in the early lesions, and there is no muscular hypertrophy, either in the muscularis mucosae or in the muscularis proper. Ganglion cells are not prominent, and there are no reports of epithelial cell metaplasia.

This type of gross and microscopic appearance is frequently seen adjacent to the more advanced granulomatous type of lesion that is described forthwith and has been extensively studied by Ammann and Bockus.[26] As they describe them, the lesions in preulcerative segments in regional enteritis are quite comparable to those in the early lesions of the disease. However, whether this actually represents early developing lesions in a region of extension of what elsewhere is a more chronic proliferative inflammatory process or whether it represents a nonspecific inflammatory response, commonly seen in the bowel wall in regions of other types of lesions, remains a moot point. These lesions have a greater polymorph exudation than is seen in the early nonulcerative lesions, and Brunner gland metaplasia, seen in approximately half

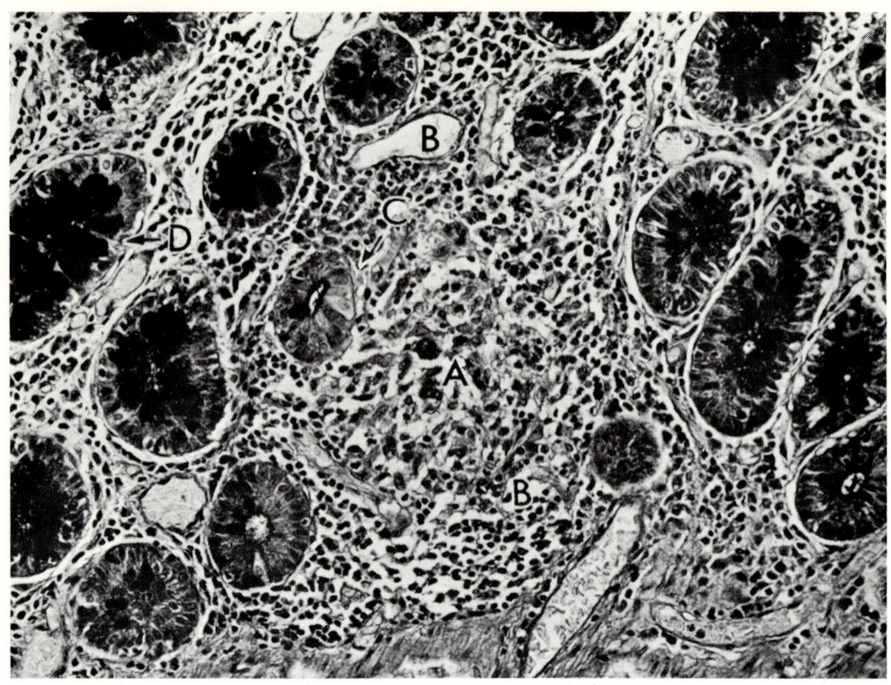

Figure 4–8 Alcian blue-PAS stained early or minimal lesion of regional enteritis. An aggregate of large histiocytes (A) is adjacent to lymphatics of the lamina propria (B). The glands (C) immediately adjacent to the lesion have a diminished mucus production when compared with more distant ones (D). The lesion is located a short distance above the muscularis mucosae (E). ×50.

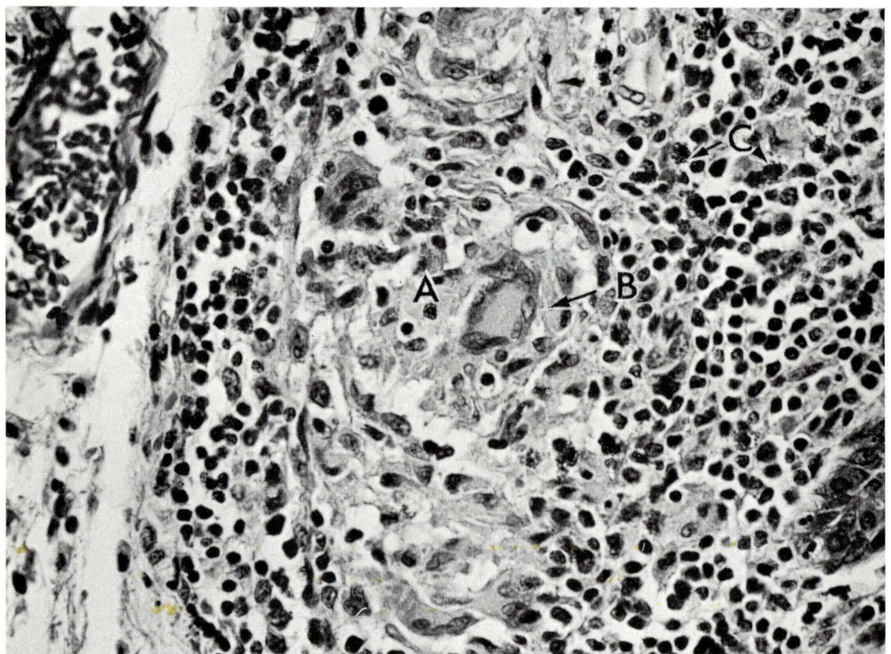

Figure 4–9 A more circumscribed granuloma consisting of enlarged histiocytes (A), giant cells (B), plasma cells, lymphocytes, and a few mast cells (C). The lesion is situated between the bases of glands. ×100.

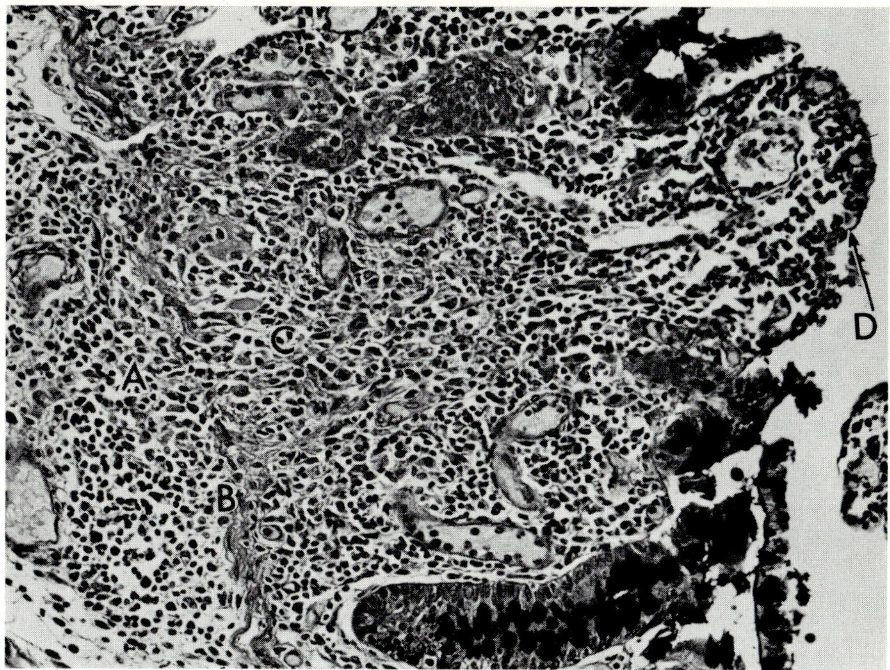

Figure 4–10 Alcian blue–PAS stain of an early or minimal lesion of regional enteritis of a specimen taken near the proximal surgical margin. An ill-defined patch of large histiocytes extends from the superficial aspect of the submucosa (A) through the muscularis mucosae (B) into the deep half of the lamina propria (C). Extensive lymphatic and capillary congestion is shown. A short blunt villus (D) is artifactually denuded. An increased number of lymphocytes is seen in the mucosa and submucosa surrounding the histiocytes. The space occupying lesion widely separates the mucosal glands and has probably caused the shortened retracted villus. ×50.

their 40 cases, has not been described in the early acute lesions. The clinical sequelae of acute ileitis are meager, and among the 15 acceptable cases reviewed by Warren and Sommers 80 per cent, or 12, regressed, 2 cases (13 per cent) progressed, and one (7 per cent) died. This is comparable to the more recent data given in Table 4-1. The surgeon generally does not remove the inflamed ileal segment in these cases, though he may do an appendectomy. The appendix usually has evidence of periappendicitis or lymphoid hyperplasia, or it may be free from lesion. Mesenteric nodes in seven cases were acutely inflamed and in four, hyperplastic.

Presumptive evidence from several studies suggests that approximately half or more of the early acute inflammatory lesions will resolve and the patient will become symptom free for several years. Because of the general nonspecific nature of the early lesions, one cannot be certain whether many of the resolving cases are actually a different disease process from regional enteritis. Also, whether some of these

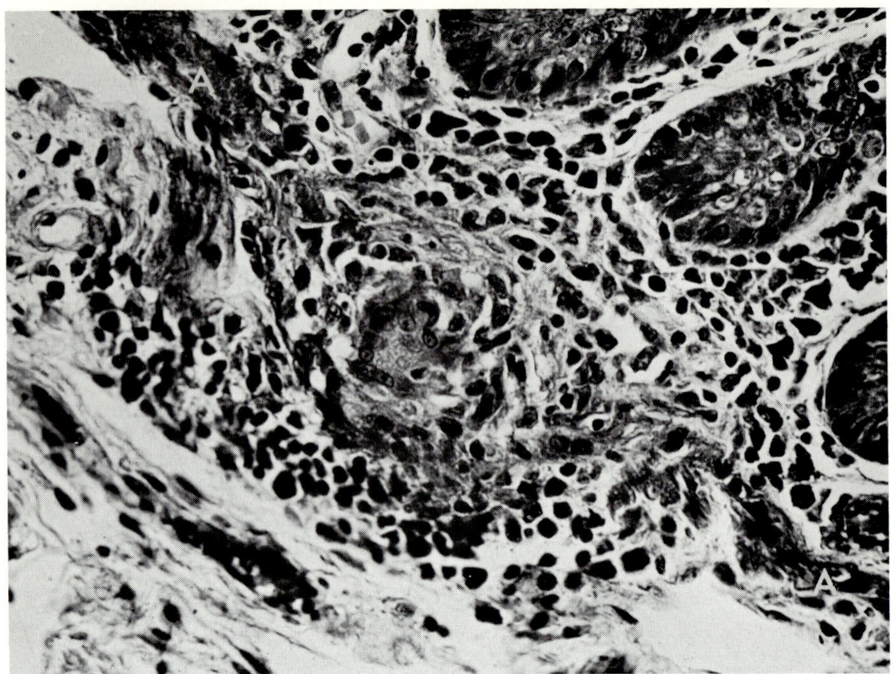

Figure 4–11 Gomori trichrome stain of a lesion similar to the preceding one revealing the relationship of the lesion to the muscularis mucosae (A). ×63.

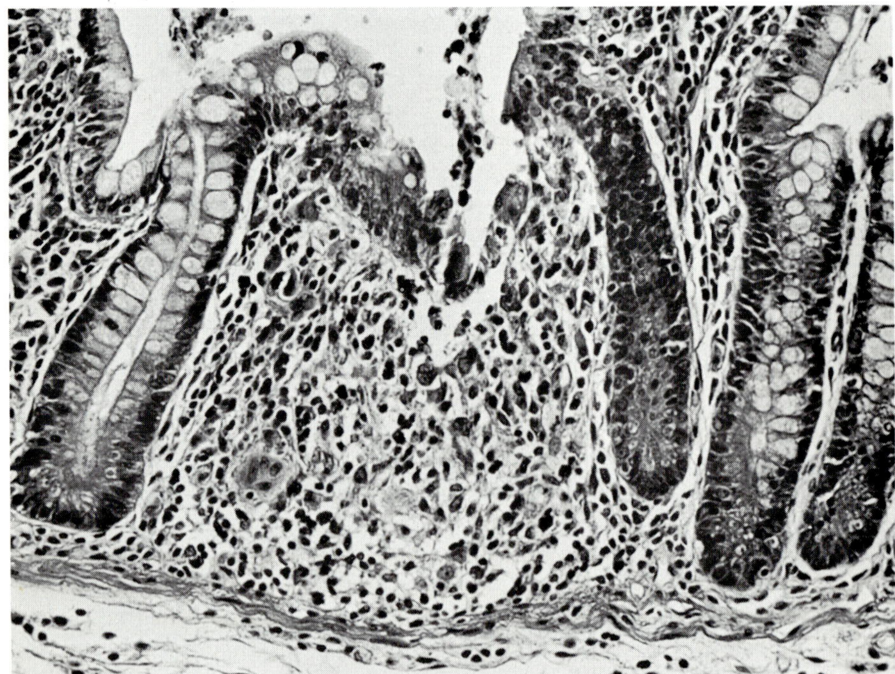

Figure 4–12 A section through the center of a serially sectioned small regional enteritis lesion revealing the lateral splaying of the glands by the thickened lamina propria. The boundaries of the patch of histiocytes are ill defined. ×63.

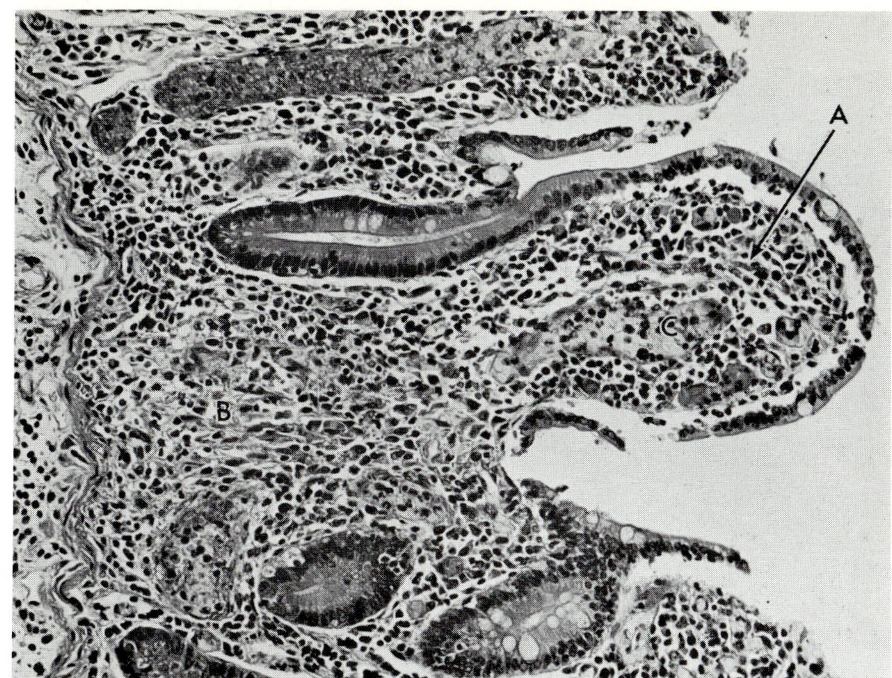

Figure 4–13 Another lesion from the same specimen demonstrating a shortened, thickened, rounded villus (A) associated with the presence of a regional enteritis lesion in the deep half of the lamina propria (B). Capillary congestion is also shown (C). ×40.

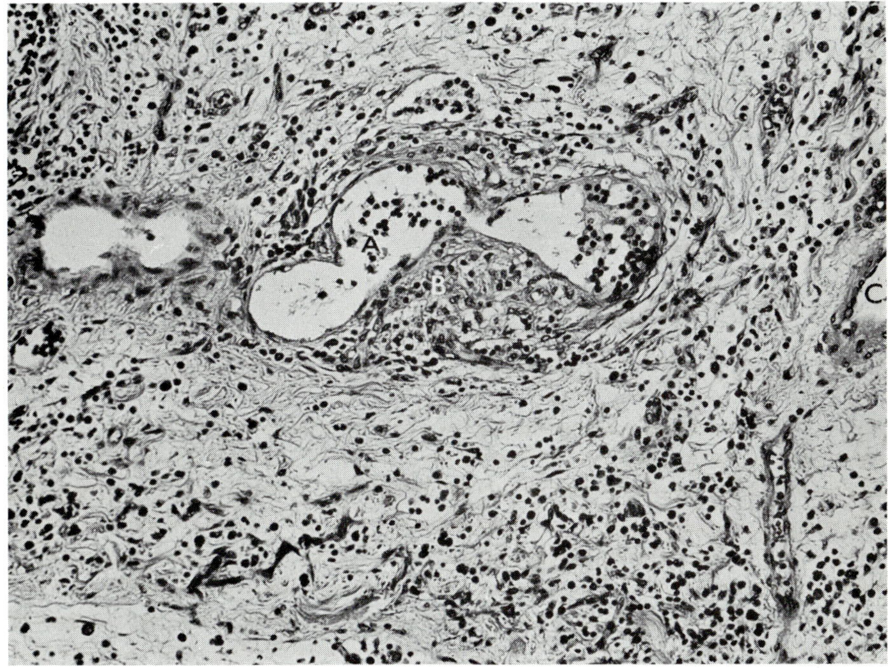

Figure 4–14 This photomicrograph is of the thickened and edematous subserosa of an early or minimal lesion. A lymphatic (A) is markedly distended, contains some lymphocytes, and has an increased number of histiocytes and lymphocytes adjacent to its wall (B). Blood vessels are nearby (C). At this stage the cellular infiltrate is diffuse and fibrosis minimal. ×51.

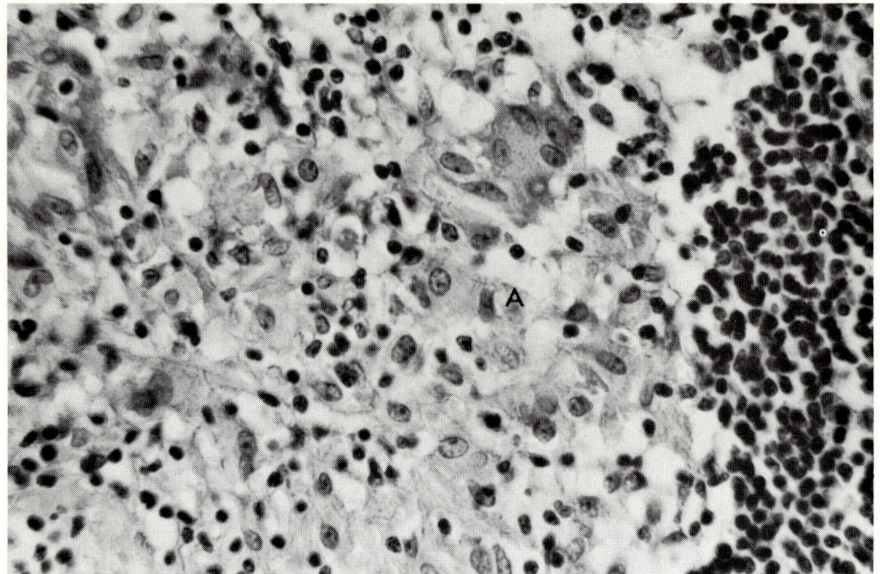

Figure 4–15   Another lesion from the subserosa of the same specimen with a more extensive granulomatous response (A). The lymphocytosis is more concentrated around the granuloma. ×100.

cases have recurrent lesions later in life is not known. Whether the acute lesion lasts for only a few days, weeks, or months is also not documented. The patients with whom the author has had experience have had a history of abdominal crampy pain of short duration, often lasting only a day or two, suggestive of intestinal obstruction, appendicitis, or other acute abdominal inflammatory disease. This implies that the lesion in many cases may be extremely transitory in nature.

INTERMEDIATE PHASE

The intermediate phase is the transition period from early acute to chronic proliferative inflammation. The sparse reports of this phase suggest that a rather rapid transition from the acute to the chronic phase occurs without any distinct morphologic or clinical events. The macroscopic features are similar to those described for the early acute stage; however, the thickening of the wall and mesentery may be more extensive, mucosal ulceration and fistulas are more frequently seen. The changes of the bowel, mesentery, and regional lymph nodes are more extensive and intense than those seen in the acute phase and consist of a mingling of the characteristics of the acute and chronic forms. Grossly, the intestine is hyperemic. The bowel is indurated, and the mucosa may be friable as a result of extensive ulceration extending through the submucosa. The mucosa often has a reticulated pattern due to coalescence of ulcers leaving scattered islands of swollen mucosa. The ulcers may in part be covered by fibrinous membrane. The inflammatory exudate is a mixture of polymorphs, lymphocytes, and plasma cells. In the mesentery and lymph nodes there is a similar but milder inflammatory reaction.

The microscopic features continue to be mainly extensive lymph channel distention, vascular congestion, and lymphedema, often more uniformly distributed throughout the involved segment than in the previous stage. A noticeable increase in goblet cell population occurs. Ulceration of the mucosa, necrosis, and polymorph infiltrate is more extensive in the mucosal region than in early lesions, the changes may occasionally extend more deeply into the muscularis, and prominent lymphedema and inflammatory exudate may be present in subserosal lesions as well. Usually the slit-like ulcers extend to the submucosa, and the mucosa adjacent to the ulcer is generally thinned overlying a dense infiltrate of plasma cells, lymphocytes, and eosinophils. In some cases a slight nodular hypertrophy of the muscularis mucosae is seen near the ulcers. Fine fibrillar fibrosis occurs in the submucosa with a diffuse infiltration of mononuclear cells and prominent hyperplasia of the lymphoid follicles. Neural changes are detectable, characterized by increased prominence of nerve fibers and ganglia that were not discernible in the early phase. There is a diffuse nodular hypertrophy of neurolemmal cells as well as an increased number and prominence of ganglion cells limited to the myenteric plexes. At this stage the muscularis is hypertrophic. Histiocytes and large mononuclears are more frequent and are extensively distributed throughout the mucosa and submucosa and between fascicles of smooth muscle and the muscular coat. Some hypertrophy of the muscularis mucosae may also be in evidence. The histiocytes are succulent in appearance with a large densely staining nucleus, and some binucleate or multinucleate cells may be found. There is a slight tendency for clusters and aggregates of histiocytes to occur, but dense granulomas are not yet formed. Some increase in collagen fibers and fibroblast proliferation, particularly in the submucosa, is now detectable. Strands of collagen fibers and fibroblasts tend to separate the bundles of the muscularis extending into the subserosa. These changes, along with the cellular exudate, are also seen particularly at sites where blood vessels course through the muscularis. Lymph follicle hyperplasia in Peyer's patches and in the involved nodes appears more prominent.

CHRONIC PROLIFERATIVE PHASE

Reports in the literature describing this phase are numerous, reflecting the fact that this is the lesion usually seen by pathologists in surgically resected specimens and at autopsy. The appearance of

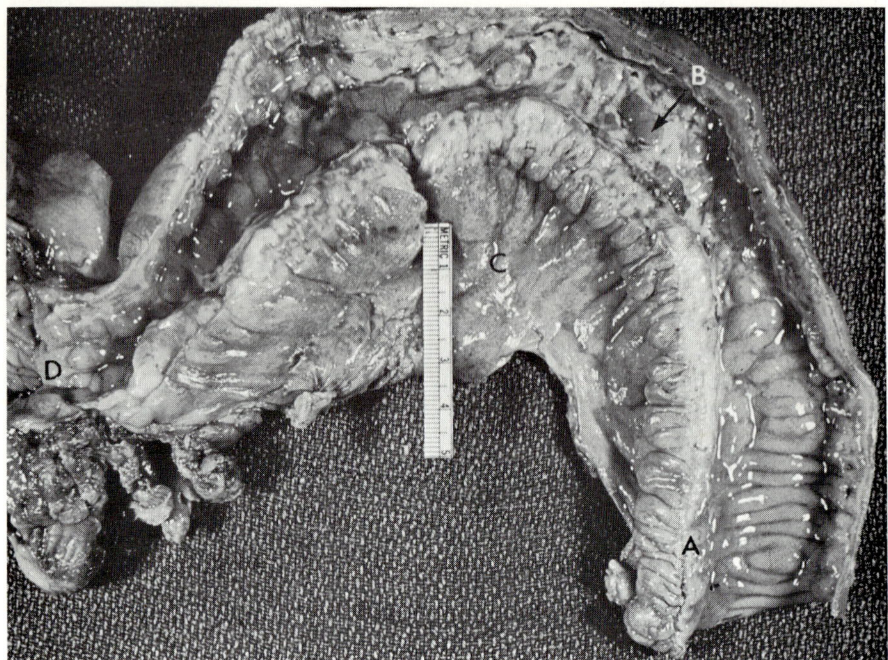

Figure 4–16   Advanced stage of regional enteritis involving terminal ileum. The wall of the ileum is markedly thickened and firm (A). Eroded mucosa has a "stony brook" appearance (B), and the mesentery is short and thick (C), producing sharp angulation of the bowel. Ileocecal valve circumference is not increased (D).

lesions in this phase, as in the preceding one, is sometimes altered because of the extensive clinical use of antibiotics and anti-inflammatory drugs such as corticosteroids. Warren and Sommers' cases (60 male and 60 female) were predominantly in the chronic phase of the disease.[19] They did not attempt to identify the percentage that were in the early phase, but 93 per cent were in the chronic phase, and they reviewed reports of 99 acute and 22 subacute cases in the literature.

The macroscopic appearance of the chronic granulomatous lesion consists of a sharply demarcated segment of intestine that is indurated, soggy, and leathery and is often compared to a garden hose in size and consistency (Frontispiece; Figs. 4-16 to 4-30). The wall is usually thickened to 1 cm. or more, and all layers are involved. The lumen may be irregularly narrowed to less than 1 cm.; usually the ileocecal valve will barely admit a probe. Ulceration in the chronic phase is not invariably present, but as a rule there are shallow ulcers along the long axis of the bowel, especially beneath the mesenteric attachment. The serosa is hyperemic, dull, and occasionally bears white pinhead nodules. Mesenteric fat partially surrounds the intestine, extending from the mesenteric attachment anteriorly and posteriorly, corresponding to the thickened and inflamed segment. The mesentery is thickened, stiff,

(Text continued on page 86.)

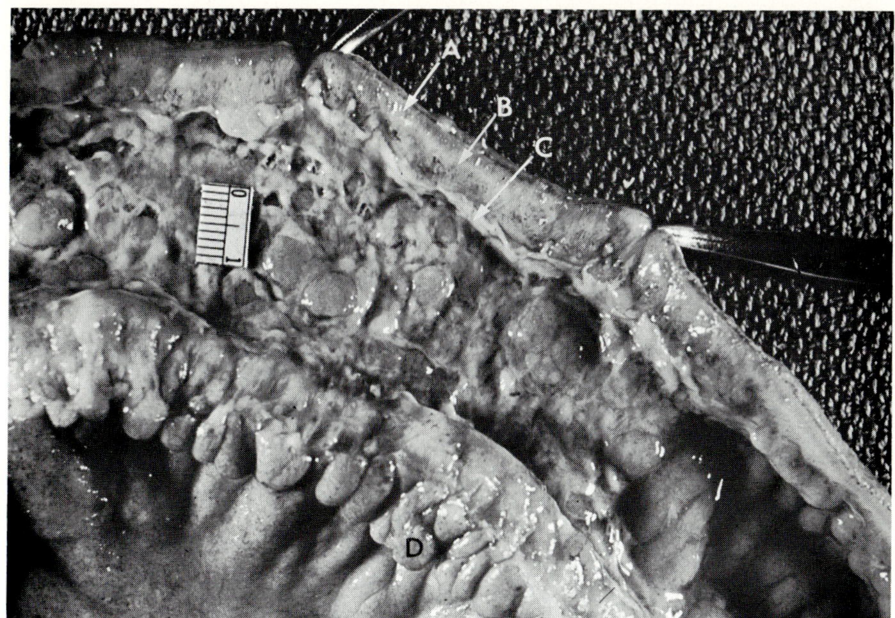

Figure 4–17 A portion of the specimen shown in Figure 4–16. The thickening of the wall involves the serosa (A), muscularis (B), and submucosa (C). The firmness of the wall is such that it stands erect and does not lie flat as does a normal ileum. Mesenteric fat (D) extends onto the bowel wall.

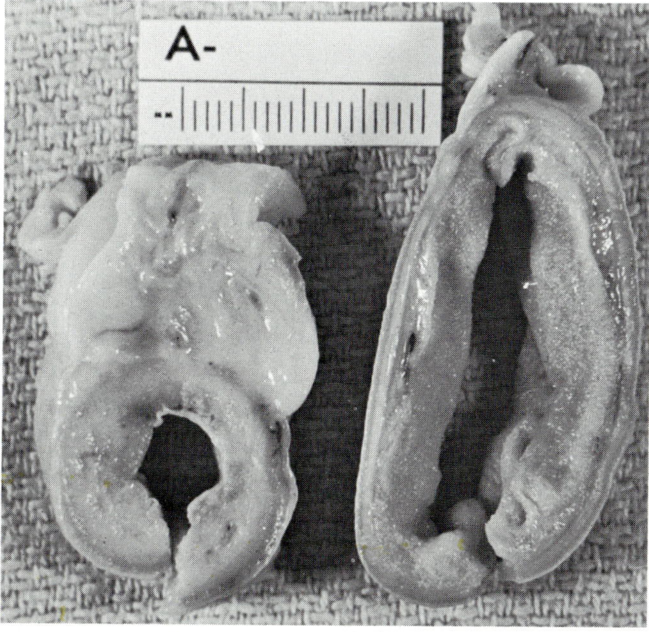

Figure 4–18 Cross section through the terminal ileum of regional enteritis (left) compared with a normal ileum (right). The mesentery of regional enteritis is markedly thickened, fibrous, and striate on cross section and extends around approximately one-third of the circumference of the bowel. The thickening of the diseased bowel involves all layers.

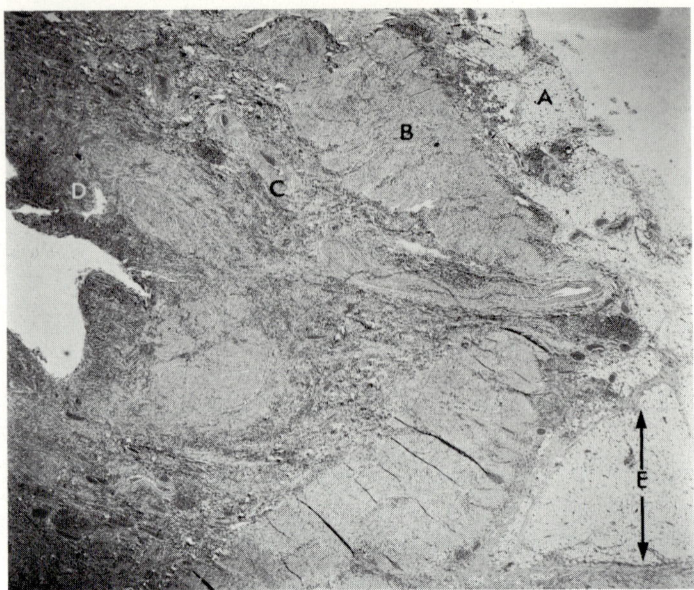

Figure 4–19   A low magnification (approximately ×4) of the lesion shown in Figure 4-18 demonstrating the proliferative and infiltrative features of the inflammatory infiltrate in the serosa (A), muscularis (B), submucosa (C), and remaining portions of the mucosa (D). Thick bands of fibrous connective tissue extend into the mesentery (E).

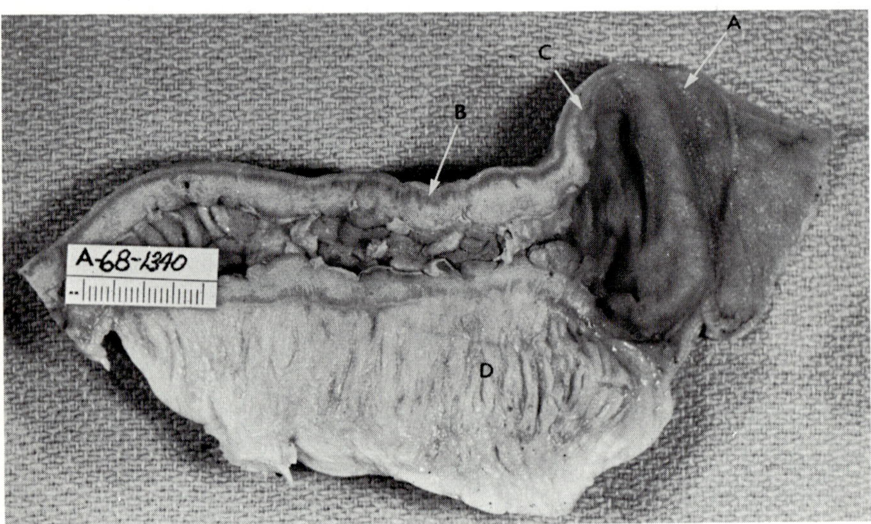

Figure 4–20   A regional enteritis lesion revealing a flaccid, thin, uninvolved portion (A) of ileum adjacent to the thick, firm, erect lesion (B). A rather narrow zone of transition is seen (C). Also prominent is the striate appearance of the transected mesentery (D).

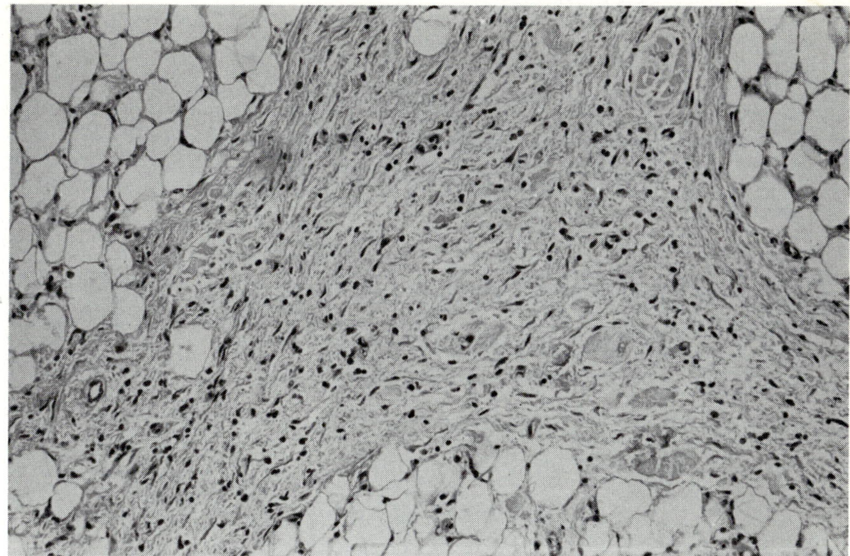

Figure 4–21   A microscopic view of a section through the mesentery shown in Figure 4-20. Thick bands of collagenous connective tissue course through the adipose tissue. ×20.

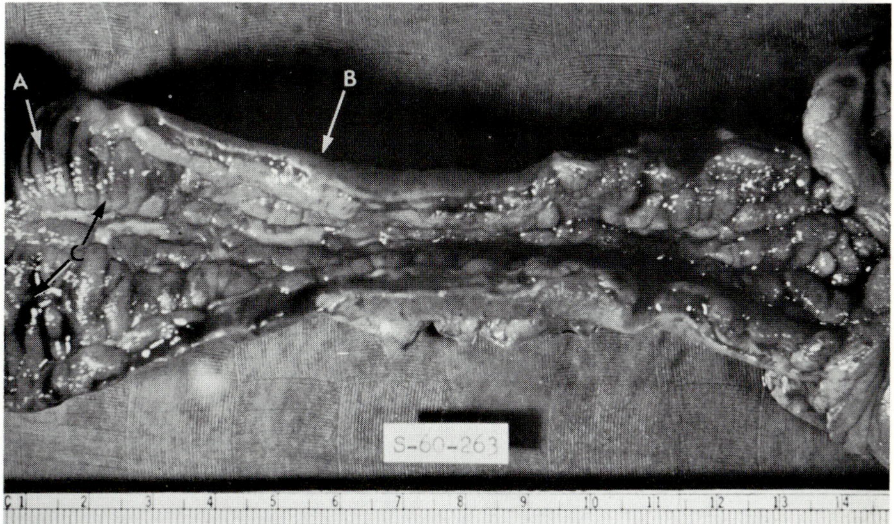

Figure 4–22   The terminal ilial lesion of relatively advanced regional enteritis emphasizing the contrast between the flaccid uninvolved bowel (A) and the firm, thick, erect involved bowel (B). Also shown is the presence of ulcers at the bases of mucosal folds (C).

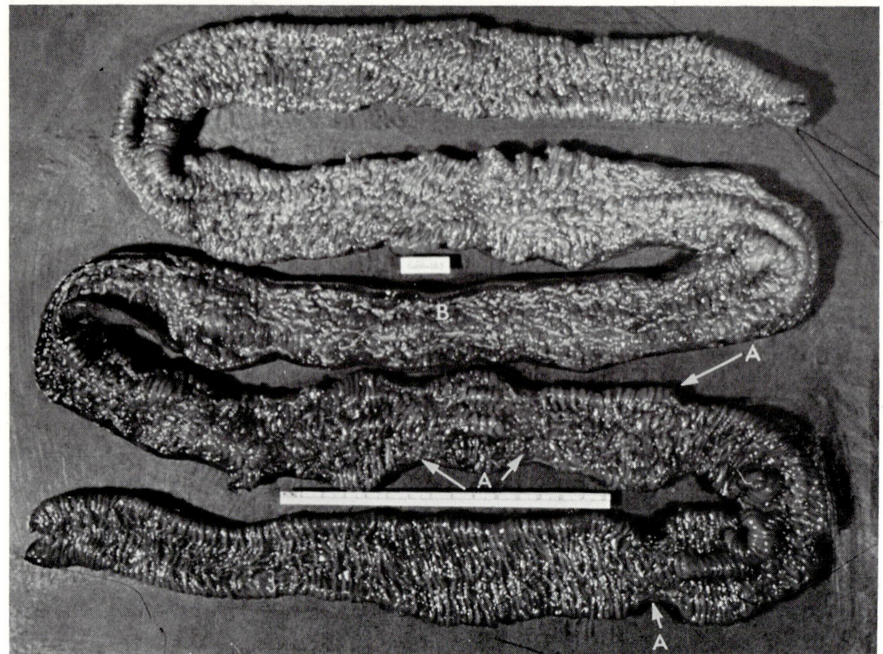

Figure 4–23   A more proximal segment of small intestine from the same patient shown in Figure 4-22 revealing the presence of multiple skip area strictures (A) and a less typical diffuse ulcerated lesion (B). See Figures 4-24, 4-25, and 4-27 for close-up views of selected areas of these lesions.

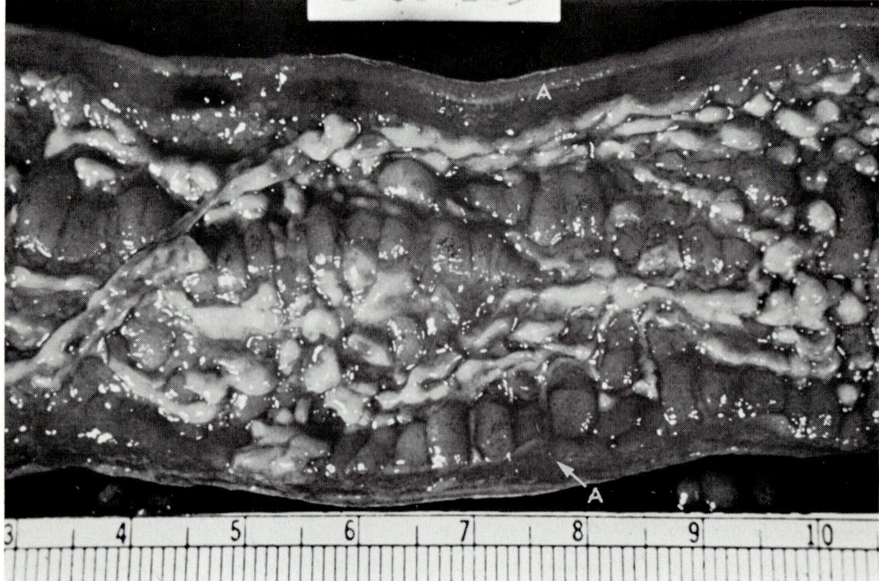

Figure 4–24   A close-up view of the elongated "skip" lesion shown in Figure 4-23. Its total length is approximately 17 cm. Shown here are the thickened bowel wall (A) and "stony brook" appearance of the ulcerated mucosa.

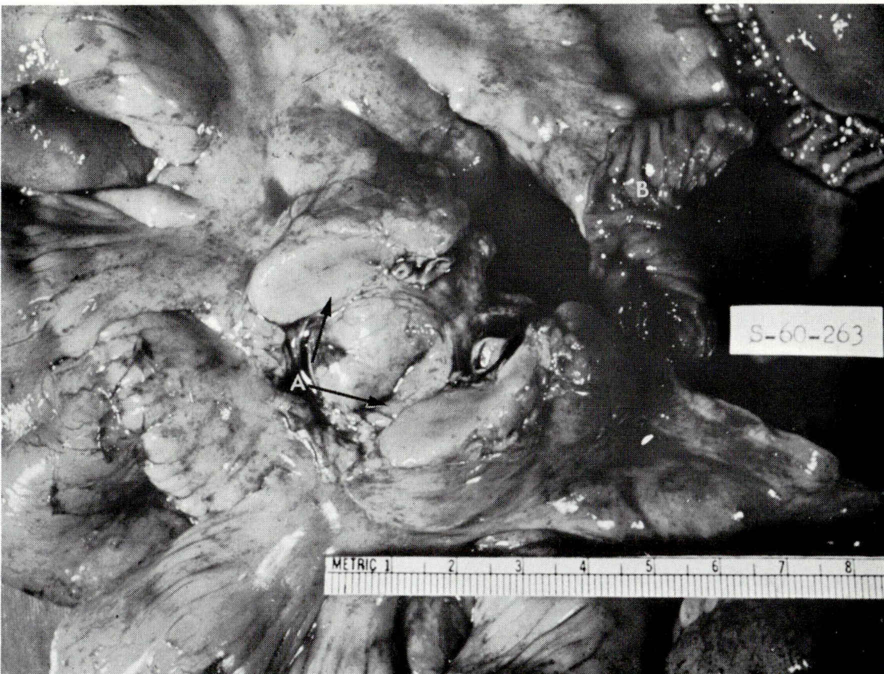

Figure 4–25   A transected enlarged mesenteric lymph node (A) from the case shown in Figures 4-22, 4-23, and 4-24. The node is enlarged to 2.5 cm., is firm, and the cut surface does not reveal distinctive markings. A portion of the mucosa is shown (B).

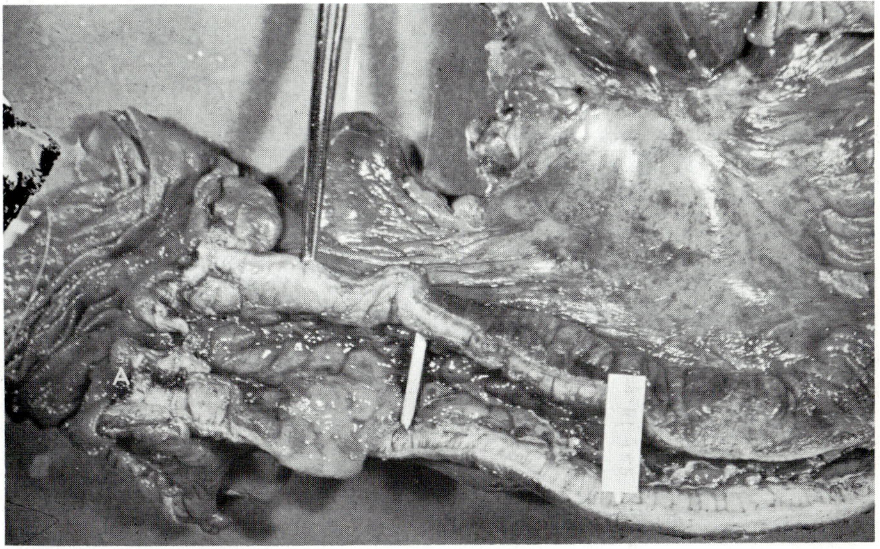

Figure 4–26   An extensive advanced terminal ileal lesion of regional enteritis revealing a sharp junction with uninvolved cecal mucosa (A) at the ileocecal valve. The diameter of the ileocecal valve is not increased.

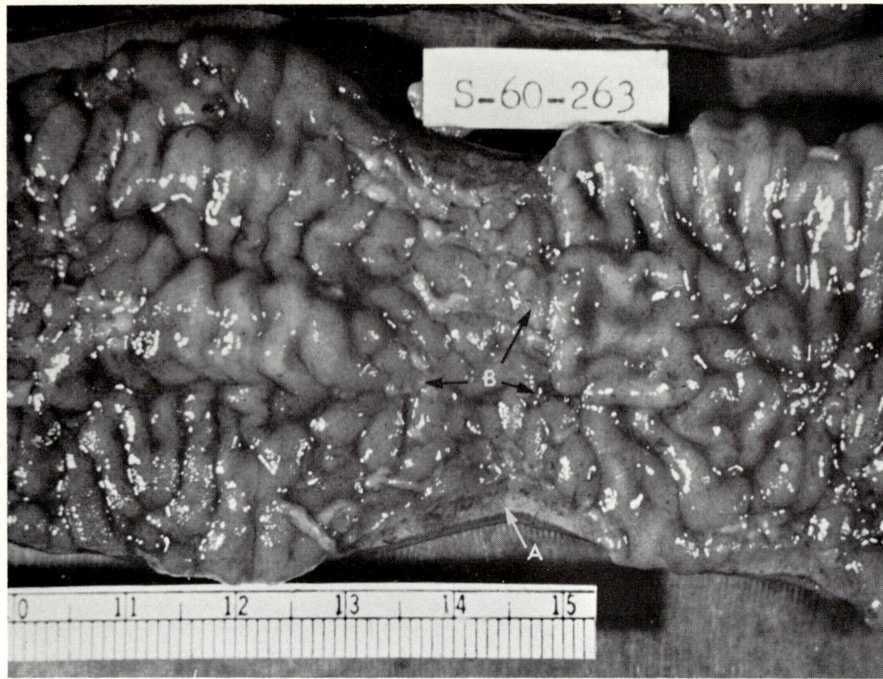

Figure 4-27 A moderately advanced "skip" lesion also shown in Figure 4-23. The bowel wall is moderately thickened (A) and the ulceration of the overlying mucosa is not extensive (B).

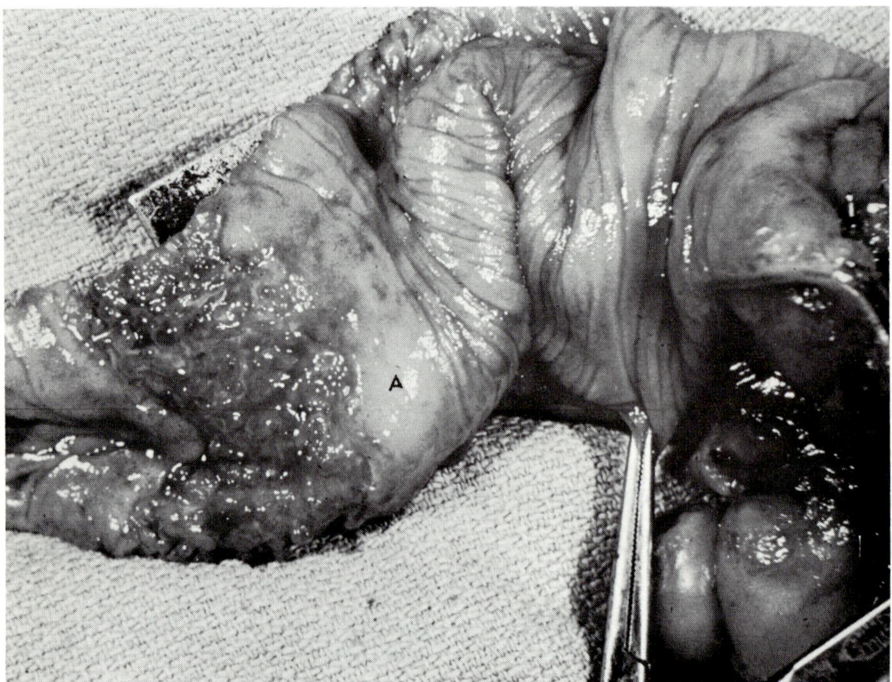

Figure 4-28 A "skip" lesion of less common appearance with a finely granular denuded mucosal surface and "ironed out" adjacent mucosal folds (A). The bowel wall was not markedly thickened.

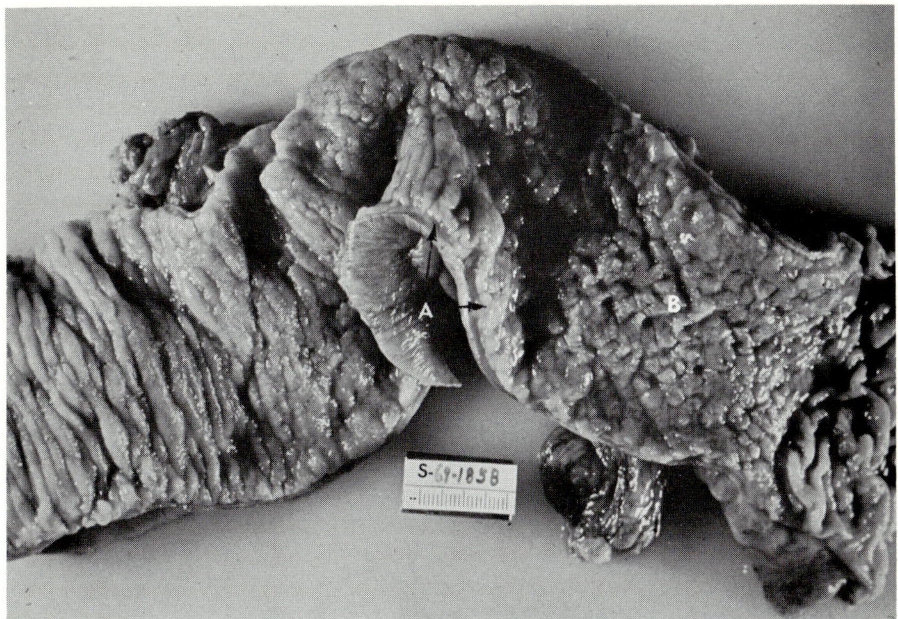

Figure 4–29 Another "skip lesion" with minimally thickened bowel wall (A) and numerous small ulcerated clefts at the bases of mucosal folds producing a shaggy or "cobblestone" appearance (B).

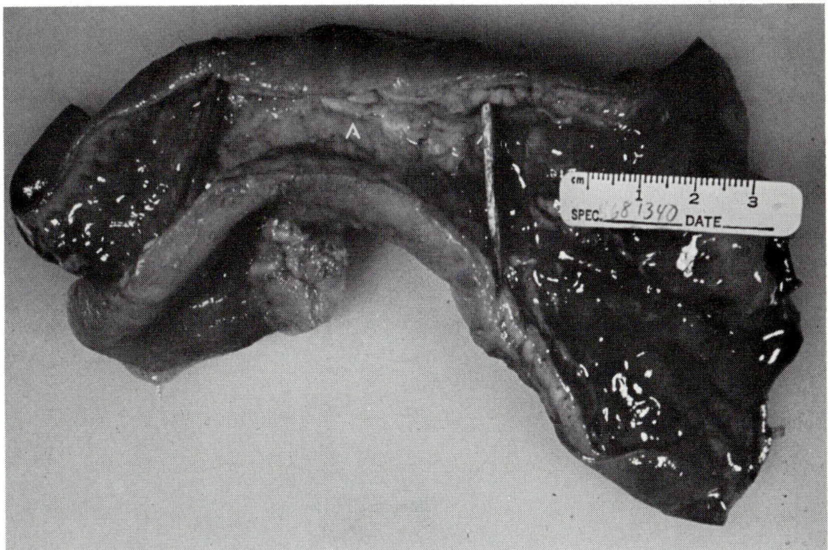

Figure 4–30 A "skip lesion" (A) in a more proximal loop of ileum than that in the preceding figure. Its gross features are comparable to those indicated for terminal ileal lesions. Contrast the gross appearance of this advanced lesion with that of a relatively early one shown in Figures 4–1 and 4–4.

short, and contains large edematous lymph nodes (Figs. 4–16, 4–18, 4-20, and 4-28). The surface of the mesentery is thickened and fibrotic, giving an irregular contour to the bowel. Dense, fibrous adhesions fixing the diseased bowel to adjacent structures are frequently seen. Proximal to the diseased portion there is dilatation and hypertrophy. Adhesions between loops of bowel are frequent, and many late cases have fistulous tracts, especially between the terminal ileum and colon. In rare instances free perforation into the abdominal cavity occurs. The frequent occurrence of granulomatous nodules distributed in a miliary fashion on the peritoneum near the primary intestinal lesion has been reported.[27] The existence of this disease process in Meckel's diverticulum has also been observed.[28] Angiography of these same lesions reveals a decreased number of vessels in the bowel wall, and the capillary phase is fainter than in nonaffected segments or is not visible at all. Venous return is diminished. Fistulous tracts are present in about one third of the late cases (Figs. 4-31 and 4-32).

The microscopic features of chronic granulomatous regional enteritis include shallow beveled mucosal ulcers coated with fibrin and inflammatory cells, especially polymorphs, principally in the mucosa (Fig. 4-33). Beneath this the submucosa is edematous and crowded with plasma cells, lymphocytes, and eosinophils. The cellular exudate infiltrates all layers and extends into the mesentery locally. Submucosal and subserosal lymphatics are dilated and the muscle layer is hypertrophied (Figs. 4-34 and 4-35). The submucus and myenteric nerve

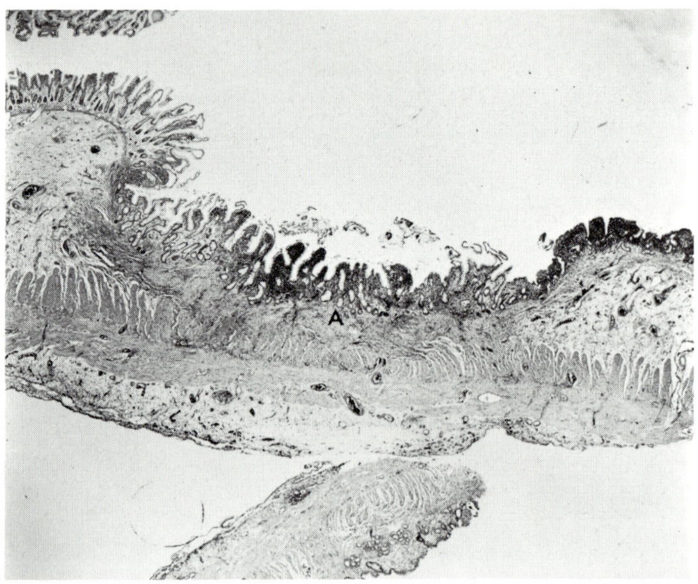

Figure 4–31 A healed regional enteritis "skip lesion" in a specimen with active lesions elsewhere. The mucosa, submucosa, and muscularis are fused together by scar tissue (A). ×10.

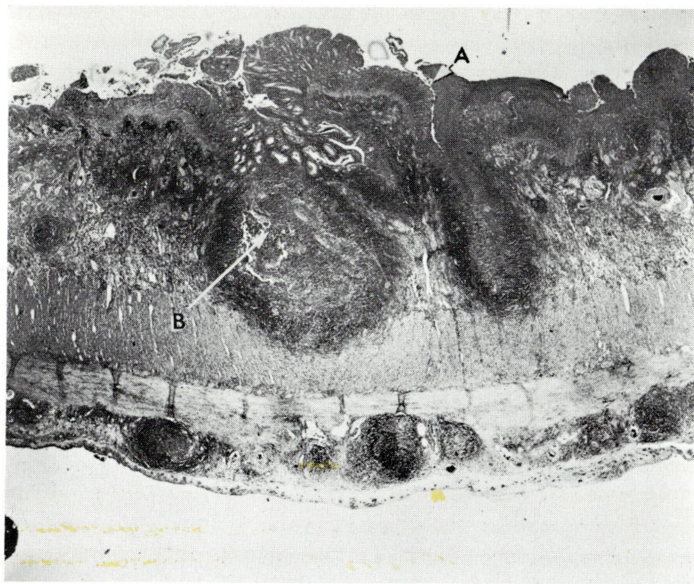

Figure 4–32 Developing fistulous tracts of the ileum longitudinally (A) and tangentially (B) sectioned and extending into the muscularis. ×5.

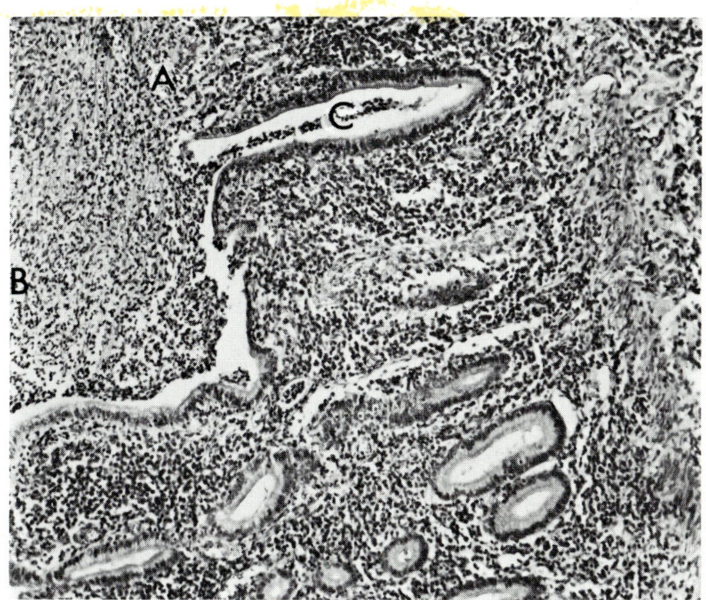

Figure 4–33 A microscopic section through the edge of a mucosal ulcer (A) with the intestinal lumen to the left (B). Note the streamer of pus extending from the lumen into a gland (C) adjacent to the ulcer. No necrosis of the epithelium of the gland is seen. To contrast the presence of pus in the lumen with a crypt abscess see Figures 2-1, 5-1, and 5-2. ×10.

plexes appear prominent. Focal granulomas are frequently observed scattered through all layers of the intestinal wall including the lymph nodes (Fig. 4-36). These granulomas consist of large histiocytes with one or more nuclei. The cytoplasm may be vacuolated, but usually does not contain foreign bodies.

The typical granulomas are composed of a cluster of hyperplastic histiocytes surrounding one or two giant cells that may resemble either the Langhans or foreign body types (Figs. 4-34, 4-37 to 4-41). The number of nuclei is usually less than is commonly seen in these types of giant cells, and those with two or three nuclei closely resemble histiocytes. They often have a reticulated or frothy cytoplasm with a scalloped border, but foreign bodies are not demonstrable within them though occasional Schaumann bodies (but not asteroids) have been reported.[27] Stains for fat or acid-fast bacilli are negative. Necrosis is not a feature of the granulomas.

In addition to the primary granulomas, one occasionally sees foreign body giant cells and an accompanying reaction in the vicinity of ulceration and secondary infection. At these foci the granulomas blend imperceptibly into the surrounding inflammatory tissue and the giant cells usually contain foreign material in their cytoplasm. One must also be wary of the foreign body reaction in the vicinity of the resection suture line in cases previously operated on and in the walls of sinus tracts. Whether an occasional giant cell may represent a foreign body response to phagocytosed structures derived from the dietary stream remains disputed. However, the majority are multinucleate histiocytes

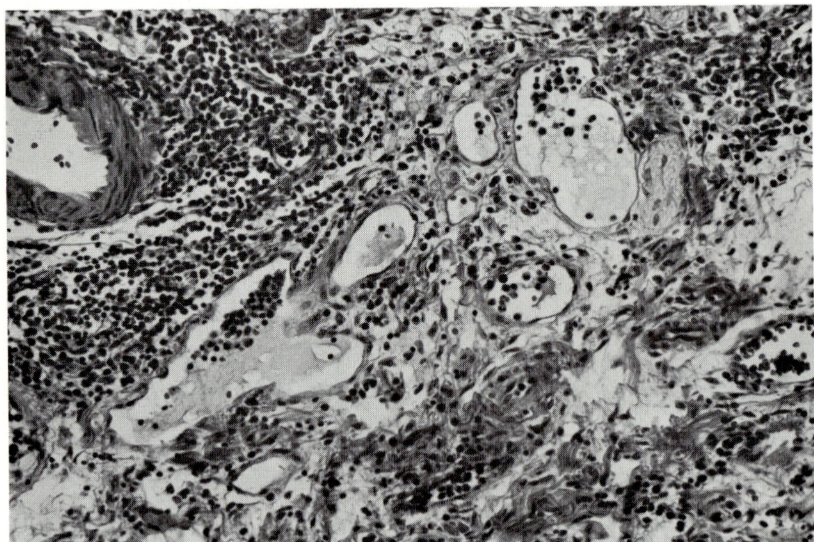

Figure 4-34 Submucosal changes in regional enteritis. The mucosa is to the left. Extensive lymphatic and blood vascular congestion is seen with a diffuse infiltration of mononuclear cells, principally lymphocytes and plasma cells. ×64.

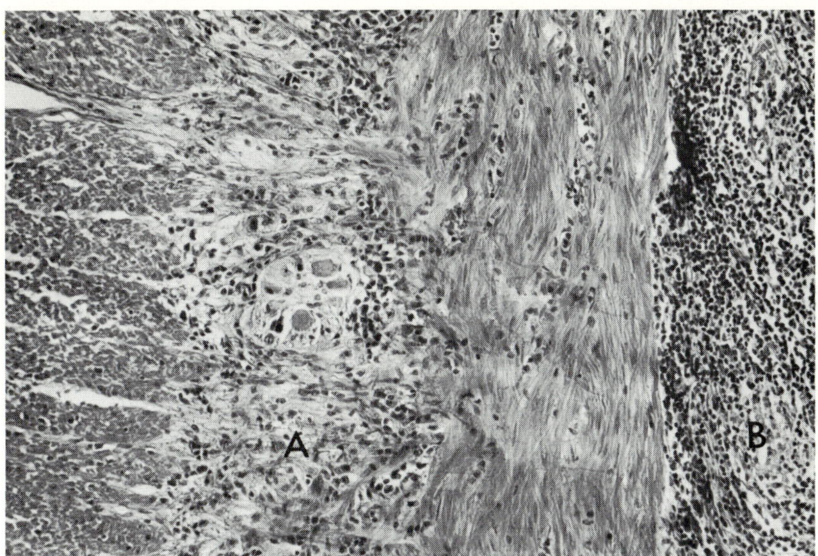

Figure 4–35 Muscularis and subserosal changes of regional enteritis. The mucosa is to the left. Along the path of blood vessels extending through the muscularis and between the circular and longitudinal layers of muscle, inflammatory cell infiltrates are found (A). Extensive mononuclear cell infiltration of the deeper layers of the subserosa (B) is also seen. ×64.

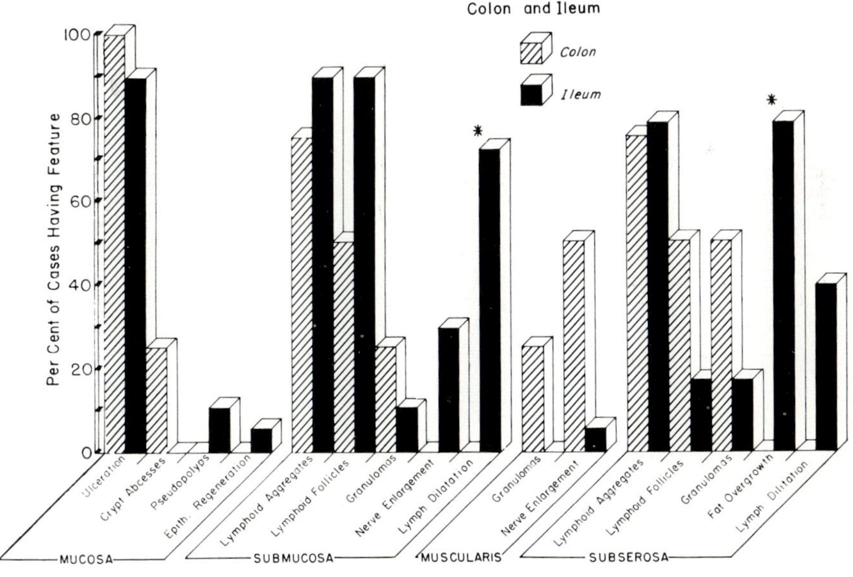

Figure 4–36 Frequency of occurrence of various histologic features in regional enteritis of the colon and of the ileum. Note that the majority of the changes are in the submucosa and subserosa, and that the pattern of the disease is similar in both sites. The asterisks indicate statistically significant differences in frequency of occurrence ($\chi^2 > 3.84$; $p < 0.05$; Yates' adjustment for continuity[2] as necessary). (W.U. Ill. #62-8955.) (Courtesy of S. L. Saltzstein and B. F. Rosenberg, Amer. J. Clin. Path. *40*:610-623, © 1963, and Williams & Wilkins Co. Baltimore.)

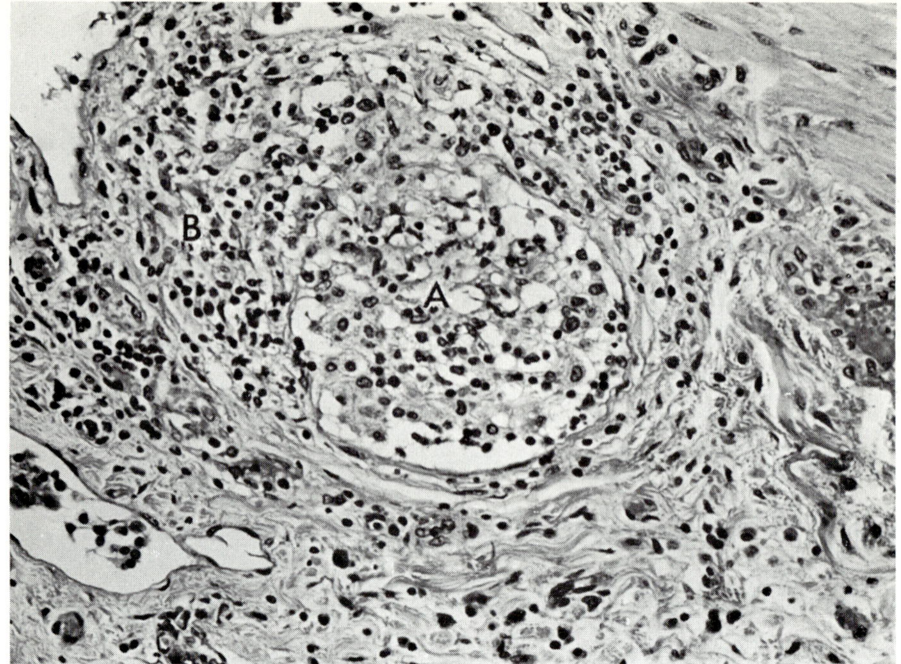

Figure 4–37 A regional enteritis granuloma located in the submucosa. A patch of histiocytes (A) is surrounded by numerous lymphocytes (B). ×64.

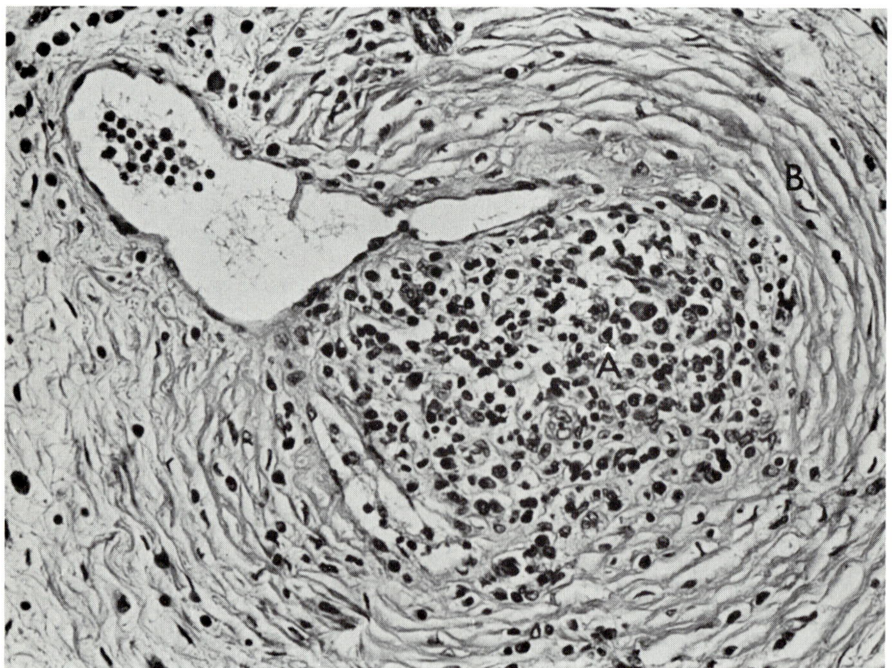

Figure 4–38 A regional enteritis granuloma mainly consisting of lymphoid cells (A) surrounding a few histiocytes. The lesion appears to be adjacent to distended lymphatic channels and is surrounded by layers of fibroblasts and collagen (B). ×64.

90

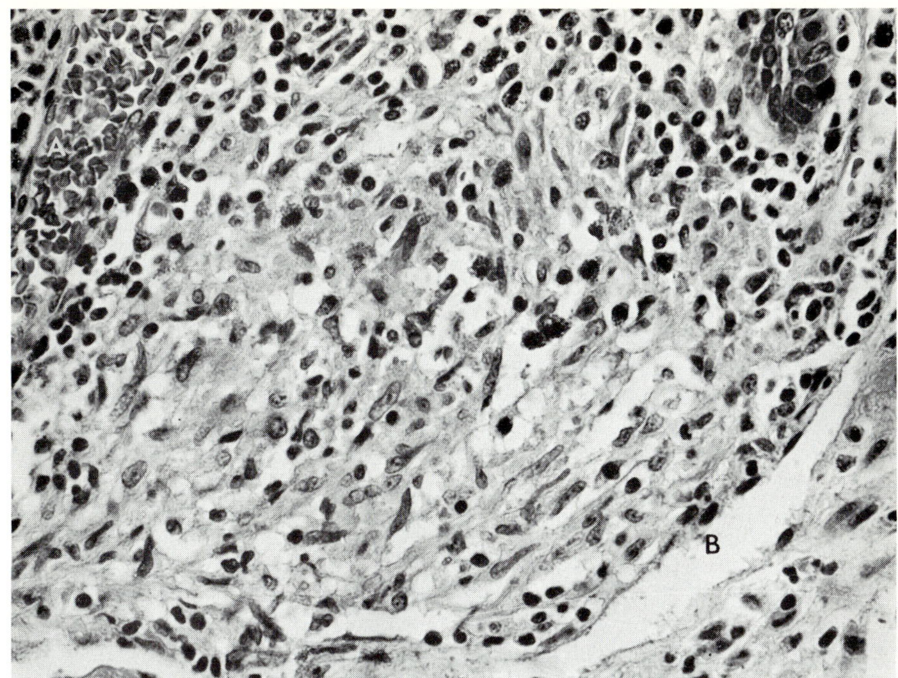

Figure 4–39 A regional enteritis granuloma of histiocytes occupies the space between a capillary (A) and a distended lymphatic (B). ×100.

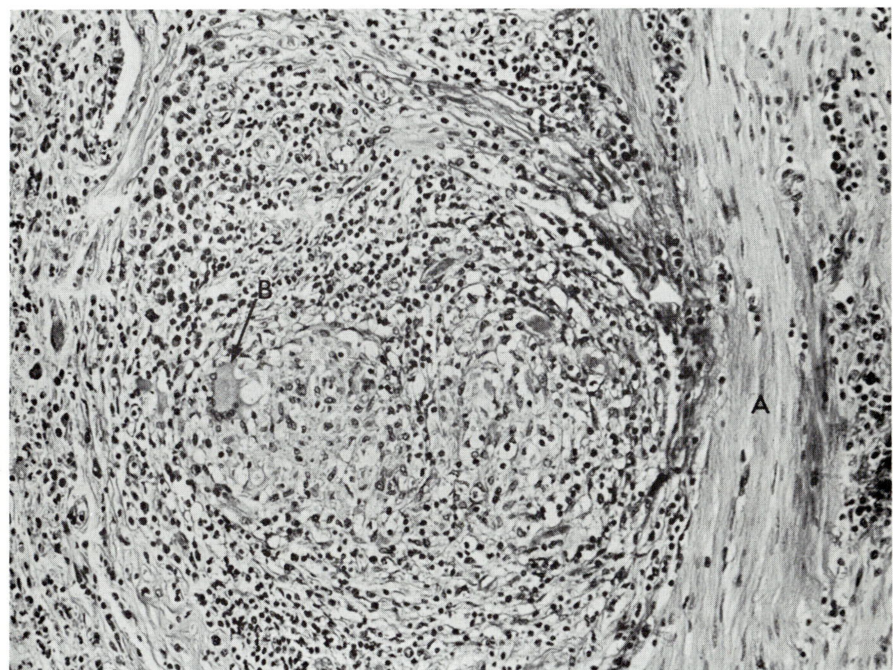

Figure 4–40 A regional enteritis granuloma adjacent to the muscularis (A). One giant cell (B) is seen near the edge of a patch of histiocytes. ×40.

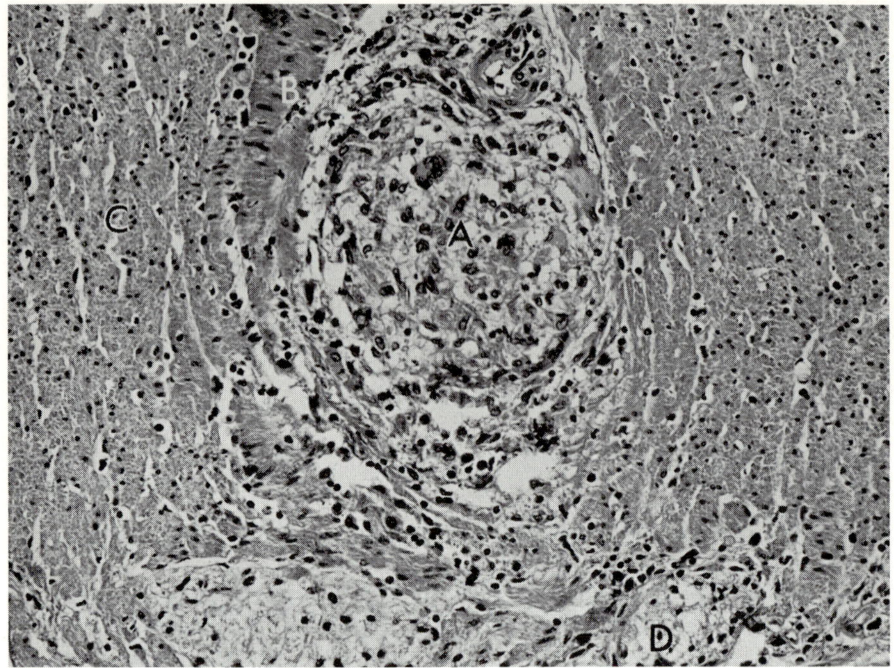

Figure 4-41   A regional enteritis granuloma (A) adjacent to a tangentially cut blood vessel (B) coursing through the muscularis (C). The adjacent subserosa is also shown (D). ×51.

of unknown cause. Though the granulomas in the late cases are usually easily found, occasionally an extensive search is necessary to find the specific ones. They are frequently surrounded and often dissected by collagen fibers, which are abundant at this stage. The collagen fibers and fibroblasts are extensively distributed throughout the deeper portions of the mucosa between layers of the fibers of the muscularis mucosae, and the submucosa may be entirely composed of collagenized connective tissue with few adipose cells remaining (Fig. 4-42).

Random sampling of the mesenteric lymph nodes will reveal the characteristic granuloma in about half of the cases (Figs. 4-43 and 4-44). When systematic sampling of lymph nodes is done the yield is much higher. Generally, the more frequent the granulomas in the intestinal wall, the more frequent they are in the lymph nodes. However, in about 20 per cent of the cases that do not have demonstrable granulomas in the intestinal wall, careful search of the lymph nodes will reveal their presence. This is a useful observation in differentiating between regional enteritis and ulcerative colitis because, in the latter disease, lymph node hyperplasia is often seen but granulomas are not found. The lymph node granulomas of regional enteritis form as enlargements of the germinal center histiocytes, and others form as accumulations of sinusoidal histiocytes (Figs. 4-43 to 4-46). This is an

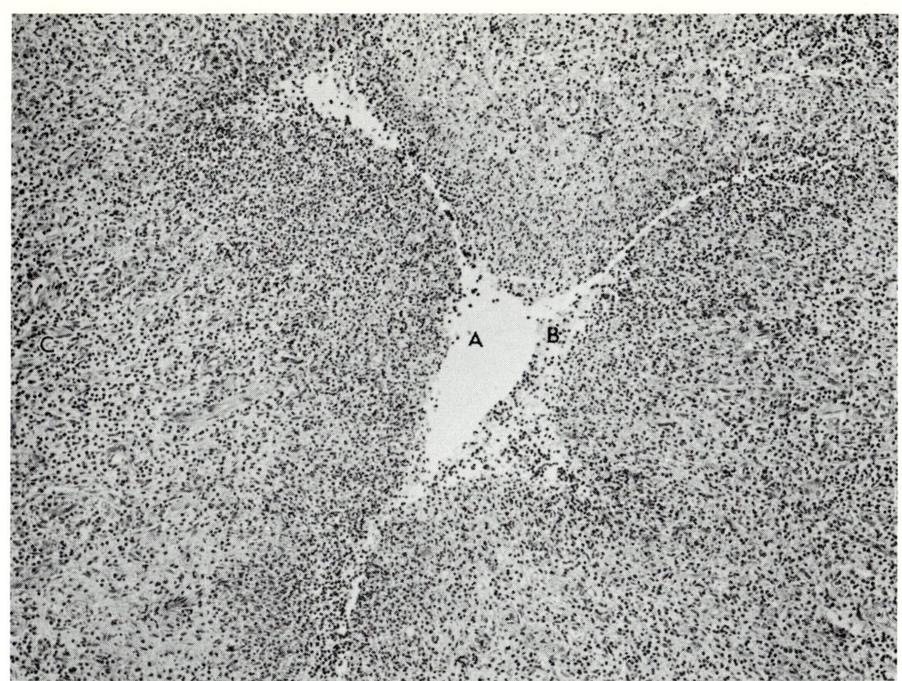

Figure 4-42 A fistulous tract (A) surrounded by necrosis (B), polymorphs, and granulation tissue (C). ×40.

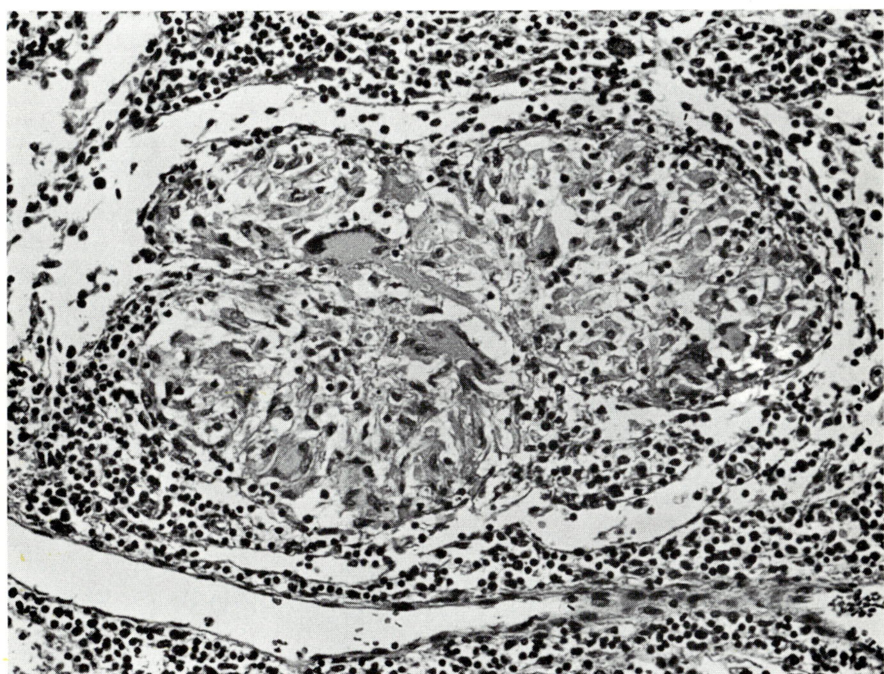

Figure 4-43 A regional enteritis granuloma within a mesenteric lymph node. The patch of histiocytes and giant cells is clearly delineated from the surrounding lymph node cortical tissue. ×51.

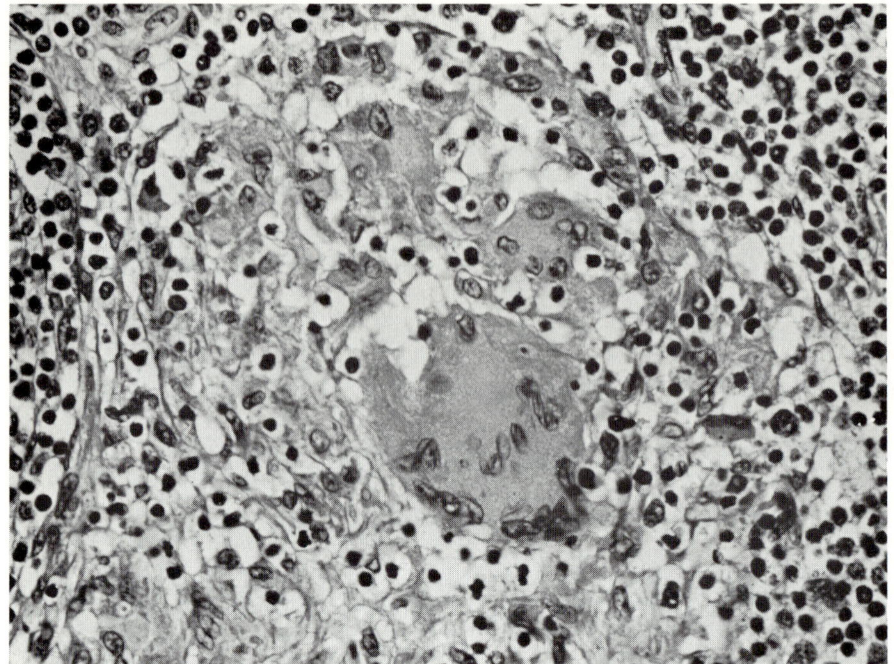

Figure 4-44   A higher magnification of a regional enteritis granuloma in the same lymph node shown in Figure 4-43. This lesion was within a sinusoid. ×100.

exceedingly important fact in considering possible etiologic factors. Reticulin fibers are increased in the germinal centers (Fig. 4-46).

The resemblance between the granulomatous phase of regional enteritis and sarcoid has long been recognized. Phear and Blackburn found no evidence of generalized sarcoidosis, and less than one third of their patients had a positive tuberculin reaction.[29, 30] More recently Williams applied the Kveim and Mantoux tests to regional enteritis patients and controls and was unable to demonstrate a relationship to either sarcoidosis or tuberculosis.[31] It is now accepted that sarcoidosis is a separate entity.

Davis counted the number of ganglion cells in the myenteric plexus of the ileum in 24 cases of regional enteritis and in an equal number of controls.[32] He recorded a threefold increase in the number of ganglion cells of the myenteric plexes of the former as contrasted with those not afflicted with regional enteritis. A comparable increase in the number of ganglion cells was also seen in the small intestine of afflicted individuals in areas not involved in the inflammatory process.

Numerous reports have recorded the features of the epithelial cells of the small intestine in those regions involved in regional enteritis.[33-36] Gastric pyloric gland metaplasia of the ileum is much more common in regional enteritis than in other small intestinal inflammatory or neoplastic diseases or in the normal state. It was rarely found in the colon

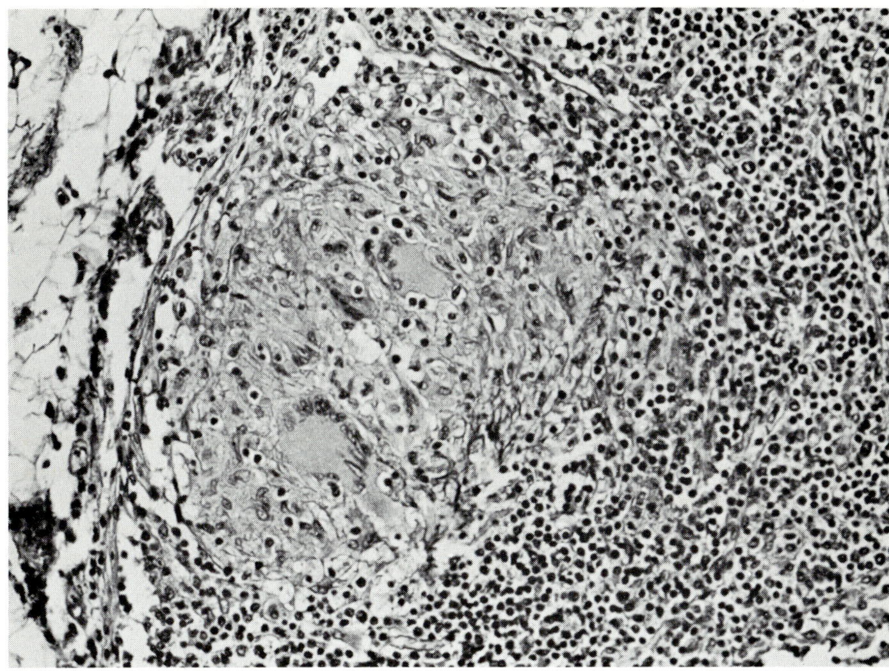

Figure 4-45 A regional enteritis granuloma in the cortex of a mesenteric lymph node is shown. Cytologic features of the histiocytes and giant cells are shown. ×50.

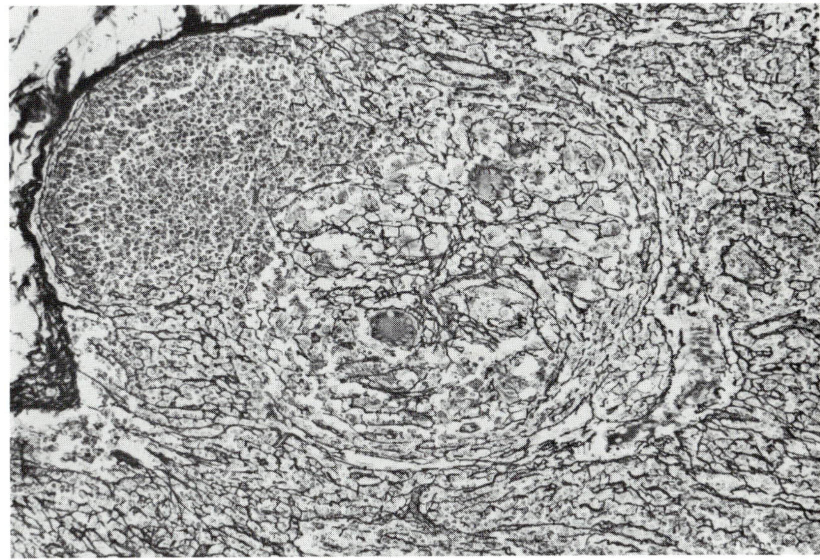

Figure 4-46 Reticulum stain of a regional enteritis granuloma in the cortex of a lymph node. There is a marked increase in the number and thickness of reticulum fibers surrounding the histiocytes and giant cells. Similar reticulum fiber formations are seen in the granulomas within the bowel wall. These lesions sharply contrast with the lymph nodes of ulcerative colitis (see Figs. 5-27, 5-28, and 5-52). ×40.

and was regarded as related to the presence of Paneth cells. Kawel and Tesluck observed the presence of Brunner gland metaplasia in 16 of 34 cases.[33] Two thirds of those having the metaplasia were recurrent cases, and these investigators considered the metaplasia to be of prognostic significance. Metaplasias usually occur after long-standing injury, therefore they may constitute a "marker" for the more severe chronic cases rather than an indication of a variation in the biologic process. Shiner examined 11 cases of regional enteritis and found villus atrophy to be a prominent feature.[34] Rippey and Sommers studied the incidence and cytologic features of plasma cells in 25 consecutive surgically resected specimens of regional enteritis and contrasted them with these cells in ulcerative colitis and in normal controls.[37] The average percentages of monocytes, mast cells, lymphocytes, and eosinophils were not greatly different in each of these groups. By counting the average percentage of cells in the mucosal lamina propria, it was observed that the predominant cell by far in regional enteritis was the plasma cell, composing about 45 per cent of the cellular exudate, whereas in ulcerative colitis, it composed 32 per cent and in normal controls, only 21 per cent. The percentages of eosinophils, lymphocytes, and monocytes in the cellular exudate in each of these three groups were about equal. Mast cells were exceedingly rare in regional enteritis and in normal controls, whereas they formed 3 per cent of the population in ulcerative colitis. The cross-sectional area of plasma cells was larger in regional enteritis than in normal controls. Ming reported a case of severe gastric metaplasia in the small intestine of a patient with regional enteritis.[36] In his case there were recognizable gastric fundic types of glands containing chief and parietal cells as well as pyloric gastric metaplasia.

Obliterative endarteritis and phlebitis are prominent blood vascular lesions seen most frequently in the outer layers of the intestinal wall and mesentery. These changes represent one of the radiologists' criteria for identifying the lesion by utilizing angiography. Because the vascular changes do not accompany early or minimal lesions, but rather accompany ulceration and secondary infection, it is most likely that they are a consequence of inflammation (as is true with a variety of inflammatory diseases) rather than an initiating factor.

DISTRIBUTION OF LESIONS

Esophagus, Stomach, and Duodenum

Several authors have reviewed the case reports of regional enteritis involving the duodenum, the stomach and duodenum, and the stomach alone.[38–41] These summaries of the literature included cases that were not histologically proved. Because of the ease with which the clinical and operating room gross findings of regional enteritis can be confused with those of other upper gastrointestinal diseases characterized by either stomach or duodenal wall thickening or both (e.g., sarcoidosis, linitis plastica type of carcinoma of the stomach, chronic duodenitis), it seemed imperative to me to develop a new list based on histologically proved lesions (Table 4-2). I have been able to find 41 reported cases of histologically proved regional enteritis of the stomach and duodenum. Duodenal involvement by regional enteritis is much more prevalent than regional enteritis of the stomach. As revealed in the table, there are 7 cases of regional enteritis of the duodenum without evidence of disease in other regions of the gastrointestinal tract, whereas 27 cases have accompanying involvement of the jejunum or ileum or both. Four cases of granulomatous gastritis, presumed to be regional enteritis occurring in isolation and without lesions in other portions of the intestinal tract, have been reported. Whether these are truly regional enteritis or whether they are actually sarcoidosis remains moot. McKusick emphasizes that the existence of sarcoid limited to the stomach need not be surprising, because the disease appears limited to other organs of the body such as the salivary gland or skin.[42] Guibert reported a case of granulomatous inflammation limited to the stomach and adjacent lymphatics, which was presumed to be sarcoid, in a 61 year old French woman.[43] To rule out sarcoid and other granulomatous diseases limited to the stomach, one would have to do thorough work-up to rule out tubercle bacilli, histologic or clinical evidence of syphilis or other granulomatous diseases in other organ sytems, and the absence of anergy to a tuberculin. Seven cases with granulomatous gastritis also had evidence of regional enteritis in other portions of the gastrointestinal tract.

The gross and microscopic features of gastroduodenal regional enteritis are similar to those in the ileum or colon. The incidence of upper gastrointestinal regional enteritis is uncertain though it must be quite rare. Perhaps the best evidence for its incidence in the duodenum was presented by Jones, who reviewed the experience of the Mayo Clinic between 1950 and 1964 and found 8 cases of duodenal involvement in 500 cases of regional enteritis, all of which were confirmed histologically.[84] This represents approximately 1.6 per cent incidence of duodenal involvement in all cases of regional enteritis. As already indicated, gastric involvement is even less common. One case of esophageal involvement has been reported.[70] As in the lower gastrointestinal tract, the histopathologic appearance depended upon the extent and stage of the disease.

In the acute stage the macroscopic appearance of the serosa was red, hyperemic, and the wall of the bowel was thickened. The mesentery contained enlarged soft edematous lymph nodes. The mucosa was ulcerated in some cases; in others it was not. Hyperplastic mucosa

TABLE 4–2   Regional Enteritis Involvement of Stomach and Duodenum

Case	First Author	Publication date	Age (Years)	Sex	Duodenum	Stomach	Jejunum	Ileum
1	Gottlieb[62]	1937	44	M	+	0	+	0
2	Ragnotti[63]	1939	50	M	+	0	+	0
3	Brown[64]	1945	29	M	+	0	0	0
4	Ross[65]	1949	21	F	0	+	0	+
5	Hawthorne[66]	1949	?	?	+	+	+	0
6	Comfort[67]	1950	26	M	+	0	+	0
7	Comfort[67]	1950	57	M	+	0	+	0
8	Comfort[67]	1950	31	F	+	0	+	0
9	Comfort[67]	1950	22	M	+	0	+	+
10	Comfort[67]	1950	49	M	+	0	+	0
11	Carlisle[68]	1952	27	M	+	0	+	+
12	Martin[69]	1953	24	F	+	+	0	+
13	Martin[69]	1953	23	F	+	+	0	+
14	Heffernon[70]	1954	48	M	+	+ (and esoph.)	+	0
15	Roberts[71]	1954	39	M	+	?	+	+
16	Brown[72]	1954	34	F	+	0	0	0
17	Richman[73]	1955	20	M	+	0	0	+
18	Richman[73]	1955	34	M	+	0	0 (and colon)	+
19	Berk[74]	1956	28	M	+	0	+	+
20	Miller[75]	1956	9	M	+	+	+	+
21	Detiege[76]	1956	22	M	+	0	0	+
22	Segal[77]	1956	24	M	+	0	0	0
23	McGarity[78]	1957	46	F	+	0	0	+
24	Anderson[79]	1957	27	M	+	0	+	+
25	Pryse-Davies[80]	1963	30	M	+	+	0 (and cecum)	+
26	Law[81]	1964	33	M	+	0	0	0
27	Rune[82]	1965	57	M	0	+	0	0
28	Fahimi[83]	1963	51	M	0	+	0	0
29	Fahimi[83]	1963	56	F	0	+	0	0
30	Fahimi[83]	1963	47	M	0	+	0	0
31	Jones[84]	1966		M	+	0	+	+
32	Jones[84]	1966		F	+	0	0	0
33	Jones[84]	1966		M	+	0	0	0
34	Jones[84]	1966		F	+	0	+	+
35	Jones[84]	1966		M	+	0	0	0
36	Jones[84]	1966		M	+	0	+	+
37	Jones[84]	1966		M	+	0	+	+
38	Jones[84]	1966		F	+	0	+	+
39	Madore[85]	1963	52	F	+	+	+	0
40	Elibol[86]	1968	31	M	+	+	+	+
41	Elibol[86]	1968	20	F	0	+	+	+

produced a cobblestone appearance. In later stages of the disease, as fibrosis became more evident, rigidity of the stomach and duodenal wall ensued. With duodenal involvement, intestinal obstruction was a frequent clinical finding. Microscopically the characteristic granulomatous changes were seen in the later stages of the disease. Caseation was absent; granulomas were also seen in the lymph follicles. There was a fairly abrupt demarcation between the involved and uninvolved segments. The presence of Schaumann bodies and asteroids within some of the giant cells in granulomatous lesions in the stomach was reported more frequently than for other parts of the gastrointestinal tract.

Whether some of these cases actually represent sarcoidosis is unproved. Fahimi and co-workers, in distinguishing between gastric involvement in regional enteritis and sarcoid, divided granulomas of the stomach into three groups.[83] Group 1 consisted of disseminated sarcoidosis with evidence of gastric involvement, and Group 2 consisted of cases of regional enteritis with the characteristic lower intestinal lesions and also granulomas in the stomach. Group 3 consisted of cases in which granulomas were limited to the stomach. They were able to find 32 cases of the latter in the medical literature. None had clinical evidence of disseminated sarcoidosis or of small bowel disease. Chest x-rays were negative in all instances. Though they were unable to rule out the presence of asymptomatic granulomas in the liver, spleen, or other internal organs, the clinical record did not reveal evidence of lesions or symptoms referable to these organs, and no such evidence has been found on follow-up. Cases of isolated granulomatous gastritis appeared to occur in an older age group than sarcoid and, indeed, in an older age group (40 to 59) than is most frequently seen with regional enteritis involving the lower gastrointestinal tract. The sex distribution was about equal for granulomatous gastritis and lower intestinal regional enteritis. The frequency of inclusion bodies noted earlier seemed to be comparable in isolated granulomatous gastritis and in disseminated sarcoidosis. It has not been reported in cases of regional enteritis with gastric involvement.

The coexistence of peptic ulcer of the duodenum in 23 per cent of young male patients with regional enteritis has been reported.[44] About half had symptoms of ulcer before the regional enteritis and half subsequent to it. Histologic proof of the nature of the ulcer was lacking though the clinical and radiographic pictures were characteristic.

Large Intestine and Appendix (Granulomatous Colitis)

It was only two years after Crohn's initial description of "regional ileitis" involving the terminal ileum only that Colp described a patient with cecal involvement.[45] Since then it has been well established that many regional enteritis patients also have lesions in the colon. As Table

TABLE 4–3   Distribution of Lesions in Regional Enteritis

First Authors	Year	Total Cases	Sites with Lesions		
			Ileum	*Colon*	*Jejunum*
Warren	1948	120	112	19 (15%)	5
Rappaport	1951	100	—	55 (55%)	—
Fone	1966	41	26	9 (22%)	2
Laipply	1957	28	26	3 (11%)	2
Cornes	1961	86	86	49 (57%)	?
Valdez-Dapena	1962	30	30	16 (53%)	?

4-3 shows, various studies reveal 10 to 55 per cent of cases of regional enteritis also have colonic involvement with or without involvement of other regions of the gastrointestinal tract. The reason for this large variation in the incidence of colonic involvement appears to be related to the care with which colonic lesions are sought. In the author's own experience, if a person searches the colon very carefully he will uncover many minute gross and microscopic lesions with or without ulceration in the cecum and other more distal regions of the colon. For obvious reasons many of the specimens examined in these series were small intestinal resections, and the entire or major portion of the colon was not removed; therefore, the opportunity of uncovering small lesions at the dissection table may have been precluded. In Meadow's study of the early lesion of regional enteritis, none of his three cases had colonic involvement, though an equal number of the intermediate or transitional stage and late stage specimens did have.[20]

When regional enteritis involves the colon, some have preferred the term regional enterocolitis; however, because of the risk of confusion with other diseases, it is preferable to utilize the designation "regional enteritis involving the colon" when the inflammatory process is granulomatous in nature. Various students of the disease use the terms ileocolitis, enterocolitis, or segmental colitis for different entities, adding to the confusion in the literature. As Table 4-3 illustrates, colonic involvement is much more frequent than jejunal involvement. The colonic lesions are usually in the cecum and ascending colon, and occur with decreasing frequency in the more distal portions of the colon. Donchess and Warren and Crohn and Rosenak confirmed the existence of colonic lesions in many cases of regional enteritis.[46, 47]

Although the colonic extension of regional enteritis is now a well-recognized clinical and pathologic entity, the existence of a regional enteritis as a cicatrizing granulomatous lesion restricted to the colon has aroused dispute. Recognition of the isolated colonic lesion of regional enteritis has been retarded by confusion in the nomenclature.

Failure to study pathologic material adequately and overreliance on clinical features rather than on the characterisitic pathologic process has contributed to the confusion. To avoid commitment some have used the term "granulomatous colitis" for lesions arising primarily in the large intestine in cases in which the small intestine was apparently normal. There are many specific agents that produce granulomatous inflammations in the colon or elsewhere in the gastrointestinal tract (e.g., tuberculosis, syphilis, actinomycosis, South American blastomycosis, histoplasmosis, schistosomiasis, lymphogranuloma venereum, foreign body material such as starch, talc, suture, lipids, barium, and mercury). Diseases of unknown etiology such as sarcoidosis and eosinophilic granuloma may also produce granulomatous lesions in the colon. While the Nickerson-Kveim test is positive in 70 per cent of patients with sarcoidosis, it is invariably negative in granulomatous ileitis or colitis.[48]

Well-documented case reports of regional enteritis limited to the colon have been published.[49–53, 57–61] Cornes and Stecher carefully studied 45 patients in whom the granulomatous inflammatory process was confined entirely to the large intestine and compared the clinical and pathologic features of their disease with those of 86 patients with regional enteritis of the classic type and 200 patients with ulcerative colitis.[53] Table 4-4, derived from their report, reveals that regional enteritis limited to the large intestine occurs in an older age group than does the classic variety and has a different sex distribution. There was a higher incidence of perianal and rectovaginal fistula. The disease had the same sex distribution as ulcerative colitis, but occurred in an older age group, and was about one sixteenth as common as ulcerative colitis. Gross and microscopic examination of the specimens showed the characteristic pathologic features of regional enteritis (Fig. 4-47).

TABLE 4–4 Large Intestinal Regional Enteritis: Age and Sex Distribution*

Age (Years)	Regional Ileitis			Ulcerative Colitis			Primary Crohn's Disease of Large Intestine		
	M	F	Total	M	F	Total	M	F	Total
0–10	2	2	4	4	3	7	0	1	1
11–20	19	10	29	8	18	26	4	5	9
21–30	17	14	31	29	42	71	3	2	5
31–40	9	2	11	20	23	43	5	0	5
41–50	5	5	10	17	20	37	1	4	5
51–60	1	0	1	2	8	10	3	2	5
61–70	0	0	0	4	2	6	2	9	11
71–80	0	0	0	0	0	0	0	4	4
Total	53	33	86	84	116	200	18	27	45

*From J. S. Cornes and M. Stecher: Primary Crohn's disease of the colon and rectum. Gut 2:189–201, 1961. Reprinted by permission of The Editor and Publishers, British Medical Journal, BMA. House, Tavistock Square, London W.C.1.

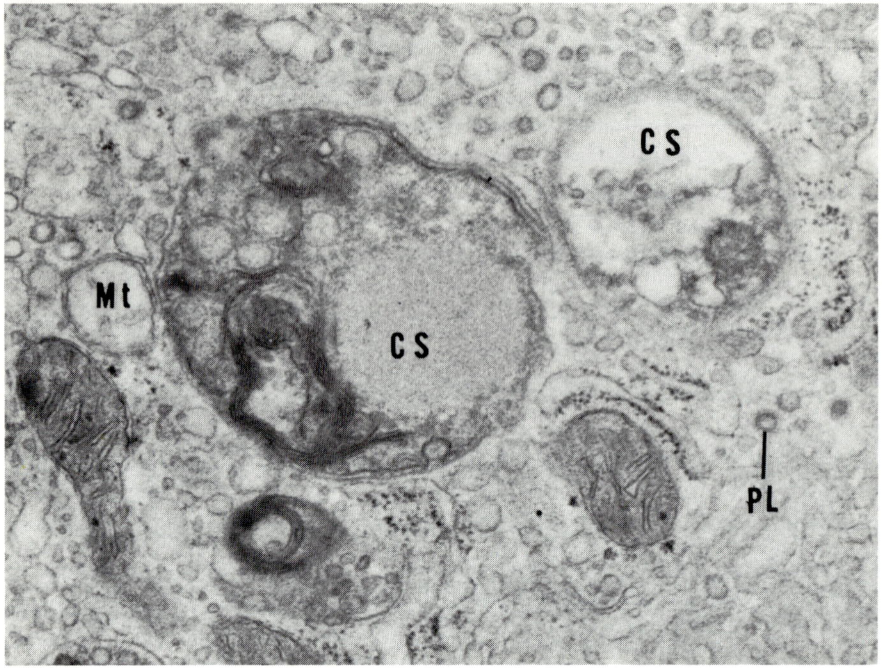

Figure 4–47   Surface epithelium in regional enteritis. Different typs of cytosegresomes (CS) are illustrated. An altered mitochondrion (Mt) and protolysosomes are present (PL). ×37,700. (Courtesy of A. Gonzalez-Licea and J. H. Yardley, *Bull. Hopkins Hosp. 118–119*:444–461, © 1966, and the Johns Hopkins Press, Baltimore, Md.)

No carcinomas of the large intestine occurred in their patients with regional enteritis of the large intestine, whereas 17 patients with ulcerative colitis had carcinoma (see Chapter Nine). They reported that the histologic appearance of the noncaseating nodules of histiocytes in this lesion could be distinguished from that seen in sarcoidosis. Lymph nodes were usually enlarged in sarcoidosis, whereas in granulomatous colitis the nodes may be of normal size or only slightly enlarged. In sarcoidosis the granulomas were usually monotonously uniform in size, shape, and stage of development; in granulomatous colitis they observed them to be variable in size, shape, and degree of maturity and often much more diffuse and not as "tight" as those seen in sarcoid. The giant cells had relatively fewer nuclei than are commonly seen in sarcoid and were frequently found in association with lymphatics. They conclude that the granulomatous lesions are part of the spectrum of distribution of regional enteritis.

Similar conclusions were reached by Lockhart-Mummery and Morson, who reported their observations on 75 cases.[52] They noted that the large intestinal lesion may be more diffuse and produce single or multiple strictures of the colon. It was associated with disease in the terminal ileum in 30 per cent of their cases; the rectum was normal in about half. They emphasized the pathologic distinctions between regional enteritis of the colon and ulcerative colitis. They indicate that the presumptive diagnosis can often be made on macroscopic evidence alone. A "garden hose" stricture similar to that in the small intestine is usually seen, and inspection of the serosa of the colon will sometimes reveal small nodular granulomas or "tubercles." There may be a patchy pericolitis due to penetration of all layers of the wall by the inflammation, just as in the small intestine. They found the mucosal surface in this disease of the large intestine similar in every way to that seen in the small bowel. The characteristic cobblestone appearance was not always present, but was a useful diagnostic feature when seen. It represents the intact mucosa being elevated by inflammatory changes and granuloma formation in the submucosa. Between the cobblestones, communicating cracks or crevices may be seen extending into the wall. They are slit-like ulcers and tend to undermine the adjacent mucosa, which in later stages may slough, leaving larger, more extensive areas of ulceration. Ulceration seemed to be a late manifestation of regional enteritis and occurred secondary to the submucosal inflammations. Even when ulceration was extensive, cracks and crevices could be demonstrated on the surface near the ulcerated areas. Frequently enlarged lymph nodes were encountered. Granulomas consisting of clusters of histiocytes and giant cells within the lymph nodes were sometimes seen. The presence of these characteristic granulomas microscopically in the bowel wall or lymph nodes was noted in about 87 per cent of their cases, when adequate sampling was done. It could be found in all layers of the wall with a predominance toward the mucosa and submucosa. Schaumann bodies were seen in about 10 per cent of the specimens. In the small intestinal lesion, the superficial ulcerated zones were covered with polymorphs, lymphocytes, and plasma cells. Beneath this in the lower layers of the mucosa and in the submucosa, lymphocytes were numerous and there were a few plasma cells and histiocytes. Focal collections of lymphocytes, often with prominent follicle formation, were sometimes scattered through all layers of the bowel wall, including the serosa. In 5 of their 75 patients the disease involved the appendix; it was in continuity with disease of the cecum in two of the cases. However, in three it was essentially a skip area of involvement.

The appendix may have lesions in about half the cases of regional enteritis. This may represent either the characteristic active lesions of regional enteritis, chronic nonspecific inflammation and fibroplasia, or chronic periappendicitis without demonstrable inflammatory changes in the inner coats of the appendix. The latter two types of lesions may either represent a "tombstone" of previous active disease of the organ or a "sympathetic" response to severe disease in an adjacent structure. Roughly half of those with appendiceal changes will have evidence of active inflammation.

Similar observations on the lesions of regional enteritis of the colon and rectum were reported from Sweden by Snellman and Westerholm and from Canada by Madore.[54, 55] Intestinal obstruction and a prominent tendency towards fistula formation and recurrence occurred in most cases. Crohn and Yarnis reported that their files include approximately 1,800 cases of ulcerative colitis and about 1,000 cases of regional enteritis and about 291 cases of segmental granulomatous disease of the colon, of which 126 also involve the ileum.[87] Hawk and others reported the experience at the Cleveland Clinic on 1,500 cases of primary ulcerative disease of the colon since 1950.[56] Approximately half were classified as regional enteritis involving the colon, which was roughly in agreement with Crohn and Yarnis.[87] They noted that deep fissures extending through the wall may be observed in about one of four cases and appear to be the basis of the frequent fistulous tracts. They also emphasize the frequent occurrence of the lesion in the ileum following colectomy. Extensive recent reports have reviewed the morphology and clinical course of ulcerative and granulomatous colitis.[89, 90]

References

1. Koster, H., Kasman, L. P., and Scheinfeld, W.: Regional ileitis. Arch. Surg. *32*:789-809, 1936.
2. Meyer, K. A., and Rosi, P. A.: Regional enteritis (non-specific). Surg. Gynec. Obstet. *62*:977-988, 1936.
3. Eliason, E. L., and Johnson, J.: Acute regional enteritis. New Int. Clin. *1*:123-133, 1940.
4. Eckel, J. H., and Ogilvie, J. B.: Regional enteritis. A report of twenty-one cases. Amer. J. Surg. *53*:345-348, 1941.
5. Sneierson, H., and Ryan, J.: Regional ileitis. Résumé of present knowledge and the addition of twenty-one cases from Broome County, New York. Amer. J. Surg. *52*:424-432, 1941.
6. Smithy, H. G.: Conservatism in the surgical management of acute regional enteritis. Surgery *13*:122-130, 1943.
7. Holloway, J. W.: Regional ileitis. Ann. Surg. *118*:329-342, 1943.
8. Pugh, H. L.: Regional enteritis. Ann. Surg. *122*:845-861, 1945.
9. Rose, T. F.: Acute regional entero-colitis with a report of three cases. Aust. New Zeal. J. Surg. *15*:184-192, 1946.
10. Homb, A.: Acute regional enteritis. Acta Chir. Scand. *94*:343-361, 1946.
11. Armitage, G., and Wilson, M.: Crohn's disease. A survey of the literature and a report on 34 cases. Brit. J. Surg. *38*:182-193, 1950.
12. O'Callaghan, R.: Acute terminal ileitis. West. J. Surg. *60*:17-19, 1952.
13. Siegel, R., and White, B. V.: Acute regional ileitis. Conn. Med. J. *17*:738-741, 1953.
14. Storrs, R. C., and Hoekelman, R. A.: Acute regional enteritis in children. New Eng. J. Med. *248*:320-322, 1953.
15. Austin, W. E.: Acute regional ileitis. Canad. Med. Ass. J. *74*:289-290, 1956.
16. Jackman, W. A.: Localized hypertrophic enteritis as a cause of intestinal obstruction. Brit. J. Surg. *22*:27-32, 1934.
17. Erb, I. H., and Farmer, A. W.: Ileocolitis. Surg. Gynec. Obstet. *61*:6-14, 1935.
18. Gump, F. E., Lepore, M., and Barker, H. G.: A revised concept of acute regional enteritis. Ann. Surg. *166*:942-946, 1967.
19. Warren, S., and Sommers, S. C.: Cicatrizing enteritis (regional enteritis) as a pathological entity: Analysis of 120 cases. Amer. J. Path. *24*:475-501, 1948.
20. Meadows, T. R., and Batsakis, J. G.: Histopathological spectrum of regional enteritis. Arch. Surg. (Chicago) *87*:976-982, 1963.
21. Austin, W. E.: Acute regional ileitis. Canad. Med. Ass. J. *74*:289-290, 1956.

22. Ficarra, B. J.: Histopathologic association between regional ileitis and giant follicular hyperplasia. Amer. J. Gastroent. *26*:590-595, 1956.
23. Crohn, B. B.: The pathology of acute regional ileitis. Amer. J. Dig. Dis. *10*:565-572, 1965.
24. Williams, W. J.: Histology of Crohn's syndrome. Gut *5*:510-516, 1964.
25. Koop, C. E., Perlingiero, J. G., and Weiss, W.: Cicatrizing enterocolitis in a newborn infant. Amer. J. Med. Sci. *214*:27-32, 1947.
26. Ammann, R. W., and Bockus, H. L.: Pathogenesis of regional enteritis based on histological study of forty cases. Arch. Intern. Med. *107*:504-513, 1961.
27. Heaton, K. W., McCarthy, C. F., and Horton, R. E.: Miliary Crohn's disease. Gut *8*:4-7, 1967.
28. Solomons, D., and Halford, M. E.: Crohn's disease of a Meckel's diverticulum occurring in a case of jejunal diverticulitis. Brit. J. Surg. *51*:910-913, 1964.
29. Phear, D. N.: The relationship between regional ileitis and sarcoidosis. Lancet *2*:1250-1251, 1958.
30. Blackburn, G., Hadfield, G., and Hunt, A. H.: Regional ileitis. St. Barth. Hosp. Rep. *72*:181-224, 1939.
31. Williams, W. J.: A study of Crohn's syndrome using tissue extracts and the Kveim and Mantoux tests. Gut *6*:503-505, 1965.
32. Davis, D. R., Dockerty, M. D., and Mayo, C. W.: The myenteric plexus in regional enteritis: A study of the number of ganglion cells in the ileum in 24 cases. Surg. Gynec. Obstet. *101*:208-216, 1955.
33. Kawel, C. A., Jr., and Tesluck, H.: Brunner-type glands in regional enteritis. Gastroenterology *28*:810-820, 1955.
34. Lee, F. D.: Pyloric metaplasia in the small intestine. J. Path. Bact. *87*:267-277, 1964.
35. Shiner, M., and Drury, R. A.: Abnormalities of the small intestinal mucosa in Crohn's disease (regional enteritis). Amer. J. Dig. Dis. *7*:744-759, 1962.
36. Ming, S. C., Simon, M., and Tandon, B. N.: Gross gastric metaplasia of ileum after regional enteritis. Gastroenterology *44*:63-68, 1963.
37. Rippey, J. H., and Sommers, S. C.: Hypertrophied plasma cells in regional enteritis. Amer. J. Dig. Dis. *12*:465-467, 1967.
38. McGarity, W. C.: Regional enteritis of the duodenum. Surg. Gynec. Obstet. *105*:203-209, 1957.
39. Jones, G. W., Jr., Dooley, M. R., and Schoenfield, L. J.: Regional enteritis with involvement of the duodenum. Gastroenterology *51*:1018-1022, 1966.
40. Pryce-Davies, J.: Gastro-duodenal Crohn's disease. J. Clin. Path. *17*:90-94, 1964.
41. Johnson, O. A., Hoskins, D. W., and Todd, J.: Crohn's disease of the stomach. Gastroenterology *50*:571-577, 1966.
42. McKusick, V. A.: Boeck's sarcoid of the stomach with comments on the etiology of regional enteritis. Gastroenterology *23*:103-113, 1953.
43. Guibert, H. L.: Maladie de Besnier-Boeck-Schaumann à localisation gastro-ganglionnaire pure. Ann. Anat. Path. (Paris) *17*:295-300, 1947.
44. Freud, W. I., and Spellberg, M. A.: The concurrence of duodenal ulcer and regional enteritis. Amer. J. Gastroent. *28*:418-422, 1957.
45. Colp, R.: A case of nonspecific granuloma of the terminal ileum and the cecum. Surg. Clin. N. Amer. *14*:443-449, 1934.
46. Donchess, J. C., and Warren, S.: Chronic cicatrizing enteritis with involvement of the cecum and the colon. Arch. Path. *18*:22-29, 1934.
47. Crohn, B. B., and Rosenak, B. D.: A combined form of ileitis and colitis. J.A.M.A. *106*:1-5, 1936.
48. Janowitz, H. D., and Present, D. H.: Granulomatous colitis—pathogenetic concepts. Gastroenterology *51*:778-787, 1966.
49. James, T. G. I.: Chronic regional colitis. Brit. J. Surg. *25*:511-516, 1938.
50. Castleman, B.: Case 30172 of the Massachusetts General Hospital. New Eng. J. Med. *230*:526-529, 1944.
51. Brooke, B. N.: Granulomatous diseases of the intestine. Lancet *2*:745-749, 1959.
52. Lockhart-Mummery, H. E., and Morson, B. C.: Crohn's disease (regional enteritis) of the large intestine and its distinction from ulcerative colitis. Gut *1*:87-105, 1960.
53. Cornes, J. S., and Stecher, M.: Primary Crohn's disease of the colon and rectum. Gut *2*:189-201, 1961.
54. Snellman, B., and Westerholm, P.: Crohn's disease of the colon and rectum. Dis. Colon Rectum *9*:427-433, 1966.

55. Madore, P., Glay, A., and Kahn, D. S.: Lesions of the gastrointestinal tract resembling regional enteritis—a granulomatous disease, a report of three cases. Canad. Med. Ass. J. *89:*1165-1170, 1963.

56. Hawk, W. A., Turnbull, R. B., Jr., and Farmer, R. G.: Regional enteritis of the colon. Distinctive features of the entity. J.A.M.A. *201:*738-746, 1967.

57. Farmer, R. G., Hawk, W. A., and Turnbull, R. B.: Regional enteritis of the colon: a clinical and pathological comparison with ulcerative colitis. Amer. J. Dig. Dis. *13:*501-514, 1968.

58. Martin, E. D., Marche, Cl., Potet, F., and Alaoui, A.: Anatomie pathologique de la rectocolite ulcéro-hemorragique. Actualités Hepatogastroent. Hôtel Dieu *4:*A165-189, 1968.

59. Laumonier, R., Potet, F., and Fondimare, A.: La maladie de Crohn du côlon. Ann. Anat. Path. (Paris) *13:*433-448, 1968.

60. Maratka, Z., Kubernatova, D., Capek, V., and Kudrmann, J.: Colite régionale ou maladie de Crohn du colon. Actualités Hepatogastroent. Hôtel Dieu *4:*A15-52, 1968.

61. Morson, B. S.: Histopathology of Crohn's disease. Proc. Roy. Soc. Med. *61:*79-81, 1968.

62. Gottlieb, C., and Alpert, S.: Regional jejunitis. Amer. J. Roentgen. *38:*881-883, 1937.

63. Ragnotti, E.: Enterite regionale. Arch. Ital. Chir. *56:*237-271, 1939.

64. Brown, S.: Chronic nonspecific regional enteritis. Amer. J. Roentgen. *54:*487-495, 1945.

65. Ross, J. R.: Cicatrizing enteritis, colitis and gastritis; case report. Gastroenterology *13:*344-350, 1949.

66. Hawthorne, H. R., and Frobese, A. S.: Chronic stenosing regional enteritis—surgical pathology and experience in surgical treatment. Ann. Surg. *130:*233-241, 1949.

67. Comfort, M. W., Weber, H. M., Baggenstoss, A. H., and Kielly, W. F.: Nonspecific granulomatous inflammation of the stomach and duodenum; its relation to regional enteritis. Amer. J. Med. Sci. *220:*616-632, 1950.

68. Carlisle, J. C., and Judd, E. S., Jr.: Regional enteritis involving the duodenum; reports of a case. Proc. Staff Meet. Mayo Clin. *27:*569-574, 1952.

69. Martin, F. R. R., and Carr, R. J.: Crohn's disease involving the stomach; a report of two cases. Brit. Med. J. *1*(suppl.):700-702, 1953.

70. Heffernon, E. W., and Kepkay, P. H.: Segmental esophagitis, gastritis and enteritis. Gastroenterology *26:*83-88, 1954.

71. Roberts, S. E., Martin, W. J., and Beahrs, O. H.: Regional enteritis involving the duodenum: Reports of a case. Proc. Staff Meet. Mayo Clin. *29:*424–427, 1954.

72. Brown, C. H., and Sims, J. R., Jr.: Regional enteritis involving the duodenum: Report of two cases. Cleveland Clin. Quart. *21:*95-102, 1954.

73. Richman, A.: Non-specific granulomatous disease of the stomach and duodenum. J. Mount Sinai Hosp. N.Y. *22:*175-183, 1955.

74. Berk, M.: Regional enteritis involving the duodenum. Report of three cases. Gastroenterology *30:*508-516, 1956.

75. Miller, P. B., Sandweiss, D. J., and Scwachman, H.: Non-specific granulomatous inflammation of the gastrointestinal tract: Report of a case. New Eng. J. Med. *255:*501-504, 1956.

76. Detiege, R., Catry, L., and Vandenbroucke, J.: Ziekte van Crohn met aantasten vanbulbusen duodenum. Belg. T. Geneesk. *12:*403–408, 1956.

77. Segal, G., and Serbin, R.: Regional enteritis involving the duodenum. Gastroenterology *30:*503-507, 1956.

78. McGarity, W. C.: Regional enteritis of the duodenum. Surg. Gynec. Obstet. *105:*203-209, 1957.

79. Anderson, D. O., Mullinger, M. A., and Bogoch, A.: Regional enteritis involving the duodenum, with clubbing of the fingers and steatorrhea. Gastroenterology *32:*917-926, 1957.

80. Pryse-Davies, J.: Gastro-duodenal Crohn's disease. J. Clin. Path. *17:*90-94, 1964.

81. Law, S. W., Searle, N. B., and Barton, N. L.: Regional enteritis of the duodenum. report of a case and reviews of the literature. Arch. Surg. (Chicago) *89:*562-569, 1964.

82. Kune, G. A., and Fullerton, J.: Crohn's disease of the stomach. Postgrad. Med. J. *41:*100-104, 1965.

83. Fahimi, H. D., Deren, J. J., and Gottlieb, L. S.: Isolated granulomatous gastritis: Its relationship to disseminated sarcoidosis and regional enteritis. Gastroenterology *45:*161–175, 1963.
84. Jones, J. H., and Lennard-Jones, J. E.: Corticosteroids and corticotrophin in the treatment of Crohn's disease. Gut *7:*181–187, 1966.
85. Madore, P., Glay, A., and Kahn, D. S.: Lesions of the gastrointestinal tract resembling regional enteritis—a granulomatous disease; a report of three cases. Canad. Med. Ass. J. *89:*1165–1170, 1963.
86. Elibol, T., Rankin, G. B., and Brown, C. H.: Crohn's disease of the stomach. Report of two cases. Gastroint. Endosc. *14:*201–204, 1968.
87. Crohn, B. B., and Yarnis, H.: Granulomatous colitis: an attempt at clarification. J. Mount Sinai Hosp. N.Y. *33:*503–513, 1966.
88. Jorgensen, T. G., Vang, O., Pedersen, G.: Thirty-three patients with acute terminal ileitis operated on for suspected appendicitis and follow-up after 5 to 22 years. Nord. Med. *82:*1415–1418, 1969.
89. Glotzer, D. J., Gardner, R. C., Goldman, H., Hinricks, R., Rosen, H., and Zetzel, L.: Comparative features and course of ulcerative and granulomatous colitis. New Eng. J. Med. *282:*582–587, 1970.
90. Zetzel, L.: Granulomatous (ileo) colitis. New Eng. J. Med. *282:*600–605, 1970.

Chapter Five

Intestinal Histopathology of Ulcerative Colitis

The recurrent acute inflammatory process of ulcerative colitis is usually limited to the mucosa and submucosa of the large intestine. Its characteristic features are an intense hyperemia, acute cryptitis, and a predominantly mucosal infiltrate of lymphocytes, mast cells, and plasma cells. Also characteristically, it does not provoke collagenogenesis in the reparative process. The inflammation progresses at a variable rate and degree of severity, usually relentlessly, with variable periods of remission and acute exacerbation. Rarely it progresses as a rapid, severe, fulminant lesion (toxic megacolon). Also uncommonly, it may be a mild, self-limited inflammation of the rectum (ulcerative proctitis). The several variants of the process are described in order.

THE INITIAL LESION

The earliest lesions of ulcerative colitis have not been identified with certainty. It is unlike regional enteritis, in which complaints suggesting acute abdominal crisis have led to surgical exploration and the fortuitous observation and biopsy of early lesions that subsequently evolved into characteristic regional enteritis. I have not seen or been able to find any such descriptions of the initial lesion of ulcerative colitis. There are no reports in the literature effectively supporting the contention that mucous colitis or some other complaint precedes ulcerative colitis. Ulcerative colitis begins abruptly without premonitory signs or symptoms that would lead one to perform a biopsy of the colon. The disease is sufficiently infrequent in the general population to make prospective study impractical, and there is as yet no way of identifying sufficiently high-risk populations to make it practical. Indeed, as Dukes points out, a further difficulty is that the parameters of the process have been ill defined.[1] The term, to some, includes almost any inflammatory process of uncertain etiology in the colon, whether localized or diffuse, mild or severe, whereas to others, it is restricted to a severe inflammation involving the whole colon. Excessive reliance on clinical patterns for classification rather than on histogenetic features has further added to the confusion.

To many students of this disease, cryptitis, or crypt abscess, is the initial and principal lesion of the disease and is pathognomonic (Frontispiece). Whether this is true or not remains unproved, though the preponderance of evidence indicates it to be an *early and characteristic* feature. *Cryptitis* is the exudation of polymorphs into the interstices of the lamina propria near the tip of a crypt of Lieberkühn in association with decreased secretion of mucus and degenerative changes of the adjacent crypt epithelium. A *crypt abscess* is a subsequent stage in the process when frank necrosis of the crypt epithelium and subjacent lamina propria ensues, resulting in a streamer of pus extending from the abscess into the lumen of the crypt and often to the surface of the mucosa (Figs. 2-1 and 5-1 to 5-7).

The importance of the identification of the initial lesion should not be underestimated, not only for diagnostic purposes, but for research as well. If cryptitis were proved to be the initial lesion, then added

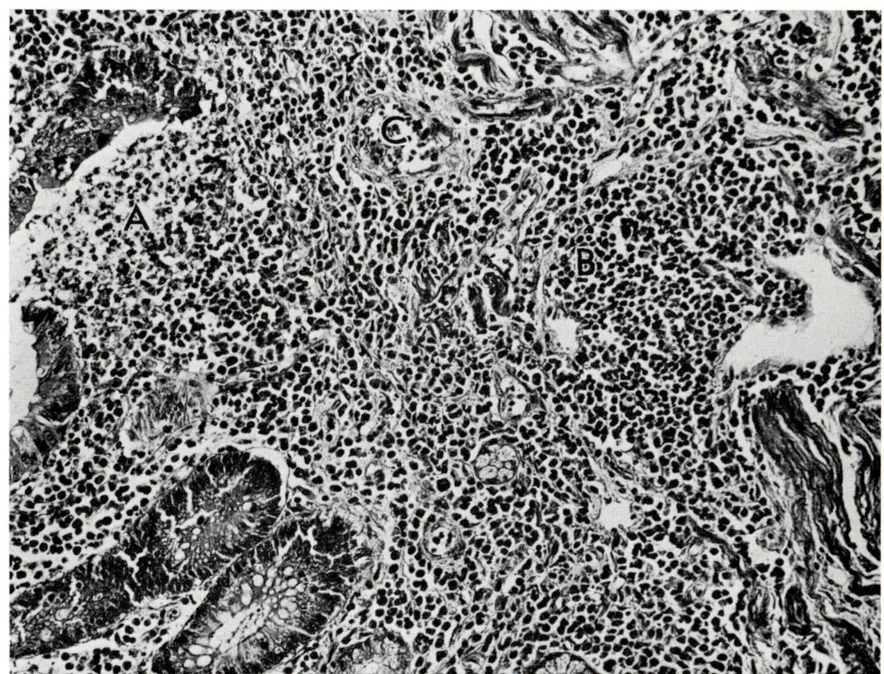

Figure 5-1 Histologic section of the mucosa and the superficial aspect of the submucosa of ulcerative colitis demonstrating the three characteristic features of the lesion. Crypt abscess (A), intensive mucosal and submucosal lymphocytosis (B), and vascular congestion (C). ×40.

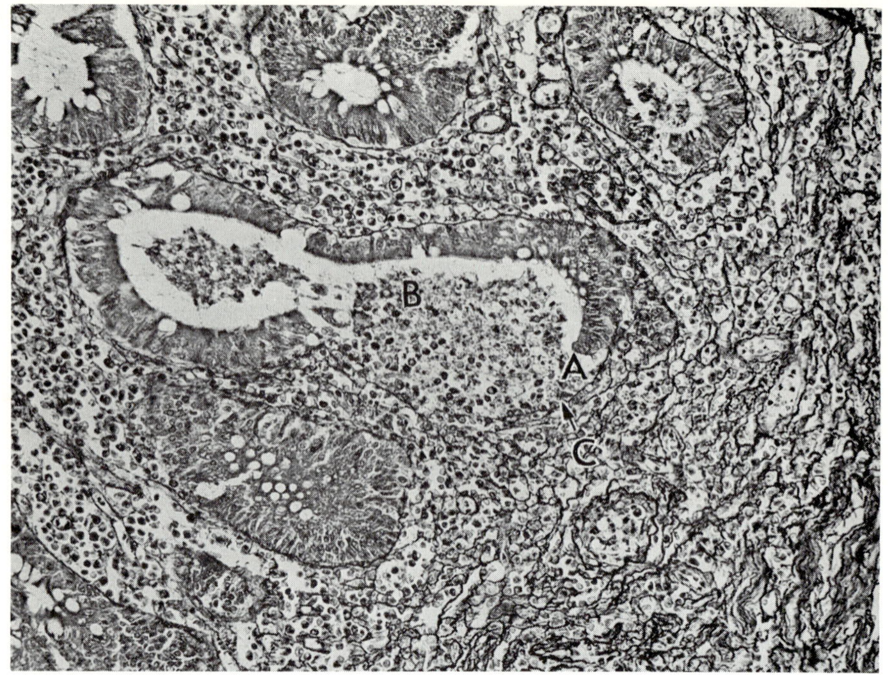

Figure 5-2   Reticulin stain of the section adjacent to the one shown in Figure 5-1. Though epithelial necrosis is seen (A) and pus extends into the gland lumen (B), there is no alteration in the amount or distribution of reticulum fibers (C). This contrasts with the pattern seen in regional enteritis (see Chapter Four). ×40.

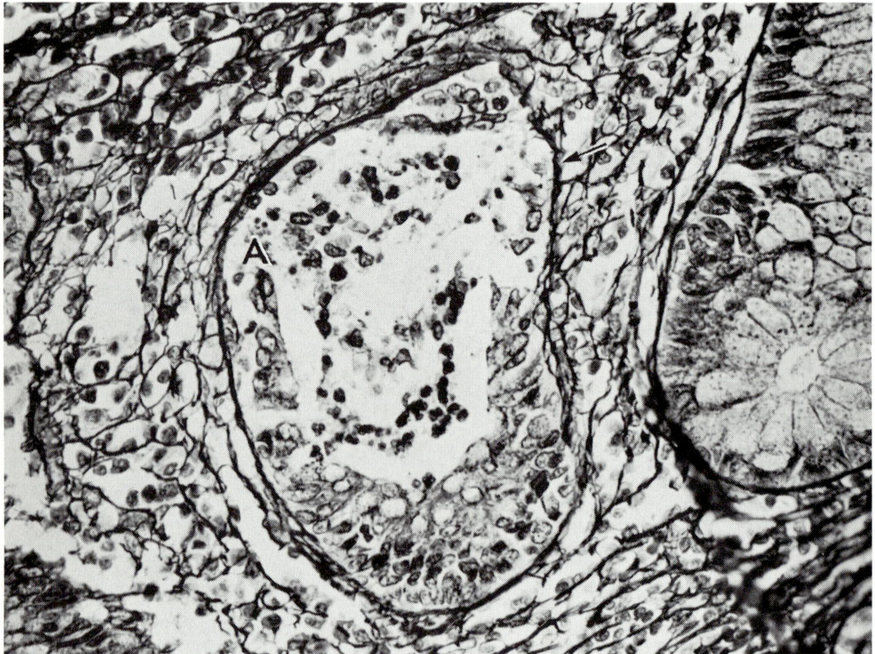

Figure 5-3   Reticulin stain of a crypt abscess. Epithelial necrosis and polymorph infiltration (A) of the tip of a crypt of Lieberkühn is shown. The reticulum fibers of the lamina propria are unaltered (arrow). Selected from serial sections. ×100.

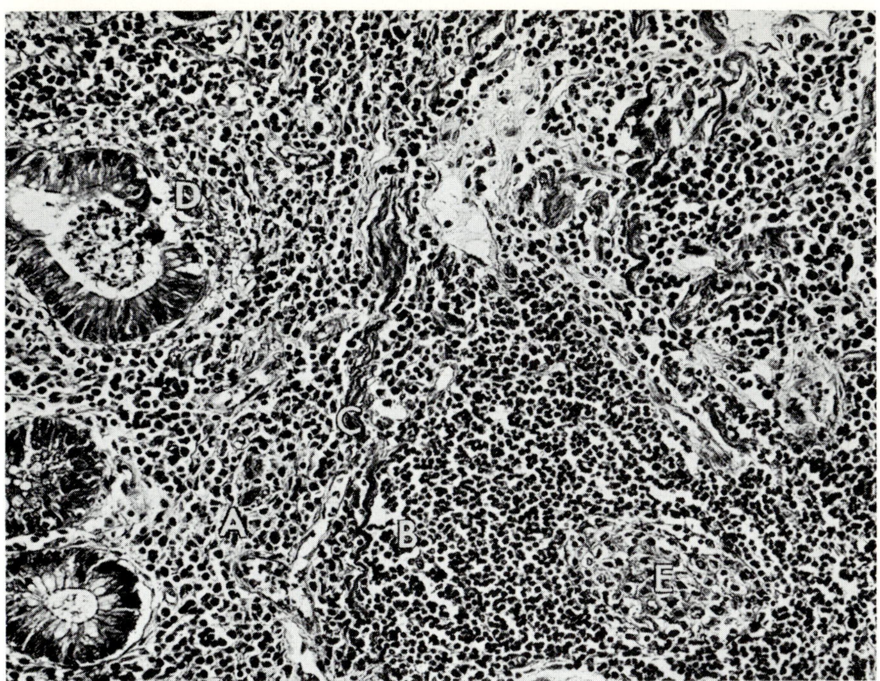

Figure 5–4   Microscopic view of the deep aspect of the mucosa (A) and superficial portion of the submucosa (B). The muscularis mucosae (C) is frayed by extensive infiltration of lymphocytes. A small early crypt abscess is seen (D). A lymphoid germinal center is also seen (E). Selected from serial sections. ×64.

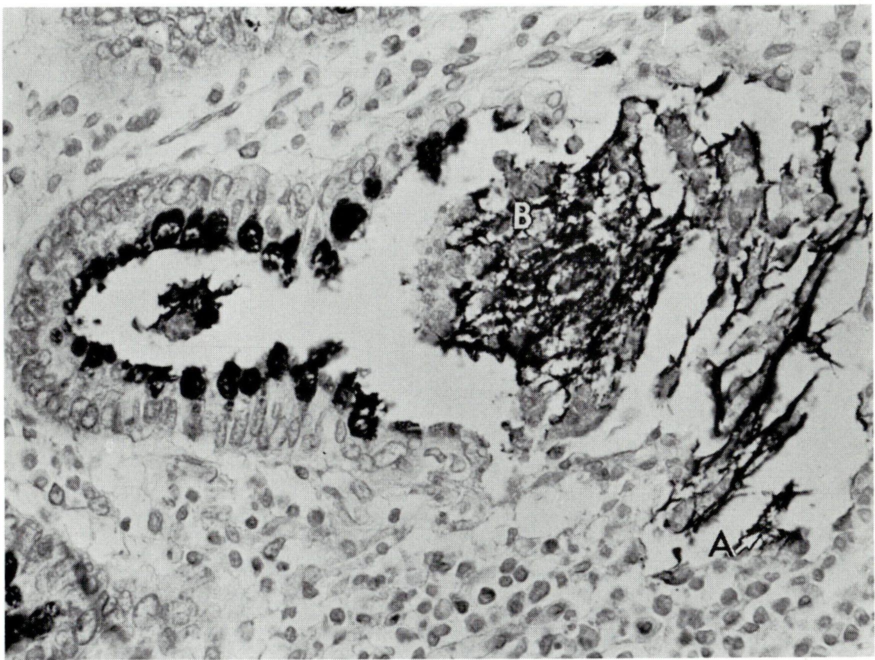

Figure 5–5   Alcian blue-PAS stain. Though mucin appears decreased in a gland with a crypt abscess, some of the mucin present leaks into the lamina propria (A). Mucus is also mixed in with the necrotic debris (B). ×125.

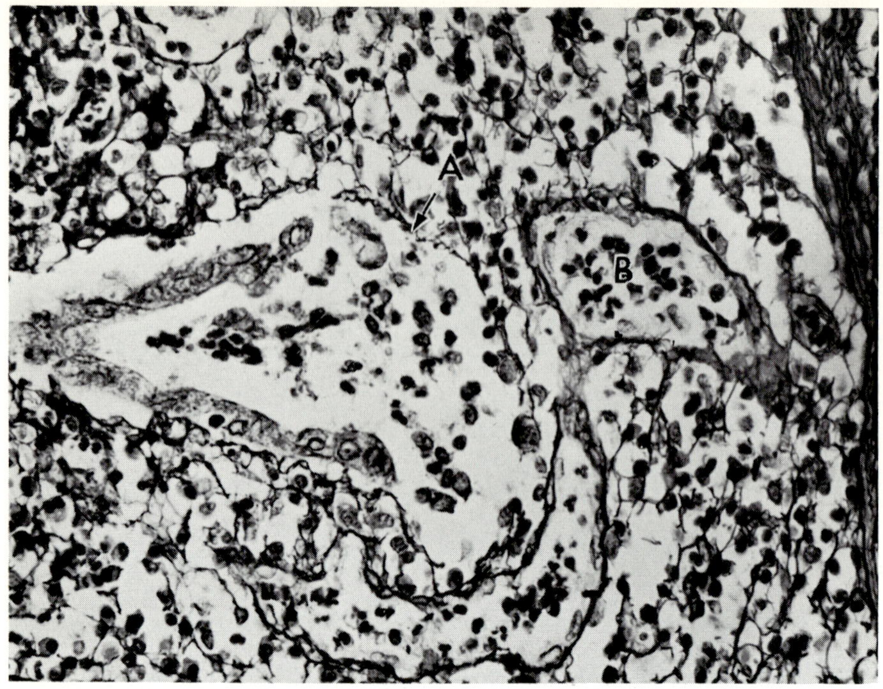

Figure 5–6 Reticulin stain. The unaltered reticulum fibers are seen surrounding a crypt abscess (A) and adjacent blood vessels (B). ×100.

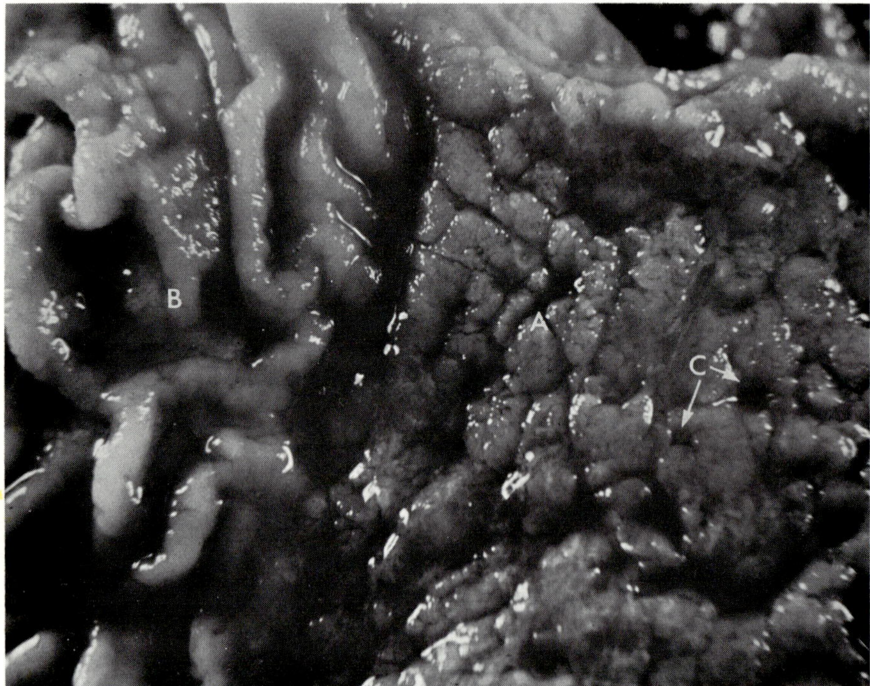

Figure 5–7 Close-up view of the colonic mucosa of ulcerative colitis showing the junction between involved (A) and uninvolved (B) regions. Punctate ulcers are seen (C) in the velvety involved region.

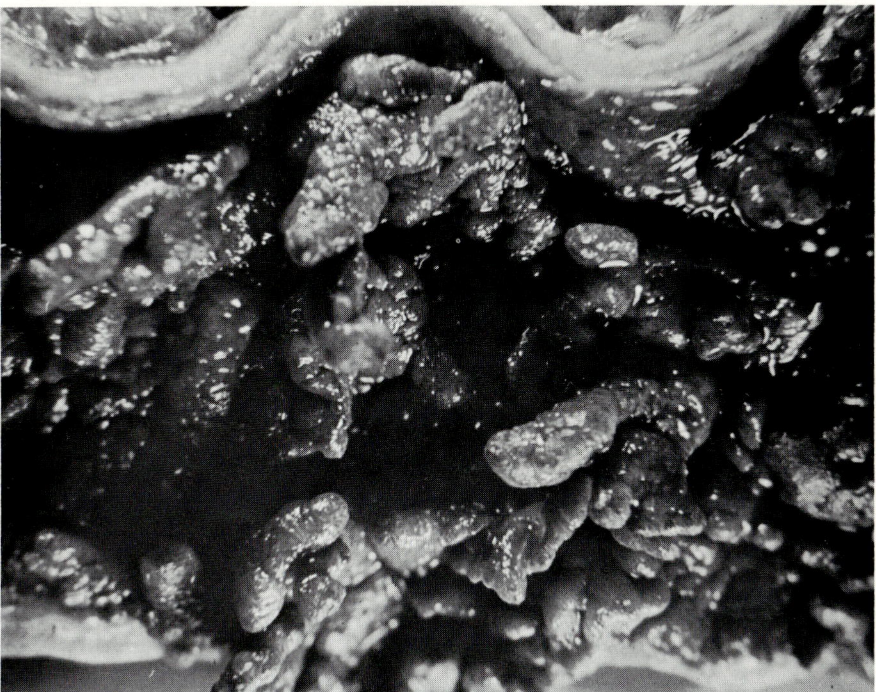

Figure 5-8   Close-up view of another region of the same specimen shown in Figure 5-7. Extreme shredding of the mucosa is seen in this severely inflamed area. The granularity of the mucosal surface is in part due to the reactive hyperplasia of the epithelium.

credence for the decreased mucosal resistance concept of its etiology would be provided. If the vascular reaction (hyperemia) or lymphocytic infiltrate or both in the lamina propria is primary, added impetus for investigation of the immune mechanism would be provided.

Lumb and co-workers attempted to identify the early lesion by studying 130 colectomy specimens of which 41 showed only partial involvement of the colon.[2] They centered their histologic investigation on those portions of the colon that appeared normal to the naked eye and observed isolated zones in which a portion of a crypt of Lieberkühn was plugged with polymorphs and surrounded by a mild degree of capillary dilatation and infiltration of the lamina propria with lymphocytes. Another group of specimens had more extensive lesions including degeneration of the crypt epithelium and microabscesses within the wall, a third group had even further extension of the lesion with acute inflammation and pus extending into the lamina propria, and a fourth group had the typical extensive ulceration. Though the first group was interpreted as the early lesion, in the time sequence, it is equally justifiable to assume that they merely represent minimal lesions of a process that had been long standing. In most of the large intestine they had not progressed to a stage of frank ulceration. Prior to the ulceration of the epithelium of the crypt, the lamina propria was already heavily infiltrated with lymphocytes. The observations of these investigators provide a magnificent record of the appearance of the mucosa with varying degrees of involvement.

Truelove and co-workers, as others have since, attempted to study the evolution of the lesions of ulcerative colitis and identify the earliest by means of serial biopsy studies of the mucosa.[3a] Lumb also utilized the biopsy method to identify the early lesions of active ulcerative colitis.[4, 5] They consider the earliest active lesions to be in the base of the crypts where polymorphs were found passing between the lining cells to accumulate inside the lumen. The basal crypt epithelium stained poorly, having vacuolated cytoplasm and nuclei with degenerative changes. As necrosis ensued, small erosions were produced that established a continuity between the lumen and the submucosa. The accumulation of polymorphs with eosinophils, red blood cells, serum, and mucus in the lumen of the crypts constitutes the crypt abscess.

That the crypt abscess is the initial and essential lesion in ulcerative colitis is doubtful for two principal reasons. Crypt abscesses are not invariably present in all cases that otherwise have the clinical and pathologic features of ulcerative colitis. Goldgraber and co-workers could find cryptitis or abscesses in only 35 per cent of their 124 patients classified as having ulcerative colitis.[6] Though their descriptions may have included cases that would not be considered ulcerative colitis as here defined, this still does emphasize the variability of their presence. It should also be noted that the crypt abscess may also be seen in other inflammatory diseases of the gastrointestinal tract, though not with the severity or frequency seen in the characteristic ulcerative colitis patient. Truelove provided a second major line of evidence to cast doubt on the primary nature of the crypt abscess in ulcerative colitis.[3b] He compared a group of serial biopsy specimens from 24 patients not suffering from ulcerative colitis with those from 42 patients with ulcerative colitis. Those from the control group were all normal except for two that had slight nonspecific histologic changes. Among the 71 specimens from patients with ulcerative colitis in a stage of active clinical disease, 67 had crypt abscesses; and more than half of the 40 specimens taken from ulcerative colitis patients who were in a stage of clinical remission and without gross evidence of inflammation on sigmoidoscopy also had crypt abscesses. The crypt abscess appeared to precede clinical relapse by a period measured in weeks. It suggests that crypt abscess formation precedes ulceration and the onset of clinical symptoms as a secondary phenomena in the disease process, and that another more subtle vascular or immunologic event probably precedes the cryptitis.

USUAL APPEARANCE OF ULCERATIVE COLITIS

More than 20 years ago Warren and Sommers recorded the morphologic observations on ulcerative colitis that have become the central reference point on which subsequent studies are based.[7] The reports of Dukes, Lumb and Protheroe, and Buie have been especially useful in clarifying details.[1, 8, 9]

On external examination of the bowel the most frequent observation of note is the decrease in total length of the colon. A normal adult has a large intestine that measures 130 to 140 cm. from the cecum to the anal ring. Large intestines with ulcerative colitis rarely exceed 110 cm. in length. The diameter is similarly reduced from a normal range of 3 to 8 cm. to approximately 2 to 4 cm. Children with ulcerative colitis have proportionately decreased bowel dimensions. This decrease in length and diameter is due to shortening of the muscle fibers, perhaps secondary to repeated spastic contractions.[35] It is not due to fibrosis or cicatrization. (It is important to measure the colon immediately after excision and prior to fixation. Erroneous measurements due to shrinkage and distortion will be made otherwise.)

The serosa usually appears normal, i.e., transparent, glistening, and without exudate (Fig. 5-9). Moderate to severe hyperemia of the

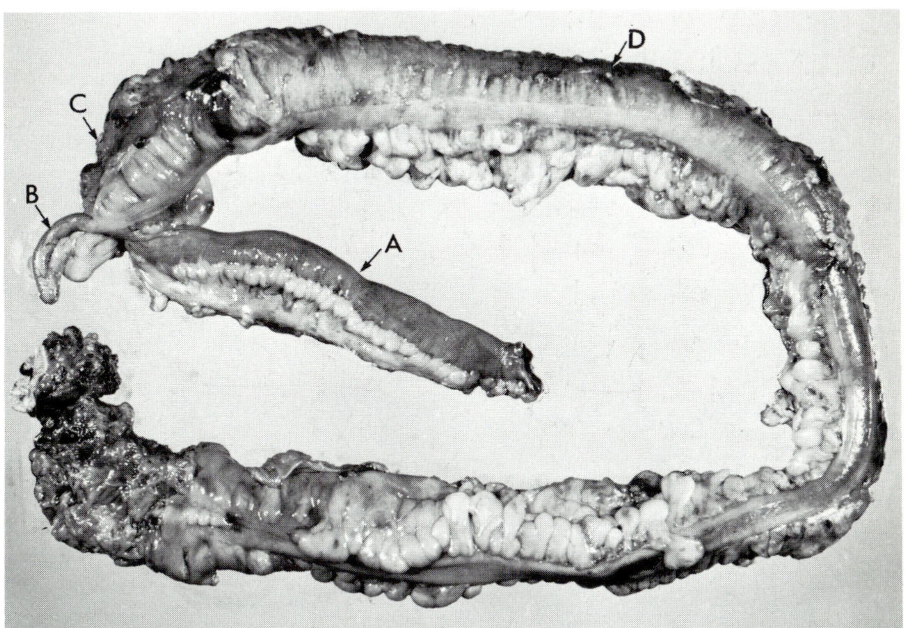

Figure 5-9 Ulcerative colitis. Unincised surgical specimen including terminal ileum (A), appendix (B), cecum (C), and colon (D). The serosal surface is free from gross morphologic change though extensive mucosal inflammation is present, as shown in Figure 5-10.

subserosal vessels in part or all of the colon may be the only tangible finding. The regional lymph nodes are sometimes enlarged and soft owing to edema and hyperplasia, but are frequently unremarkable. The texture and thickness to palpation of the colonic wall is usually within normal limits. Involvement of the terminal ileum or appendix is not discernible on surface examination.

Incision of the colon along its long axis reveals a startling degree of change in contrast to its innocuous appearance on external examination (Fig. 5-10). The bowel lumen usually contains a variable amount of watery blood, necrotic debris, and liquid feces. The mucosal lining of the colon is deep red-purple ("red velvet") with marked capillary hyperemia and congestion. It appears wet and glistening, with foci of blood and mucus. The mucosal ulcers may vary greatly in number, size, shape, extent, and distribution, depending on the stage and severity of the process (Figs. 5-11 and 5-12). The smallest ones are punctate, may be covered with pus, and may be identified only on close examination with a magnifying glass (Fig. 5-13). At the opposite extreme, ulceration may be so extensive as to extend over the entire mucosal surface. Frequently they form longitudinal furrows overlying the teniae coli, with intervening edematous pseudopolypoid fragments of mucosa remaining (Figs. 5-14, 5-15 and 5-17). When the ulcers are

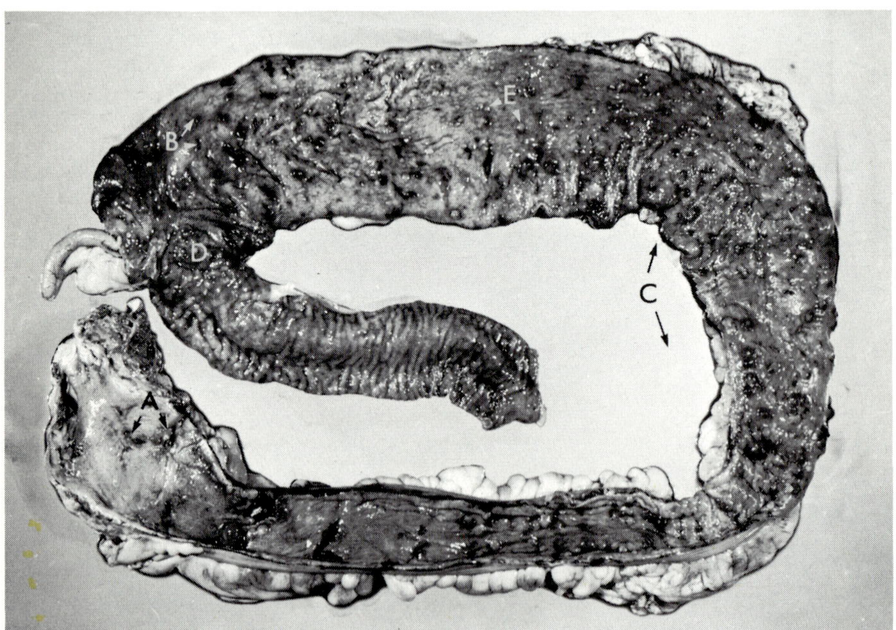

Figure 5-10   Ulcerative colitis. The specimen shown in Figure 5-9 has been incised to show the mucosal surface. Numerous mucosal ulcers are scattered from rectum (A) to cecum (B) and are particularly numerous in this case in the transverse colon region (C). "Backwash" lesions (D) are also present in the terminal ileum. Also visible are some polyps (E), which are also shown in Figures 9-3 and 9-4.

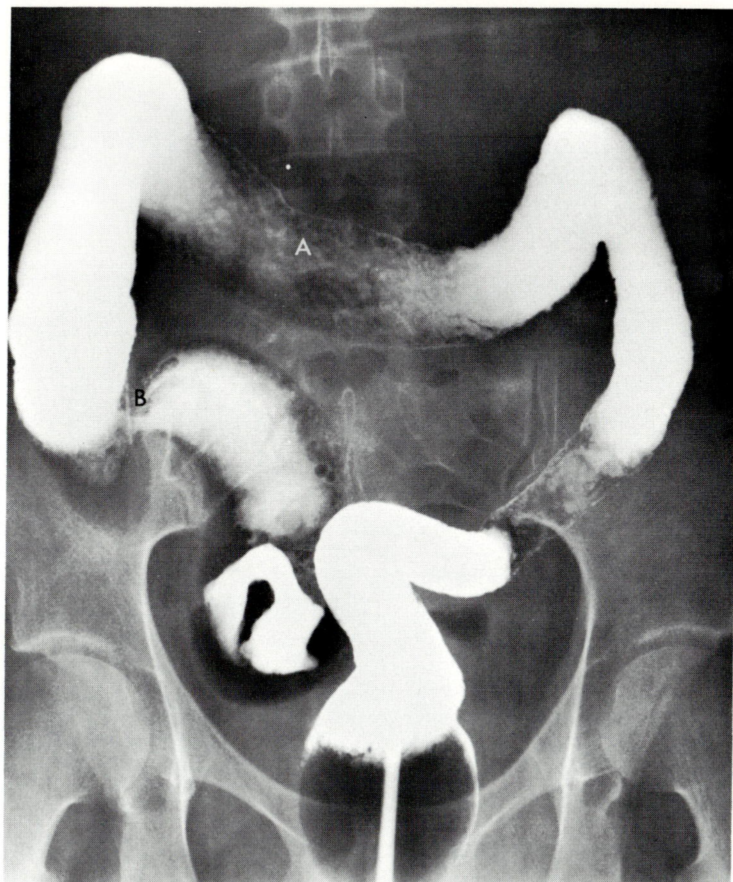

Figure 5–11 Ulcerative colitis radiograph. Barium enema before evacuation. The total length of the colon is shortened and appears diffuse. Mucosal irregularity is shown (A). Similar mucosal changes are also seen in the terminal ileum (B). Note the wide lumen in the ileocecal valve region. (Courtesy of Dr. M. M. Figley, Professor and Chairman, Department of Radiology, University of Washington School of Medicine.)

small and the surrounding mucosa edematous, careful examination may be necessary to reveal the presence of the ulcer beneath overhanging edges of mucosa (Fig. 5-18).

The "backwash" lesions in the terminal ileum sometimes accompanying ulcerative colitis have been the object of careful study too. The ileal changes extend proximally from the cecum in continuity with the latter and do not occur unless the right colon and cecum are affected. The spread in the ileum is continuous, and skip areas are not found. The ileocecal valve is invariably loose, patulous, and incompetent. No tendency to obstruction has been found. Counsell reports the incidence of ileal involvement to be 17 per cent of 107 cases, and in his review of the literature it varied from 1 to 39 per cent.[10] He confirmed that the

(Text continued on page 122.)

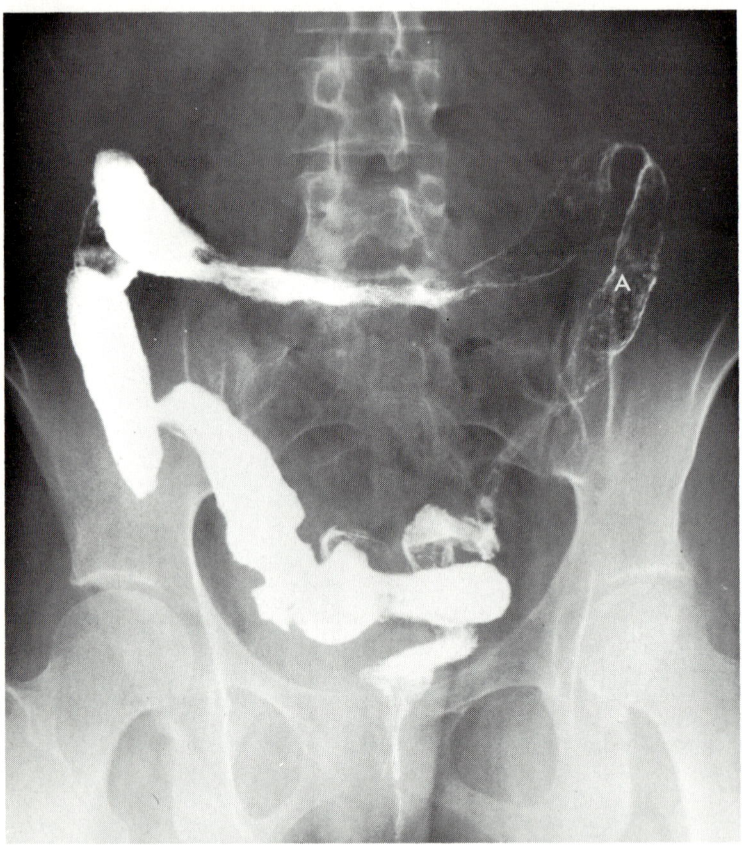

Figure 5–12   Ulcerative colitis. Radiograph of a postevacuation barium enema in the same case as shown in Figure 5–11. Diffuse mucosal irregularity is again demonstrated (A). (Courtesy of Dr. M. M. Figley, Professor and Chairman, Department of Radiology, University of Washington School of Medicine.)

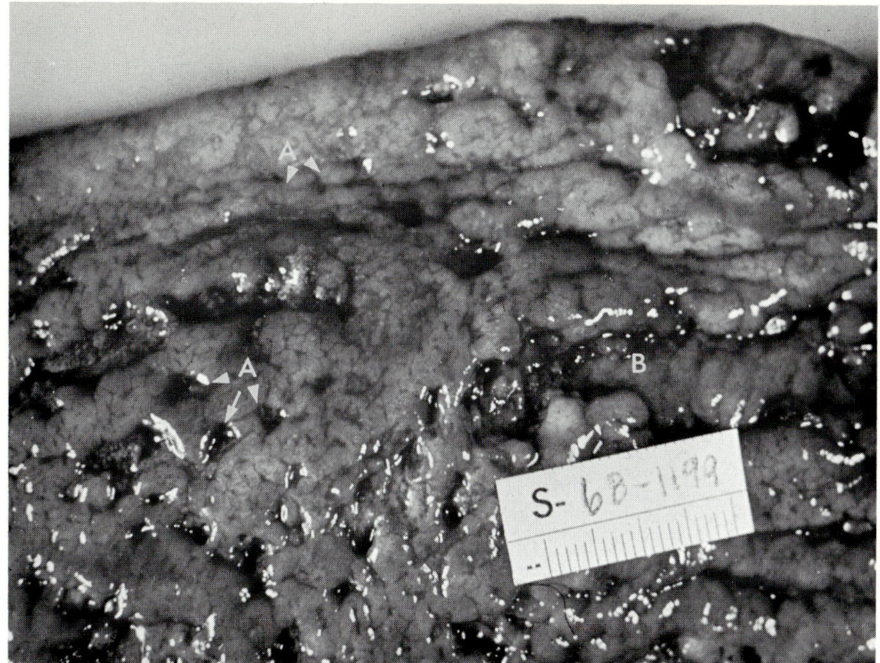

Figure 5–13 Close-up view of a region of the colonic mucosa in ulcerative colitis. Small "punched out" ulcers (A) are scattered throughout. Some regions of confluence and furrowing (B) are seen.

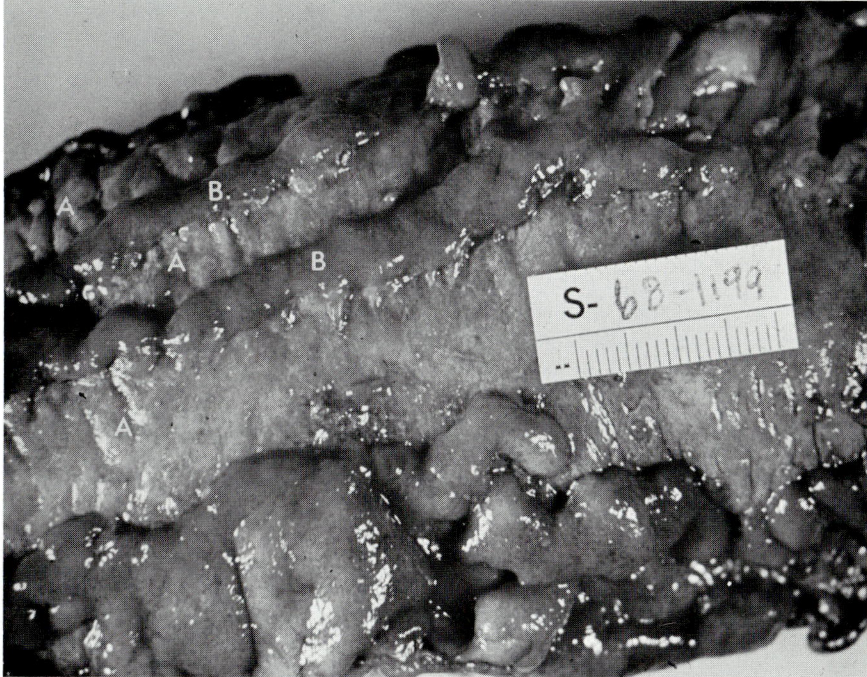

Figure 5–14 Close-up view of another region of colonic mucosa from the same specimen shown in Figure 5-13. Extensive confluence of the ulcers has produced furrows parallel to the long axis of the bowel (A) and separation by intervening strips of mucosa (B). Extensive undermining of the remaining mucosa is shown.

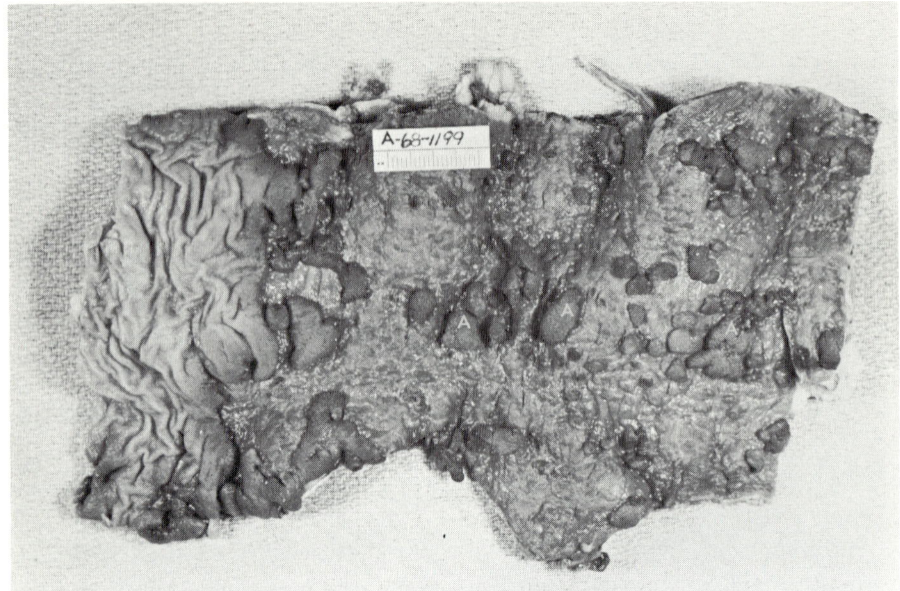

Figure 5–15 Close-up view of a region of the colon in ulcerative colitis with extensive confluence of the ulcerations almost completely denuding the surface and leaving only traces of the longitudinal strips of mucosa (A).

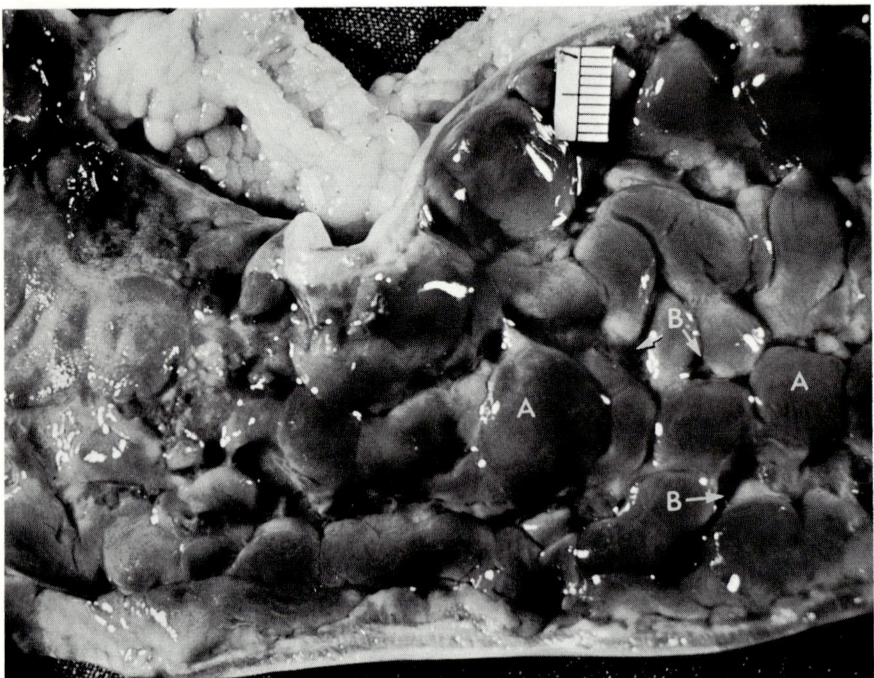

Figure 5–16 Close-up view of another colon with ulcerative colitis in which the mucosa is extremely edematous (A) and there are overlapping small ulcers (B).

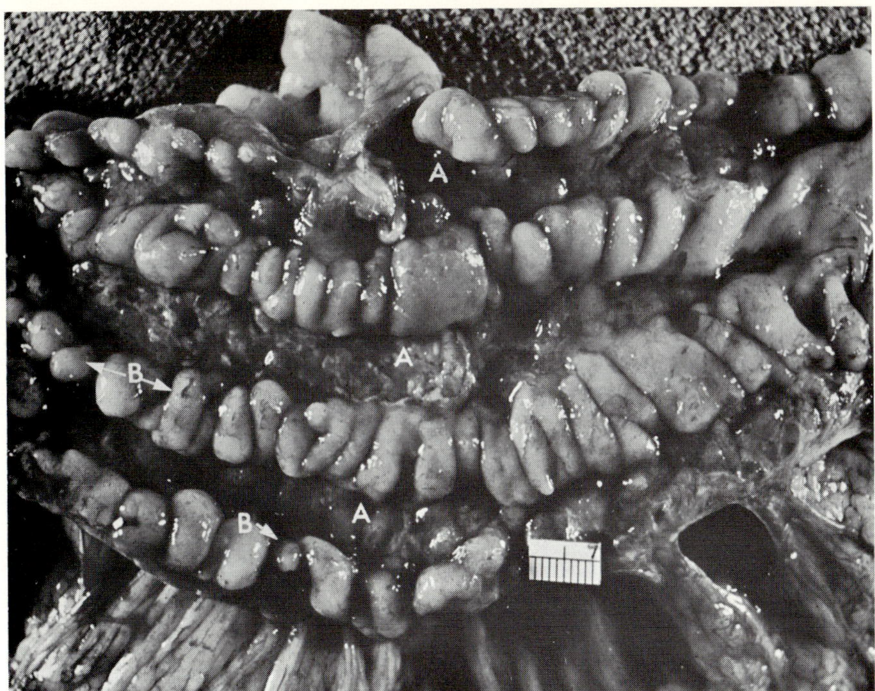

Figure 5–17 Close-up view of an advanced phase of ulceration in which confluence has produced longitudinal furrows (A) and in some regions has transected them (B). See also Frontispiece.

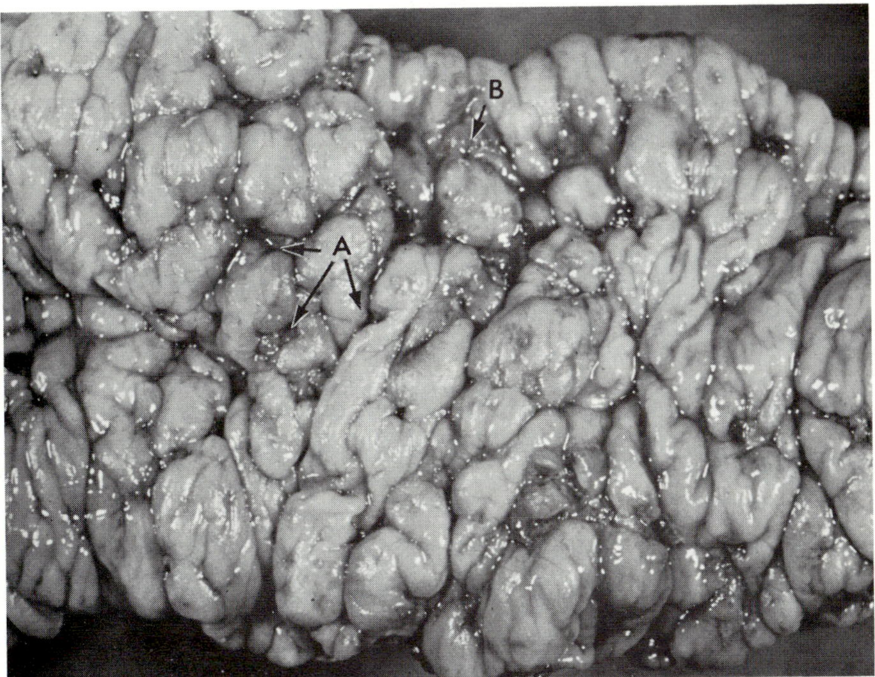

Figure 5–18 Close-up view of an earlier phase of ulceration revealing a mixture of punctate ulcers (A) and some beginning confluence (B). Mucosa is markedly edematous.

ileocecal valve was incompetent in all moderate or severe cases, and when the ileal involvement was slight the incompetence of the valve was not obvious. The longest segment of ileal involvement in his series was 14 inches. Ileal ulcerations were variable in size, but were always superficial and without perforation and obstruction. The morphologic features of the ileal lesion were comparable to those in the colon in ulcerative colitis and not to those of regional enteritis. Surgical excision of the colon is followed by a subsidence of the ileal lesion. The ileal "backwash" lesion is usually not discernible on external examination of the specimen (Fig. 5–9).

Macroscopic Observations

The macroscopic appearance of the large intestinal lesion varies with the stage of the disease and the activity of the process. The early acute progressive lesions have a deeply congested "red velvet" appearing mucosa with numerous punctate erosions but no grossly visible frank ulcerations at this time (Fig. 5–13). Careful inspection may yield barely visible microabscesses in the mucosa, which later in the progression of the disease may coalesce, forming widespread shallow ulcers, often linear with the long axis of the bowel. Coalescence of the microabscesses may undermine portions of viable mucosa, producing ragged tags or remnants of mucosa attached on only one aspect to the underlying tissue (Figs. 5–19, 5–20, and 5–21). Polypoid and pseudopolypoid overgrowth may occur and present varying mixtures of hyperemia, edema, and inflammatory cell infiltration surrounded by undermined mucosa or adenomatous hyperplasia of the mucosal elements (Figs. 5–10, 5–11, 5–12, 5–18, and 5–21). The submucosa may be slightly thickened by edema, but in the vast majority of cases the muscularis appears completely uninvolved.

The gross appearance of the more protracted ulcerative colitis lesions has many of the features of the acute lesion just described with the addition of chronic changes. Generally this phase of the disease process is entered into after two or three years of relatively active disease. At this stage, smooth velvety patches of relatively normal appearing epithelium alternate with ragged ulcers and deeper furrows (Figs. 5–17 and 5–22). Pseudopolyps may be more prominent in the form of bulbous epithelial ridges between excavated denuded ulcers. Focal thickening of the mucosa and submucosa may be seen at this stage of the disease. Scarification when present is focal in nature, producing fibrous bands that distort specific folds of the bowel or may produce some focal strictures in areas of maximal damage. In the late or quiescent stage of ulcerative colitis, when healing of much or all of the ulcerated lesion has occurred, the lumen and total bowel diameter may be diminished and there may be some increase in mesenteric fat.

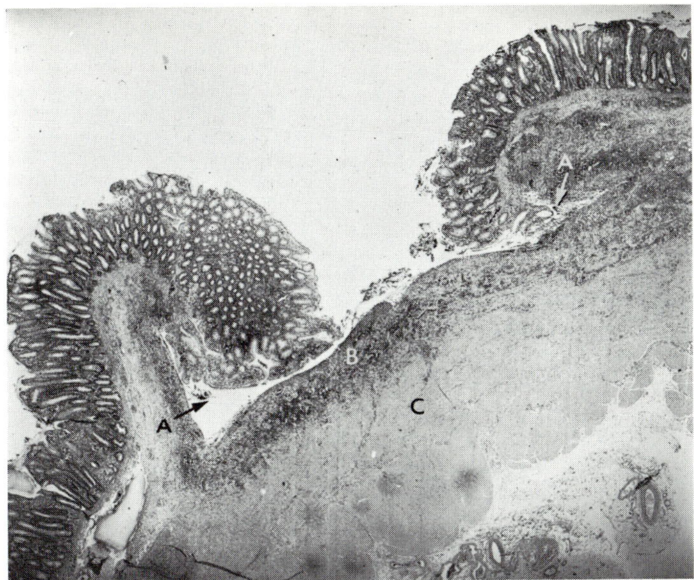

Figure 5–19   Cross section of a longitudinal furrow revealing the extensive undermining of remaining mucosa (A). Inflammatory changes (B) are superficial to the muscularis (C). ×10.

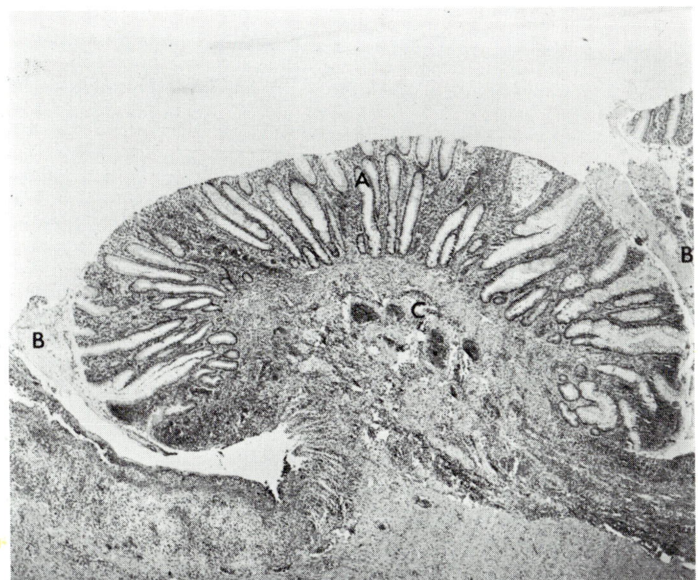

Figure 5–20   Cross section of a remaining strip of mucosa (A) between two longitudinal furrows (B). Undermining of the mucosa is shown. Vascular congestion with edema (C) is seen in the remaining mucosa. ×10.

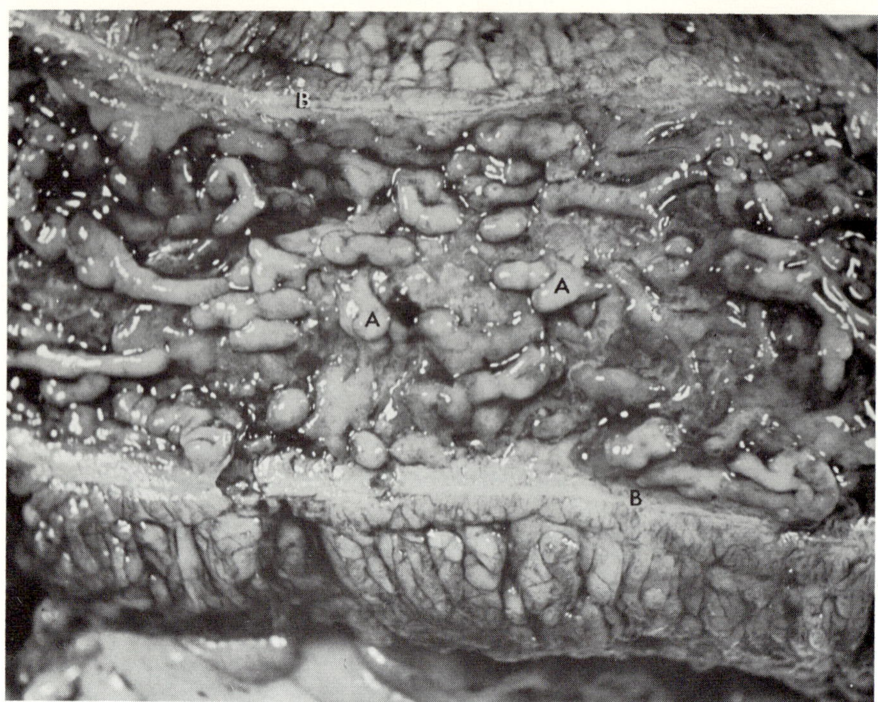

Figure 5-21 Close-up view of a portion of colon with extensive ulceration. Erosion is so extensive that the remaining mucosal tissue appears shredded. Many of the remaining tags of mucosa are attached in only one region. This, coupled with edema, produces a pseudopolyp (A). In spite of the extensive mucosal inflammation, the colonic wall is not thickened (B).

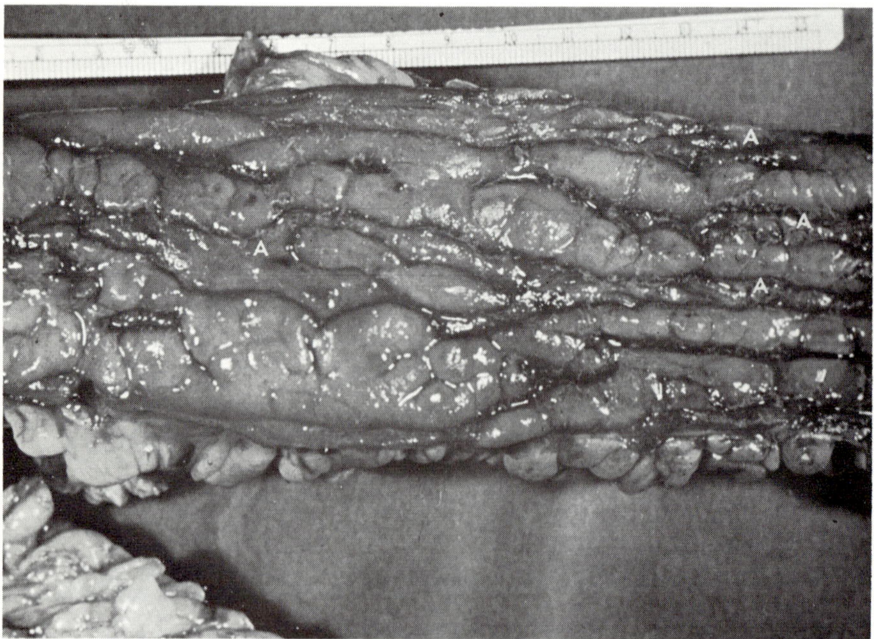

Figure 5-22 Close-up view of a portion of colon with ulcerative colitis mucosal erosions (A).

124

The circumference averages about 3.5 cm., with the lumen averaging about 1 to 2 cm. The mucosal surface appears thin and slightly irregular in contrast with the normal smooth velvety appearance. This irregularity, in some instances, may be due to the presence of small fibrous bands distorting portions of the lumen; in other instances it may be due to hyperplastic foci of regenerative pseudopolypoid tags, and in still other regions, to large aggregates of lymphoid follicles that have formed in the mucosa and submucosa. The serosa and regional lymph nodes are usually normal in appearance even in the late stages of the disease.

Late Quiescent Stage

The late or quiescent stage of the disease reveals reparative and regenerative features predominantly (Figs. 5-23 and 5-24). Mucosal regeneration may be present in most regions of the lining of the bowel, though deep focal ulcers may remain. In areas of regeneration the mucosa is thin and atrophic and lighter in color ("pearly-white") than that seen normally. Even in this stage of the disease the muscularis and serosa are usually not involved and the external surface appearance of the bowel is unremarkable except for the changes in size.

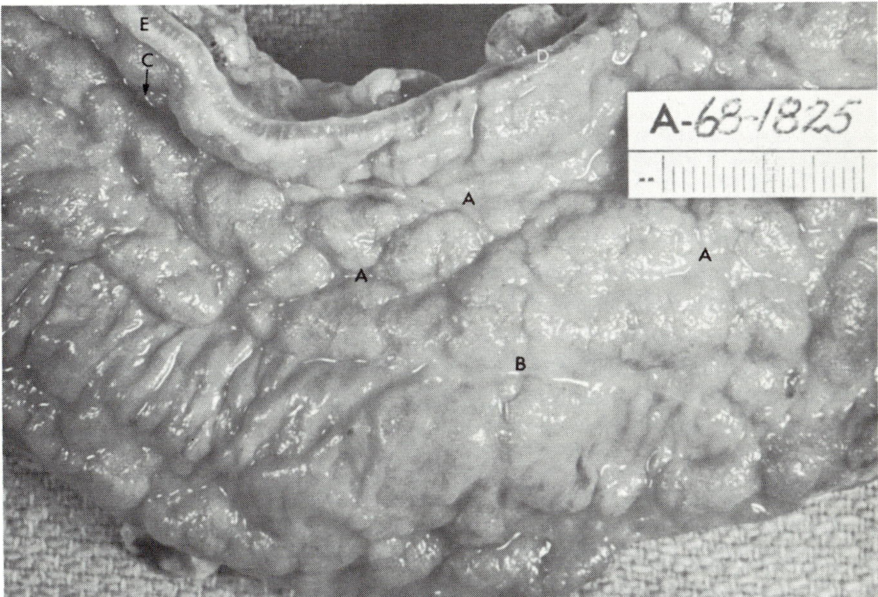

Figure 5-23 A region of ulcerative colitis that is mostly healed. Former ulcers (A) and furrows (B) have been re-epithelialized. Evidence of active ulceration is seen nearby (C). The cut surface of the wall does not appear thickened in the healed region (D), whereas the mucosal area does appear thick adjacent to the active lesions (E).

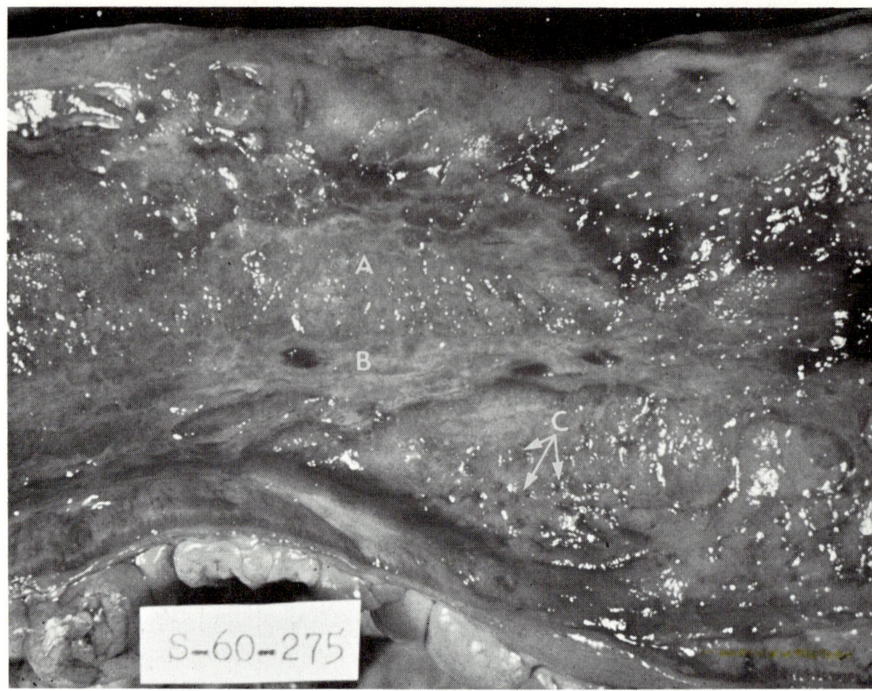

Figure 5-24 Old "burned out" ulcerative colitis seen from the mucosal surface. Thick and thin areas of mucosa result in broad elevations (A) and depressions (B) and minute pock marks (C). These irregularities are due to alternate regions of mucosal atrophy, hyperplasia, and minimal mucosal fibrosis.

Microscopic Observations

The microscopic findings in ulcerative colitis consist of three major components that vary in prominence depending on the stage of the disease. These are: (1) vascular congestion; (2) an intense infiltration of the mucosa and submucosa with lymphocytes, monocytes, plasma and mast cells, and some eosinophils; and (3) an acute inflammatory process with some reparative and regenerative change. Microscopic examination nearly always proves that the ulcerative colitis is much more widespread and severe than can be seen by the naked eye. As already noted, the earliest lesions have apparently not been identified. In those cases in which duration of symptoms has been brief, most regions of the mucosa and submucosa have mucosal and superficial submucosal vascular congestion to an astonishing degree. This is accompanied by a dense infiltration of the mucosa and superficial aspect of the submucosa with lymphocytes, plasma cells, and occasional eosinophils (Figs. 5-1 to 5-6). Polymorphs are seldom in evidence at this stage and when they do occur are associated with the crypt abscesses. Both acute and chronic types of cellular exudation occur virtually from the outset, and conversely, after years of disease, these cellular features may be present as well. Regenerative features tend to predominate in the later stages of disease. Intense infiltration of the lamina propria of the mucosa and the submucosa by lymphocytes, monocytes, and plasma and mast cells is diffuse throughout all involved regions of the bowel, and in some cases lymph follicle formation may be a striking feature (Figs. 5–25 to 5-28). Scant, if any, changes are seen in the muscularis and serosa.

Cryptitis and crypt abscesses are another early feature of the lesion. At the base of the crypts of Lieberkühn, neutrophils may be seen between epithelial cells of the base of the crypts and accumulated in the lumen. The epithelial cells are somewhat more basophilic than the uninvolved crypt cells. Their cytoplasm may be irregular and vacuolated and the nuclei pyknotic. Necrosis of the epithelial cells ensues and a small ulceration in the base of the crypt is seen. Thus, a continuity between the lumen and the lamina propria occurs. More neutrophils, some extravasated red blood cells, serum, and mucus accumulate at the site of the ulceration within the lumen of the crypt, producing the characteristic feature of the crypt abscess. As the exudation increases, a streamer of pus may be seen extending through the lumen of the crypt to the mucosal surface (Fig. 2-1). Frequently many in-

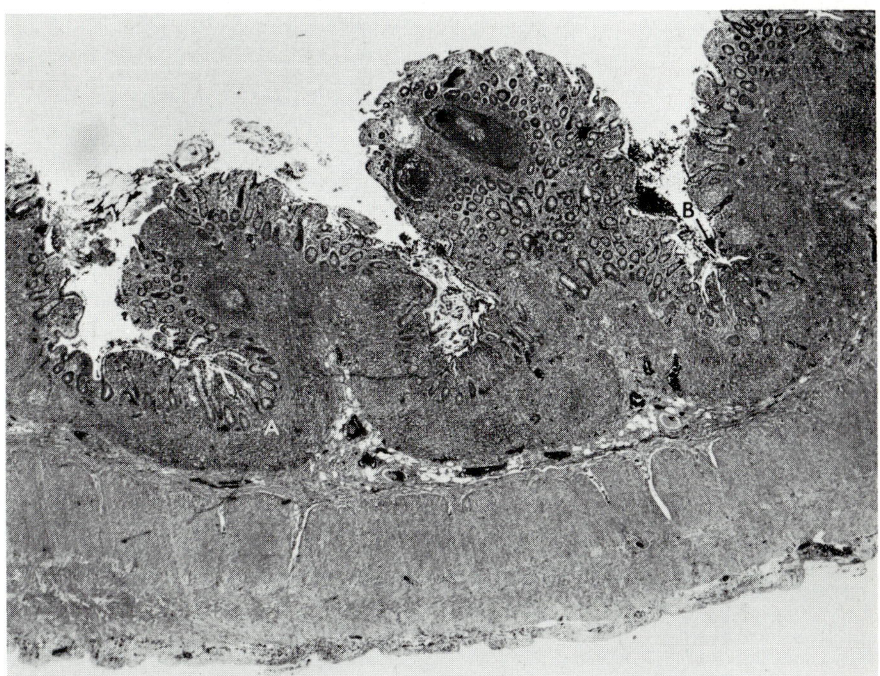

Figure 5–25 Cross section of all layers of the colonic wall revealing an intense mucosal lymphocytosis (A). Small ulcers are also seen (B). ×4.

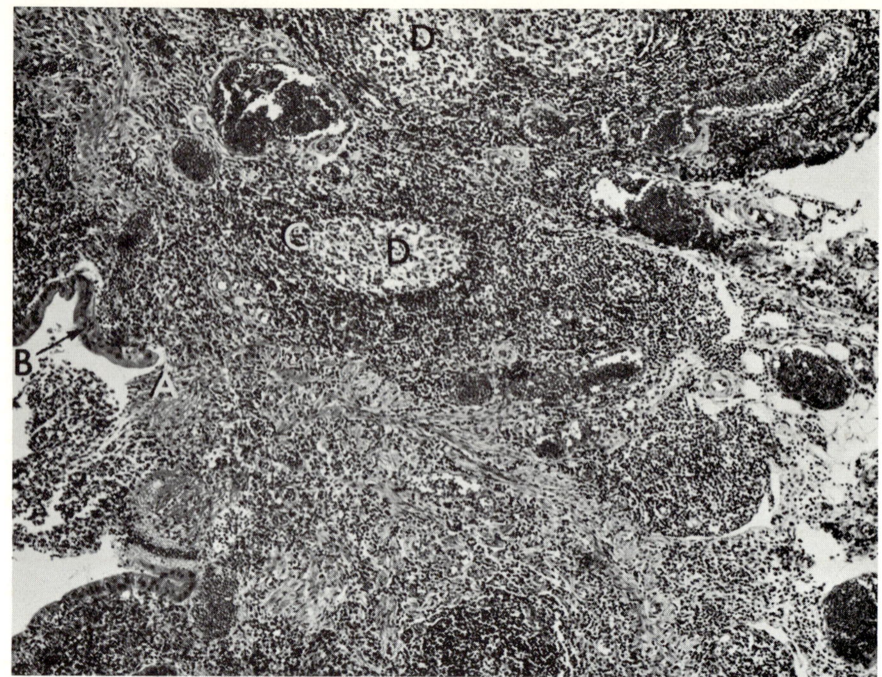

Figure 5-26 Mucosa and submucosa of the colon demonstrating a small mucosal ulcer (A), epithelial atypism (B), and intense lymphocytosis (C) with lymphoid germinal centers (D) within the mucosa and the superficial portion of the submucosa. ×20.

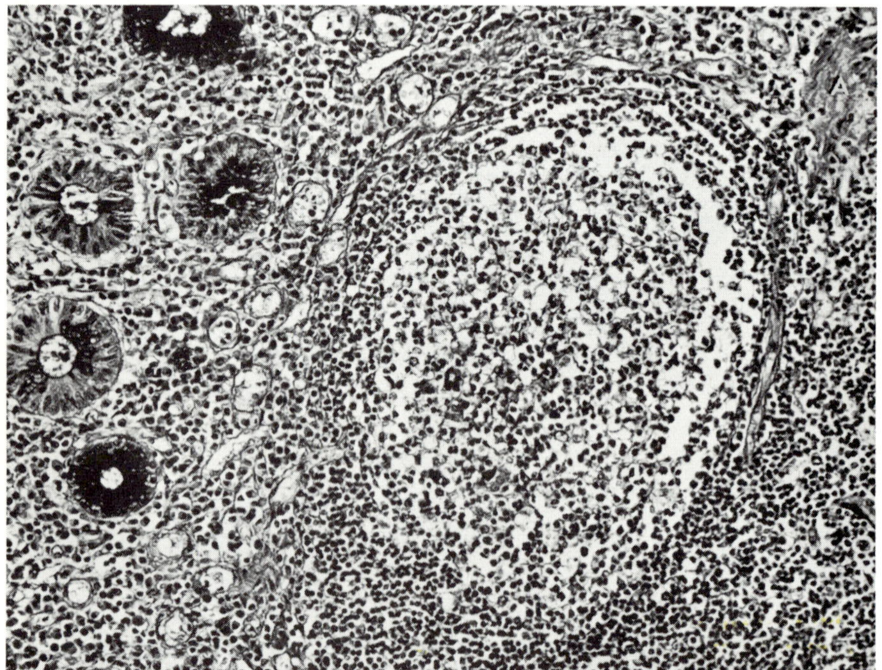

Figure 5-27 Alcian blue-PAS stain. Colon with ulcerative colitis. A lymphoid follicle is shown deep in the lamina propria adjacent to the muscularis mucosae (A). ×40.

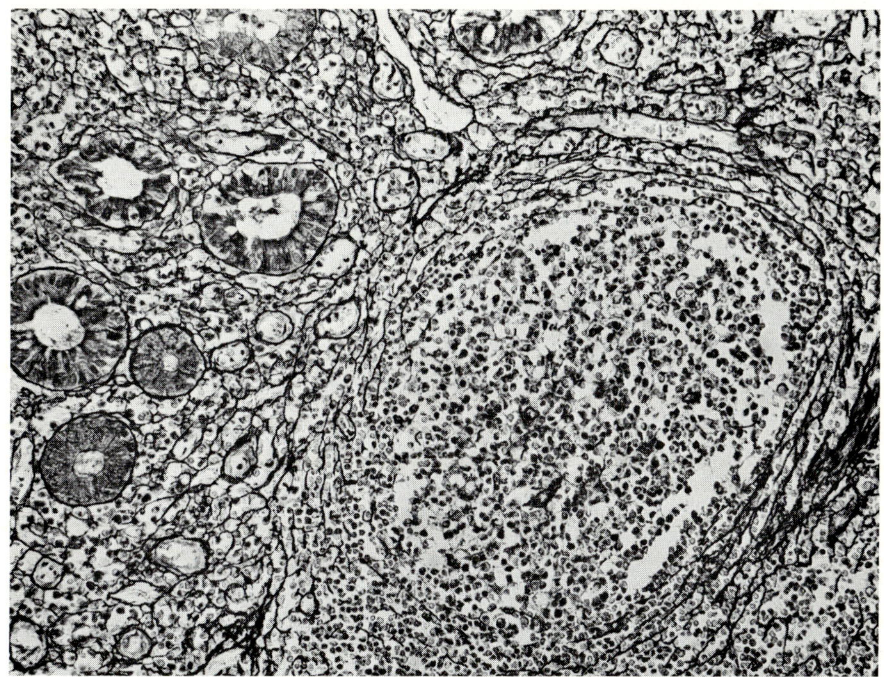

Figure 5–28   Reticulin stain. Adjacent section to that shown in Figure 5-27. The distribution of the reticulum fibers around the germinal follicle is similar to that of a normal germinal follicle and contrasts sharply with that of regional enteritis (Fig. 4-43). ×40.

volved crypts may be found in clusters, whereas others appear to be scattered at random throughout the mucosa. In some crypts, tangentially cut, the pus may be seen in the lumen without the epithelial ulceration. However, serial sections to demonstrate the base of the crypt usually reveal the erosion.

At this stage the inflammatory exudate of neutrophils appears exclusively in the vicinity of the base of the crypts, and the more extensive and diffuse lymphocytic infiltrate has few polymorphs. The deeper zones of the lamina propria, muscularis, mucosa, and submucosa have lymphocytes, plasma cells, and eosinophils in predominance. Necrosis and polymorph infiltration increasingly extend into the lamina propria from the crypt ulcer with the progression of the disease and may extend extensively laterally above the muscularis mucosa, undermining the epithelium, with subsequent devitalization and sloughing. In the majority of cases the ulcerations so produced are localized to a depth at or above the level of the muscularis mucosae. The lamina propria occupies a greater proportion of the mucosa than normal, widely separating the crypts. The intensive infiltrate of lymphocytes, the presence of edema associated with the abscess formation, and massive capillary engorgement are the causes of the separation.

Bleeding into the ruptured crypts and ulcers may produce punctate hemorrhages on the luminal surface. Features of regeneration and repair may also be visible in these early lesions. Regenerating epithelial cells in the walls of the crypts may be found. A surprisingly scant fibroblastic proliferation ensues, and few collagen fibers may be demonstrated even by special stains. Epithelial regeneration consisting of flattened, more deeply basophilic and eosinophilic cells may extend out in the ulcerated area from surviving epithelium. At this stage, exudation of mucus is increased from the surface epithelium.

In intermediate and more prolonged phases of the disease, the same features may be present, but in different proportion. The lymphocyte–plasma cell–eosinophil exudate may remain prevalent throughout the course of the disease; however, the number of crypt abscesses generally is reduced, and there is an increasing preponderance of reparative features. Gaps in the muscularis mucosae are filled with small fibrous scars.

In the late and quiescent stage of disease the microscopic appearance may show an intact mucosa with considerable alteration in its architecture (Figs. 5-23, 5-24, 5-29, 5-30, and 5-31). The number of crypts appears decreased, and the mucosa is generally atrophic, with shortened crypts more widely separated and a thickening of the lamina propria. The regular arrangement of the crypts may be distorted, and occasional nests of epithelial cell inclusions in the lamina propria and

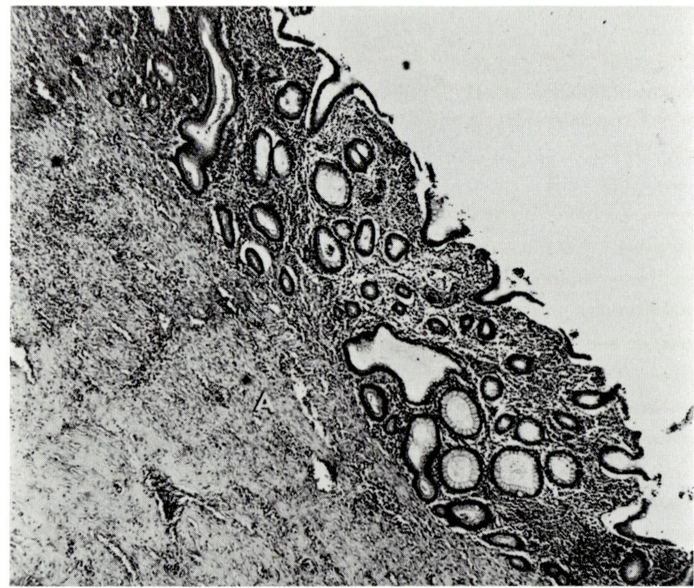

Figure 5-29 Microscopic view of alternately atrophic and hyperplastic mucosa that rests on muscularis (A) rather than on submucosa. The glands are of variable size, shape, and length, and the secretory activity varies from gland to gland. ×45.

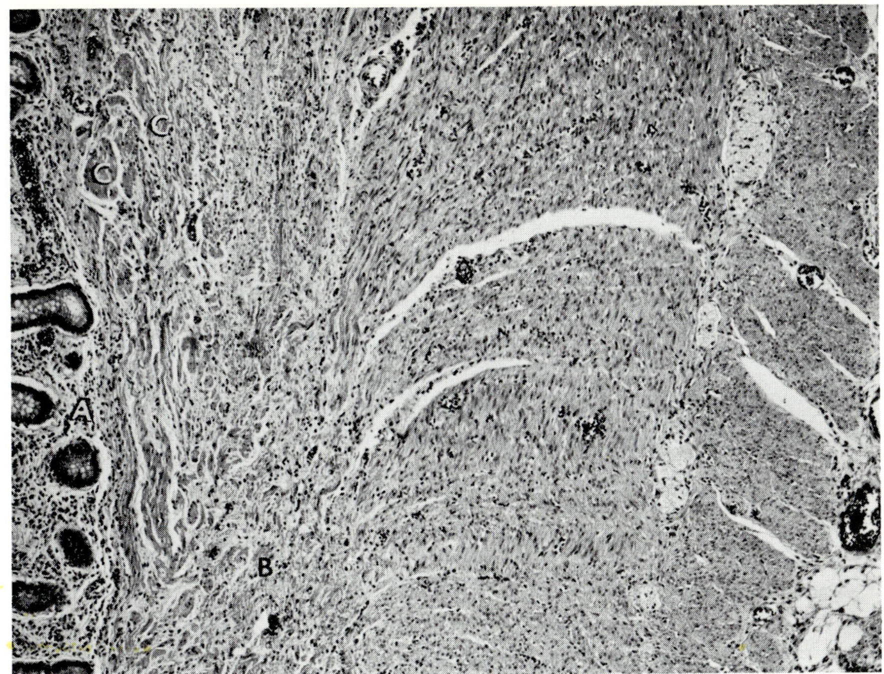

Figure 5–30 Healed ulcerative colitis lesion. The tips of the mucosal glands (left) and the lamina propria (A) are attached to the muscularis (B) without intervening submucosa. Frayed ends of the muscularis mucosae are focally hyperplastic (C). No fibrosis or inflammatory changes are seen in the muscularis or subserosa. ×10.

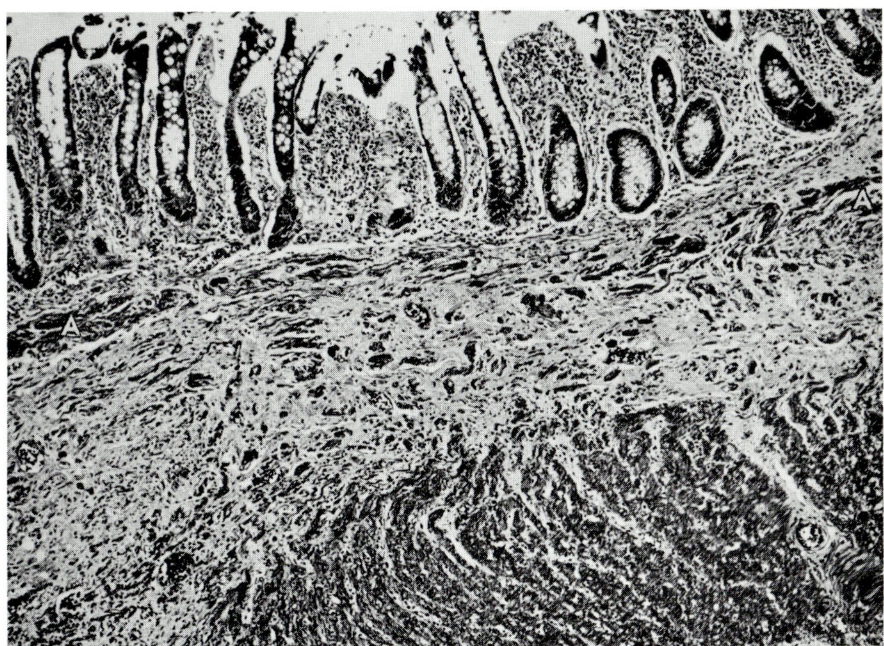

Figure 5–31 Gomori trichrome stain. A healed ulcerative colitis lesion stained to demonstrate the frayed muscularis mucosae (A). ×10.

131

submucosa may be found (Figs. 5–32 and 5–33). These appear to be regenerated epithelial nests that have lined the walls of abscesses extending more deeply into the submucosa. Numerous foci of fibrosis are seen in which fragments of the muscularis mucosae are embedded. The scars rarely extend into the submucosa. In any particular specimen one may see all phases of the disease process ranging from early to late lesions. Thus, a colon that is in the healed late quiescent stage but has undergone recent activation may have features of the acute progressive lesion superimposed on the late quiescent changes (Figs. 5–23 and 5–34).

Usually, as indicated earlier, the crypt abscesses tend to spread laterally superficial to the muscularis mucosae, producing vast areas of denudation. On occasion the submucosa may also be penetrated, and on rare occasions the abscess formation process may extend deeply through the muscularis, often along the course of penetrating blood vessels, producing abscesses through the wall and perforation. In these instances the fibrin and the polymorph exudate may appear on the adjacent portions of the serosa.

When the abscessing process extends to the submucosa, with the

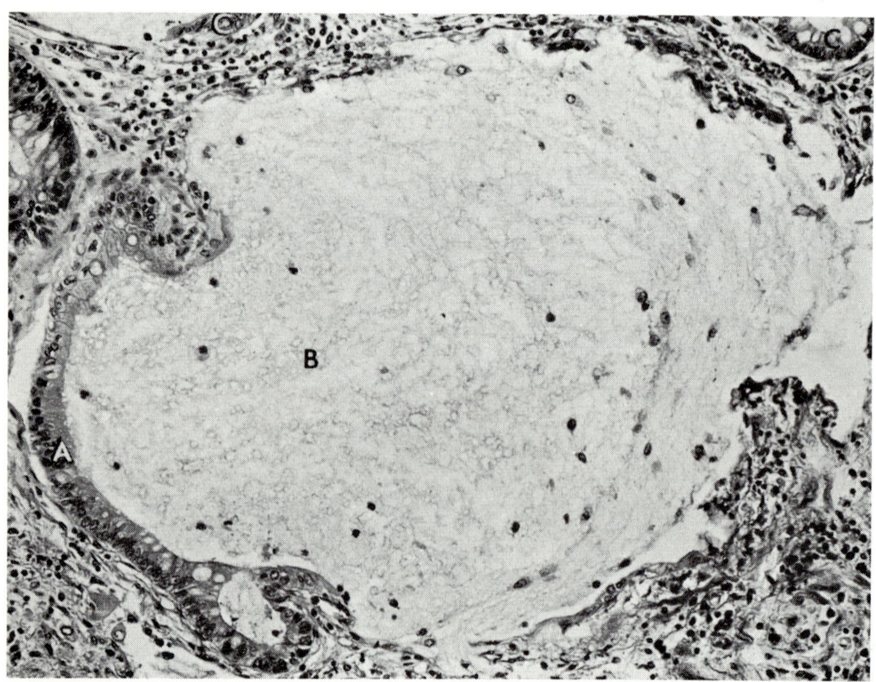

Figure 5–32   Entrapped mucosal epithelium (A) in the submucosa forms a mucous cyst (B) that is not completely epithelialized. Portions of other entrapped epithelium are seen (C). ×40.

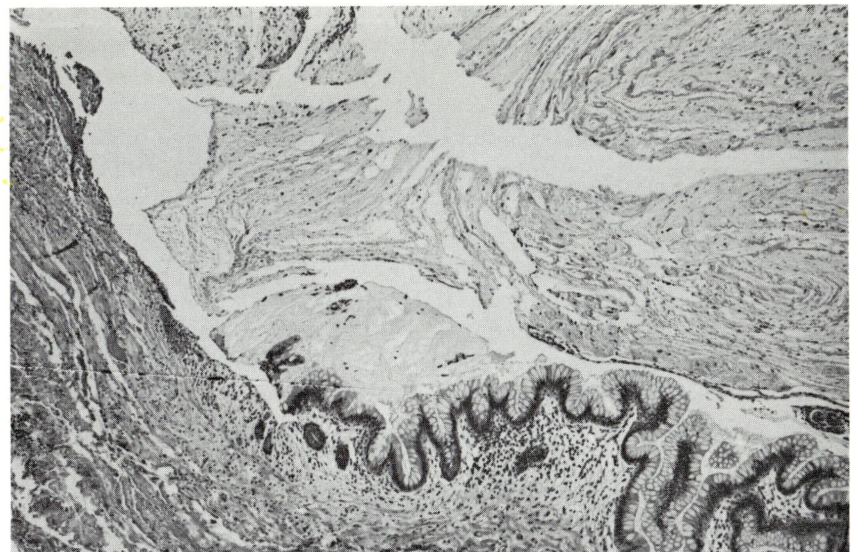

Figure 5-33   A portion of the wall of a large submucosal cyst that is partially epithelialized. Note that the epithelium rests on a lamina propria–like connective tissue that is chronically inflamed. ×40.

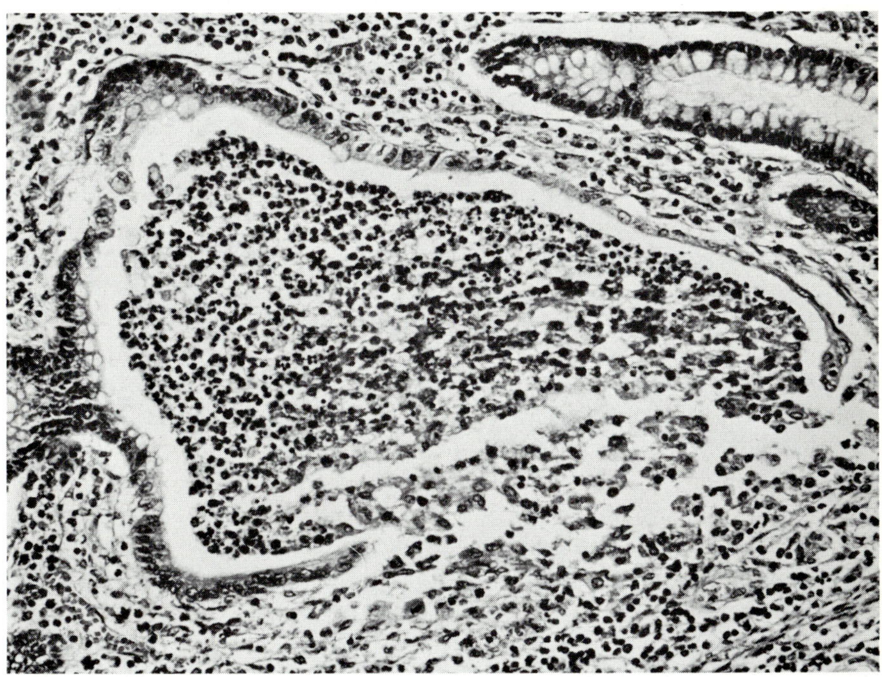

Figure 5-34   A characteristic crypt abscess from a case of inactive ulcerative colitis. ×51.

consequent minimal fibrous healing coupled with muscle spasm, strictures and possible obstruction of the bowel may ensue.[35] The mucosa at the edge of an ulcer may become undermined, lose part of its attachment, and thus give rise to a polypoid mucosal tag. Occasionally the confluence of undermined adjacent ulcers may produce a bridge of mucosa over a larger ulcer. Regenerating epithelium attempting to epithelialize the wall of an abscessed tract extending down into the submucosa may produce a permanent malformation after the focus of inflammation has healed, an epithelial tunnel into the submucosa or mucosal bridges covered on all surfaces by mucus secreting intestinal epithelium. Epithelial regeneration into mucosal, submucosal, and rarely deeper abscesses may result in entrapment of epithelial cells within the wall as connective tissue of the lamina propria and surface epithelium re-establish continuity. The entrapped epithelial nest may produce mucus filled cysts (Figs. 5-32 and 5-33). This is one explanation of the genesis of colitis cystica profunda. Hypertrophic segments of the muscularis mucosae may sometimes be seen. This is not, however, as general a feature as in regional enteritis.

Colitis cystica profunda is a lesion worthy of further consideration because of the frequency with which it is confused with well-differentiated or mucous adenocarcinoma. In one study of 24 patients with submucosal cysts of the colon and rectum, about three fourths had the process confined to one distinct region, whereas the others had widely scattered lesions.[12] It seems probable that inflammation of the mucosa from virtually any cause may produce the lesion as long as the inflammation is accompanied by sufficient necrosis to extend into the submucosa and create an excavation of which the surface supports the regenerating epithelium. Perhaps others occur congenitally as a result of embryologic rests.[12] For obvious reasons, when colitis cystica profunda occurs as a result of ulcerative colitis the lesions are quite often widespread in the large intestine.

With both carcinoma and colitis cystica profunda proved to be sequelae to some cases of ulcerative colitis, these sequelae pose an important problem in histopathologic differential diagnosis for the pathologist. Except for the usual cellular criteria for distinguishing neoplastic from hyperplastic and normal cells, anaplasia or cellular atypia has not been described in colitis cystica profunda. Also, the benign cysts are surrounded by an inflammatory infiltrate extending from the mucosal source of the cyst. Occasionally mucous cysts lack epithelium, presumably secondary to pressure atrophy and necrosis. Not infrequently the benign cysts have secondary glands formed within their walls. Perhaps their most distinctive feature is the broad band of fibrous connective tissue encircling them in an orderly fashion. The cyst epithelium usually rests on an orderly patterned and loose, almost myxoid, layer of connective tissue. Benign cysts have not been reported within the muscularis or serosa; however, one must keep in mind that in those rare instances of ectopic epithelium due to defective embryogenesis, segments of reduplicated intestinal wall could occur outside the muscularis. In these instances the cystic reduplication would probably have its own muscular coat.

Ultrastructure of Ulcerative Colitis

Gonzales-Licea and Yardley compared the ultrastructural features of seven cases of ulcerative colitis with six cases of control diseases.[13] They observed that the microvilli of the epithelial cells in ulcerative colitis were shorter and more scanty than normal when the cells had other ultrastructural changes (Figs. 5-35, 5-36, and 5-37). These epithelial cells also showed dilatation of the endoplasmic reticulum, including the formation of large cysternae. The mitochondria in ulcerative colitis were sometimes swollen and rounded, and the cristae were small and scanty (Figs. 5-38 and 5-39). Several types of lysosome-related structures were observed in the epithelium as well. These were widely scattered in both crypt and superficial cells (Figs. 5-40 and 5-41). Epithelial cells containing these changes were intermixed with normal healthy-looking ones (Figs. 5-42 and 5-43). Separation of the epithelial cells because of ballooning of the intercellular space between both the superficial and crypt epithelial cells was seen in all but one case of ulcerative colitis (Fig. 5–44). The separations were most prominent near the base where they were associated with loss of intercellular interdigitation. The separation sometimes extended up to the terminal bar. Inflammatory cells were observed infiltrating between the epithelial cells in all the ulcerative colitis specimens (Figs. 5-45 and 5-46).

(Text continued on page 142.)

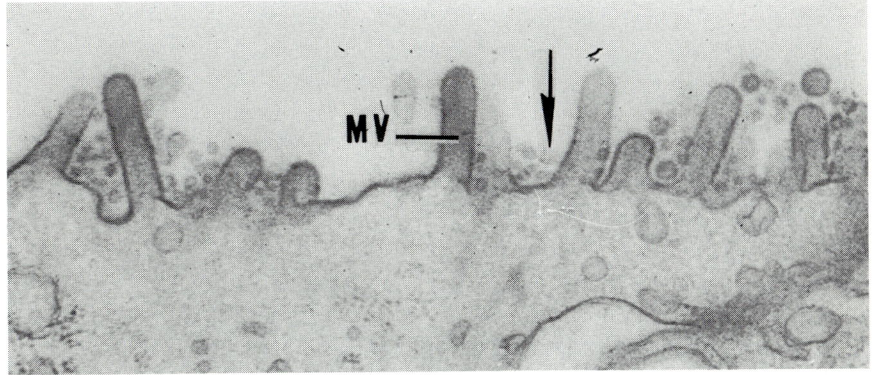

Figure 5-35 Ulcerative colitis. Surface epithelium. An epithelial cell showing altered microvilli (MV) that are shorter than normal and scanty. Small round bodies are present (arrow). ×47,100. (Courtesy of A. Gonzalez-Licea and J. H. Yardley, Bull. Hopkins Hosp. *118-119:*444-461, © 1966, and the Johns Hopkins Press, Baltimore, Md.)

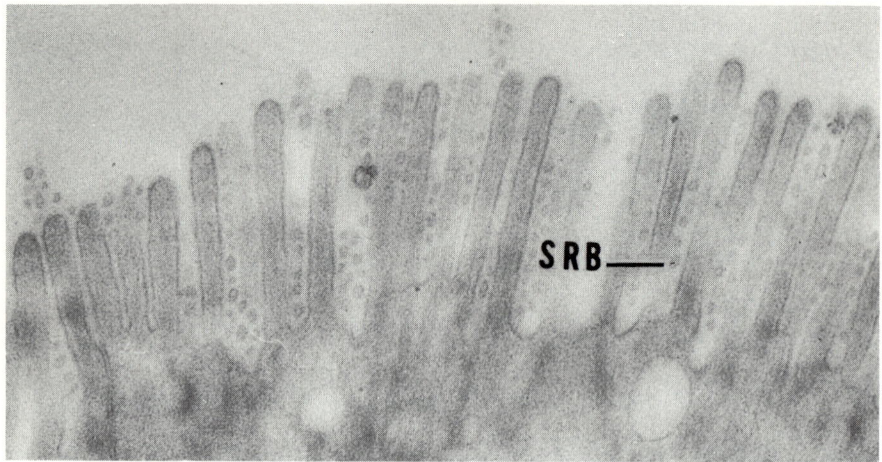

Figure 5-36   Familial polyposis. Surface epithelium. Many small round bodies (SRB) are seen between the microvilli; this phenomenon occurred in all ulcerative colitis and control cases. ×47,000. (Courtesy of A. Gonzalez-Licea and J. H. Yardley, Bull. Hopkins Hosp. *118-119:*444–461, © 1966, and the Johns Hopkins Press, Baltimore, Md.)

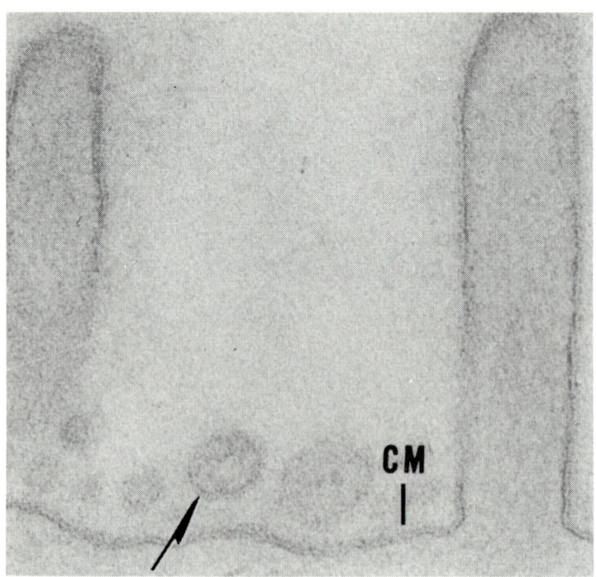

Figure 5-37   Ulcerative colitis. Crypt epithelium. Detail of small round bodies; they occasionally show a poorly defined double membrane (arrow). The cell membrane (CM) is also indicated. ×95,000. (Courtesy of A. Gonzalez-Licea and J. H. Yardley, Bull. Hopkins Hosp. *118–119:*444–461, © 1966, and the Johns Hopkins Press, Baltimore, Md.)

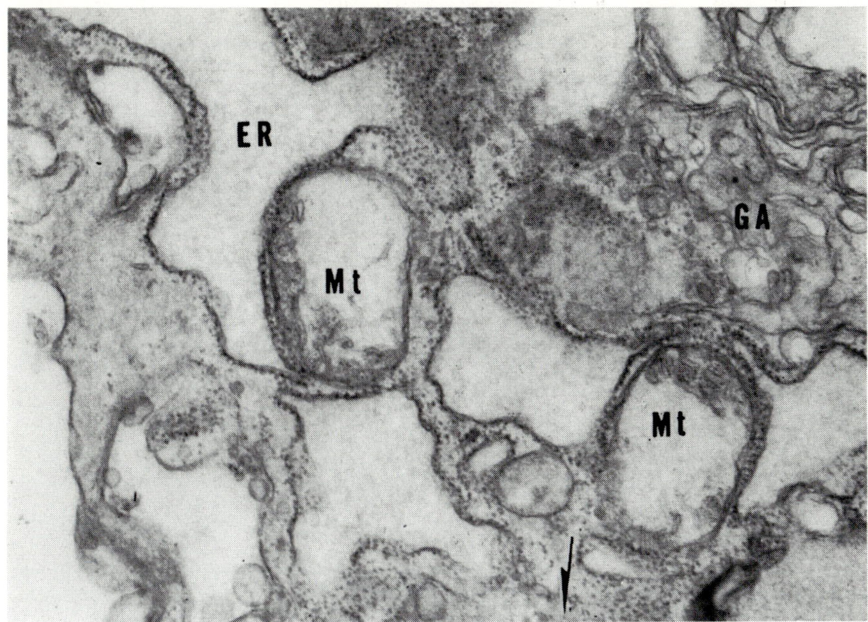

Figure 5–38   Ulcerative colitis. Surface epithelium The granular endoplasmic reticulum (ER) is dilated, as can be seen by comparison with the normal-looking ER (arrow). Two altered mitochondria (Mt) and a Golgi profile (GA) are also indicated. ×37,700. (Courtesy of A. Gonzalez-Licea and J. H. Yardley, Bull. Hopkins Hosp. *118–119*:444–461, © 1966, and the Johns Hopkins Press, Baltimore, Md.)

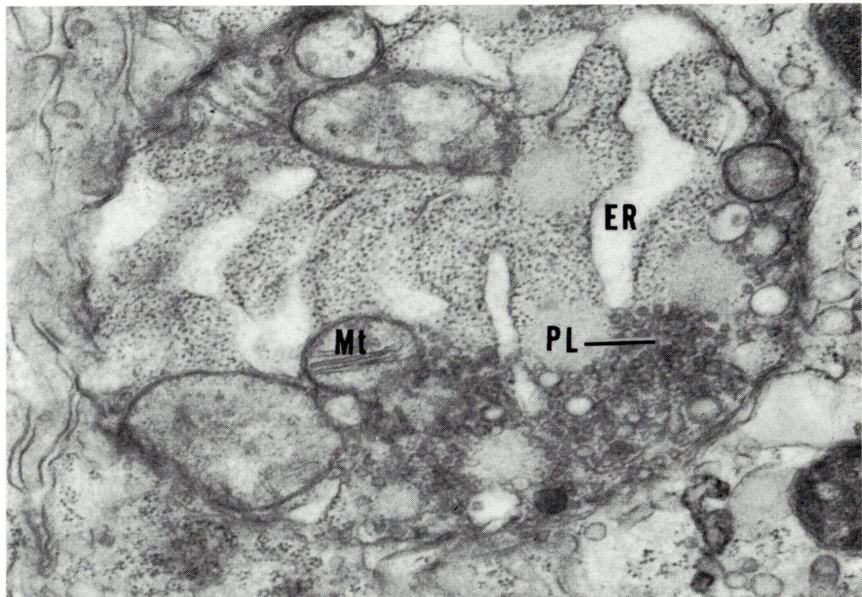

Figure 5–39   Ulcerative colitis. Crypt epithelium. A membrane-bounded cytosegresome is shown. It contains mitochondria (Mt), endoplasmic reticulum profiles (ER), and protolysosomes (PL). ×37,700. (Courtesy of A. Gonzalez-Licea and J. H. Yardley, Bull. Hopkins Hosp. *118-119*:444–461, © 1966, and the Johns Hopkins Press, Baltimore, Md.)

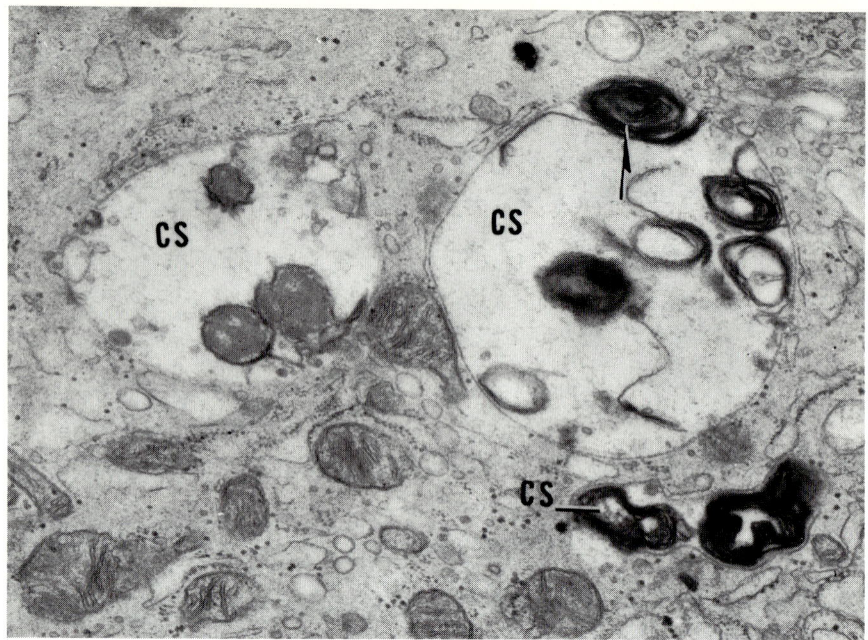

Figure 5–40 Ulcerative colitis. Surface epithelium. Three cytosegresomes (CS) containing myelin figures (arrow). These were a common finding. Mitochondria can also be seen. ×21,200. (Courtesy of A. Gonzalez-Licea and J. H. Yardley, Bull. Hopkins Hosp. *118-119*:444–461, © 1966, and the Johns Hopkins Press, Baltimore, Md.)

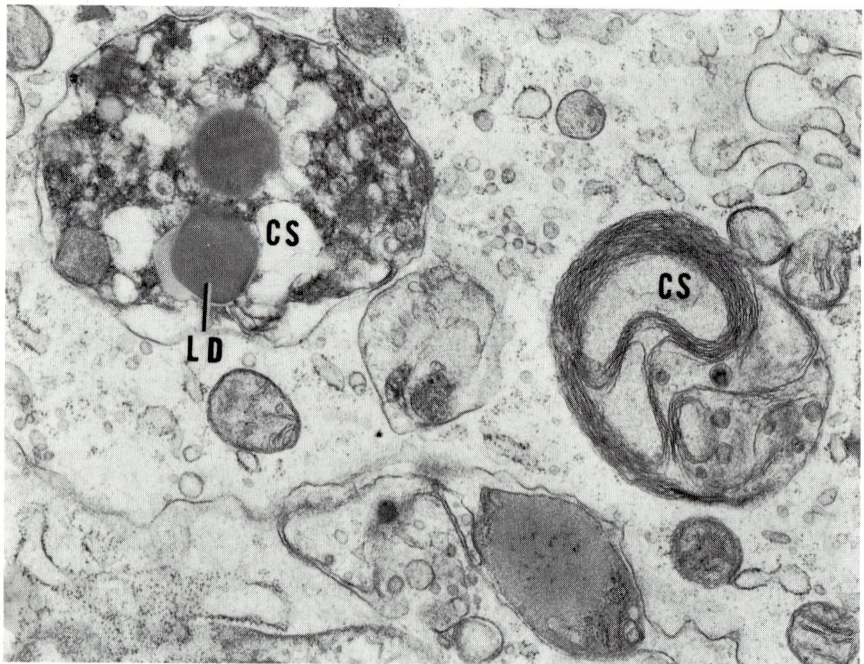

Figure 5–41 Shigellosis. Crypt epithelium. Various types of cytosegresomes (CS) are also seen here. Well-developed myelin figures, such as also occurred in ulcerative colitis, are seen to the right. Lipid droplets (LD) are noted within another cytosegresome. ×28,200. (Courtesy of A. Gonzalez-Licea and J. H. Yardley, Bull. Hopkins Hosp. *118-119*:444–461, © 1966, and the Johns Hopkins Press, Baltimore, Md.)

138

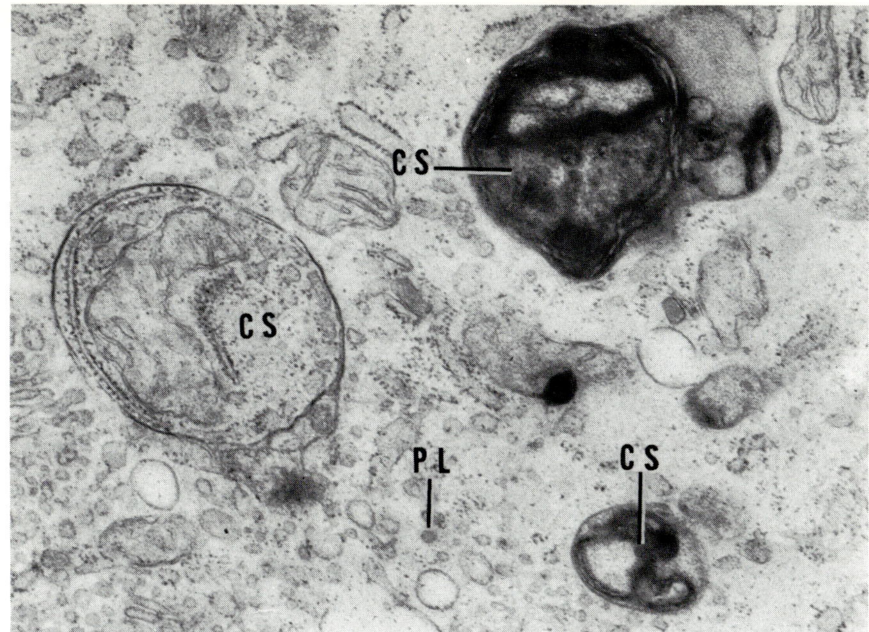

Figure 5–42 Postradiation proctitis. Surface epithelium. Three types of cytosegresomes (CS) are seen. Endoplasmic reticulum profiles and mitochondria are easily identified within the cytosegresome to the left. Also mitochondria and protolysosomes (PL) are seen. ×37,700. (Courtesy of A. Gonzalez-Licea and J. H. Yardley, Bull. Hopkins Hosp. *118–119:*444–461, © 1966, and the Johns Hopkins Press, Baltimore, Md.)

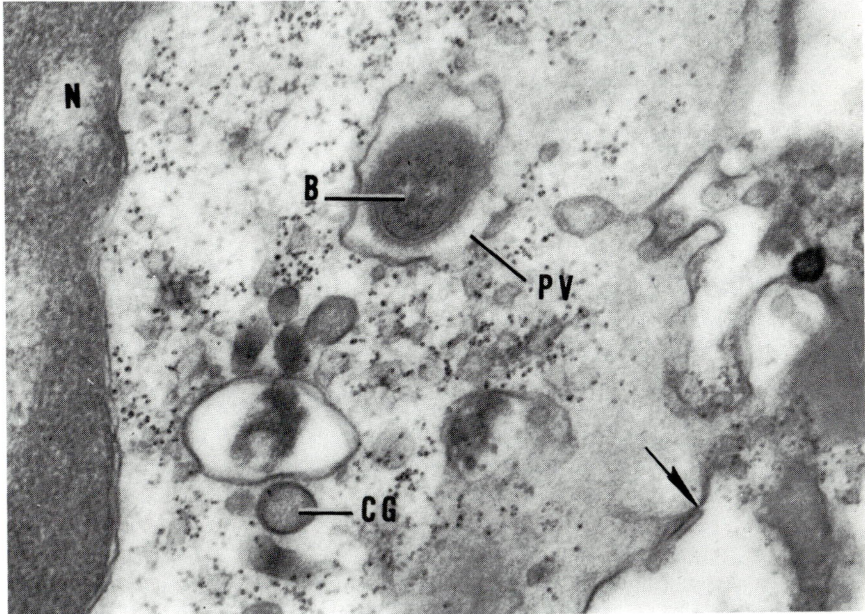

Figure 5–43 Ulcerative colitis. A polymorphonuclear leukocyte located in the bowel lumen showing a bacterium (B) within a phagocytic vacuole (PV). Cytoplasmic granules are shown (CG). Other phagocytic vacuoles, a portion of the nucleus (N), and cytoplasmic cell membrane (arrow) are also seen. ×47,100. (Courtesy of A. Gonzalez-Licea and J. H. Yardley, Bull. Hopkins Hosp. *118-119:*444–461, 1966, and the Johns Hopkins Press, Baltimore, Md.)

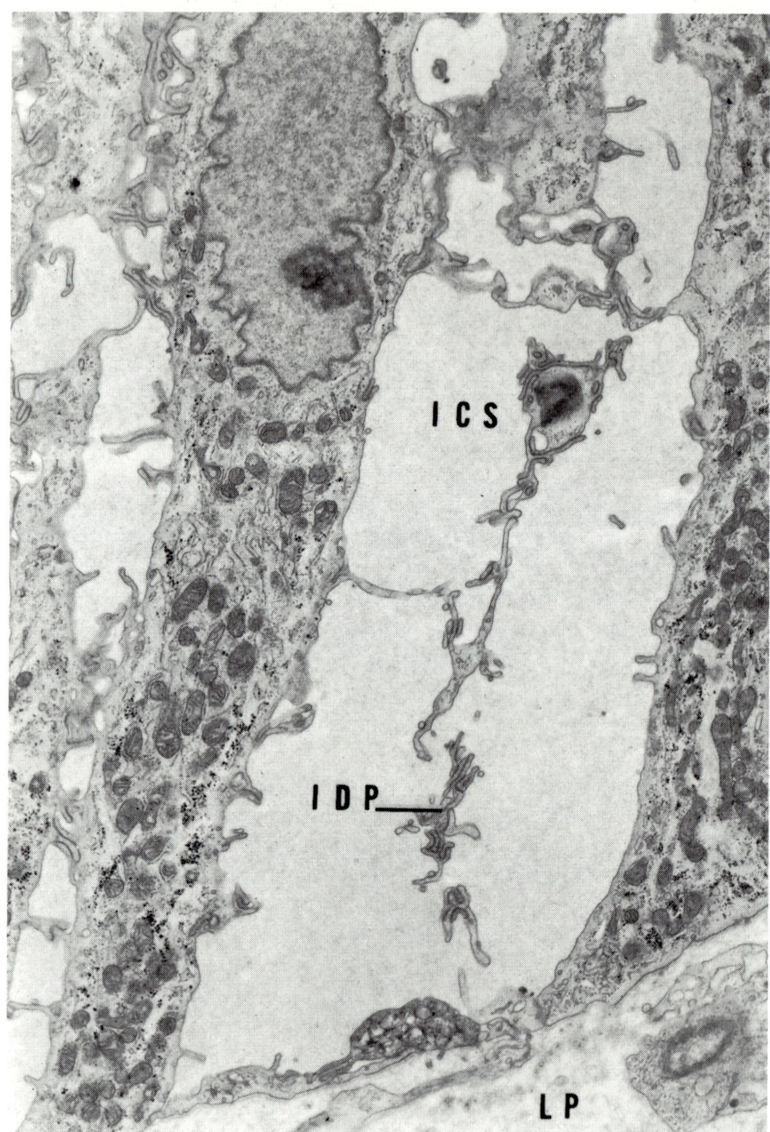

Figure 5–44 Ulcerative colitis. Surface epithelium. Note the separation of the epithelial cells owing to ballooning of the intercellular space (ICS). A delicate cell process, remnants of the interdigitations, are also seen (IDP); the lamina propria (LP) is identified. ×8,500. (Courtesy of A. Gonzalez-Licea and J. H. Yardley, Bull. Hopkins Hosp. *118-119:*444–461, © 1966, and the Johns Hopkins Press, Baltimore, Md.)

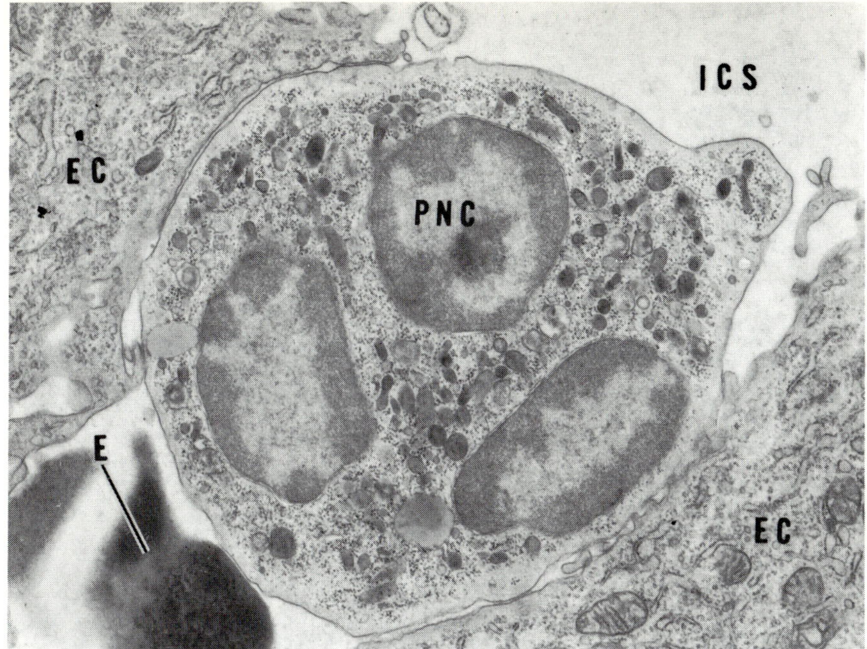

Figure 5-45 Ulcerative colitis. Surface epithelium. A polymorphonuclear leukocyte, neutrophil type (PNC), is located in the intercellular space (ICS) between two epithelial mucosal cells (EC). A portion of an erythrocyte is also identified (E). ×13,300. (Courtesy of A. Gonzalez-Licea and J. H. Yardley, Bull. Hopkins Hosp. *118–119*:444–461, © 1966, and the Johns Hopkins Press, Baltimore, Md.)

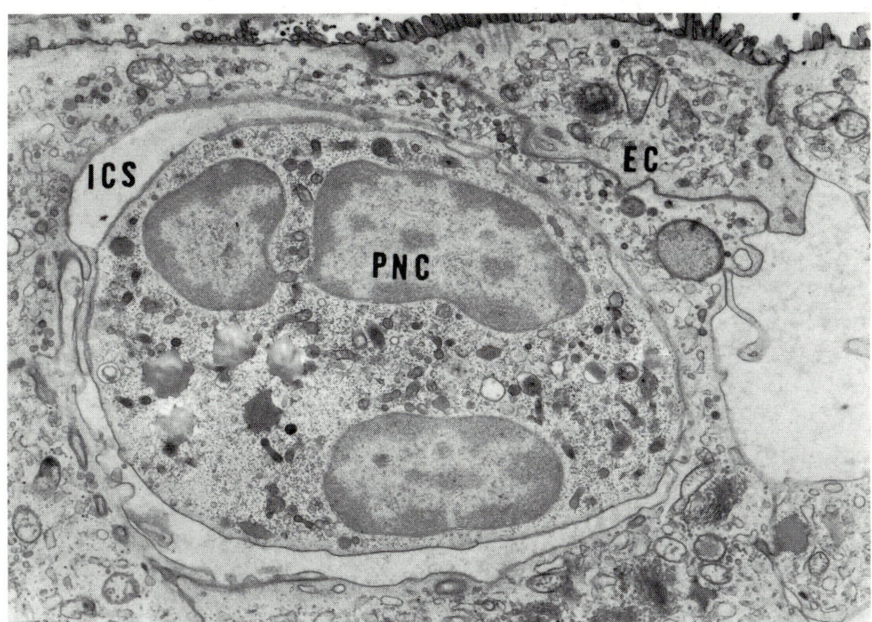

Figure 5-46 Shigellosis. Crypt epithelium. A leukocyte (PNC) of the type that is seen in Figure 5-45 is similarly located in the intercellular space (ICS) between the epithelial mucosal cells (EC). The crypt lumen is located at the top. ×6,680. (Courtesy of A. Gonzalez-Licea and J. H. Yardley, Bull. Hopkins Hosp. *118–119*:444–461, © 1966, and the Johns Hopkins Press, Baltimore, Md.)

Neutrophils predominated; however, eosinophils, monocytes, and immature lymphocytes were occasionally seen. Polymorphs were seen in the basement membrane, and in some places degenerative changes were similar to those described for other diseases. Polys were also seen within the crypts as were lymphocytes, erythrocytes, and mucous epithelial cells. No microorganisms were found. Breaks in the basal lamina were associated with sites of polymorph transmigration. Lymphocytes, polymorphs, macrophages, and collagen fibers in the lamina propria were increased in ulcerative colitis. None of these elements, however, showed distinctive features. These observations confirm those previously established by light microscopy regarding ulcerative colitis; no unique features were uncovered.

The Inflammatory Process in Ulcerative Colitis

Other investigators have studied the specific features of the inflammatory process of ulcerative colitis. Bassler emphasized the importance of the intramural abscess in the colon as a complication of ulcerative colitis and its role in the production of late perforation and generalized peritonitis.[14] Jacobson studied the epithelial basement membrane by light microscopy in 136 ulcerative colitis patients and in 28 normal controls, utilizing the freeze-dry technique on biopsy specimens.[15] He concluded that all specimens from the ulcerative colitis patients had areas of destroyed or thinned basement membrane as revealed by the PAS reaction, changes that conflict with those observed by Yardley under electron microscopy.

Paneth cell metaplasia has been reported as a constant feature of the crypts in ulcerative colitis by Watson and co-workers.[16, 17] They observed that Paneth cells, exceedingly sparse in the normal colon, were increased as much as three hundred fold in cases of ulcerative colitis, which they consider to be a result rather than a cause of the lesion. The cells were present in the greatest numbers in the ascending, transverse, and descending colon and were much less common in the sigmoid and rectal regions. They indicate that no other condition of the large bowel has been found to be so constantly associated with Paneth cell metaplasia. Paneth cells of the small intestine have been shown to have increased amounts of lysosomal enzymes.[34] Esterases, aminopeptidases, succinic and isocitric and lactic dehydrogenases, and NaDH diaphorase have been demonstrated in their secretory granules. Indeed, they form a widely scattered digestive gland. McAuley and Sommers did differential leukocyte counts on the inflammatory exudate in 25 cases of ulcerative colitis and demonstrated that mast cells occurred significantly more frequently in this condition than in other colonic inflammations.[18] In ulcerative colitis 0.5 per cent of the cells of the exudate were mast cells compared with 0.04 per cent in the controls. Söltoft recently reported his quantitative immunofluorescent microscopy studies on biopsies of lesions from ulcerative colitis and regional enteritis and of tissue from normal controls.[42] Ulcerative colitis and regional enteritis specimens contained a greater number of plasma cells than the controls and, in addition, the ulcerative colitis group had a higher proportion of cells containing IgM and IgG.

Storsteen and co-workers quantitated the frequently observed hyperplasia and hypertrophy of the myenteric plexus in ulcerative colitis.[19] They found approximately a threefold increase in the number of ganglion cells in cases of chronic ulcerative colitis and had no explanation for its significance. It should be noted that an apparent increase of nerve ganglia in the bowel wall occurs in a variety of intestinal inflammations, including regional enteritis and appendicitis.

Histochemical studies on the mucosal lesions have yielded some interesting observations that deserve further investigation. Greco et al. studied the goblet cell mucin production in 10 ulcerative colitis patients and 13 normal controls.[20] They observed slight to severe alteration in the pattern of mucin production. Neutral mucins were decreased, whereas sulfomucins and acidic mucins in general were increased. Hellstrom and Fischer also used a battery of mucin stains to demonstrate a decrease in the production of epithelial mucins in ulcerative colitis in contrast to regional enteritis and emphasize the use of this difference as a point in differential histodiagnosis. My own unpublished observations indicate that there is a decrease in mucin in the immediate vicinity of cryptitis and crypt abscesses, though it may be actually increased in less inflamed regions. I did not observe any alteration in the histochemical nature of the mucins as revealed by the Alcian blue–PAS, colloidal iron, and aldehyde fuchsin reactions. Hradsky et al. and Binder reported an increased activity of acid phosphatase, esterase, and aminopeptidase enzyme activity in the epithelium of ulcerative colitis lesions.[22, 33] Malic, succinic, and lactic dehydrogenase activity was unchanged. The changes observed are most likely nonspecific responses to inflammation. Unfortunately, no other patients with other colonic inflammatory disease were used as controls. Jankey and Price studied the enzyme histochemistry of the small intestinal mucosa in ulcerative colitis.[32] They were unable to demonstrate changes that might, through faulty digestion or absorption, facilitate the entry of unusual bowel contents into the colon. Spencer and co-workers found the mean renewal time for rectal epithelium prolonged in patients with active ulcerative colitis, which contrasted sharply with renewal times in granulomatous colitis, ulcerative colitis in remission, and normal controls.[43]

Lunderquist, utilizing angiography in the study of ulcerative colitis, observed an altered vascular pattern.[23] Most noteworthy was a decreased perfusion of the mucosa and a blunt obstruction to the flow of contrast media. This now common radiologic observation raises anew the possibility of important vascular changes in the pathogenesis of the lesions.

TOXIC MEGACOLON

Toxic megacolon is a term sometimes used to describe the extreme dilatation that occurs in some patients with acute fulminating ulcerative colitis. This is in sharp contrast to the unimpressive external appearance of the colon in the common form of ulcerative colitis. The cause of the dilatation is unknown though it is tempting to speculate that it may be a loss of motility and relaxation of the muscularis with consequent distention due to accumulation of exudate, necrotic debris, blood, and feces. The lesion is so severe that it is life-threatening, usually because of exsanguination into the colonic lumen. In several large series of cases the death rate often approached 50 per cent during the acute attack.[24-27, 36] With either medical or surgical management or both the prognosis is improved somewhat, especially with surgical excision of the colon. Toxic megacolon occurs at the onset or during the course of about 1 in 10 to 20 cases of ulcerative colitis. It occurs as the initial attack as frequently as it does as a relapse. It affects both sexes equally and may occur at any age. Clinically it is characterized by the sudden onset of severe diarrhea, shortly followed by tachycardia, fever, extreme weakness, and apathy in those with excessive loss of fluid and electrolytes. Mild colicky abdominal pain and tenderness in the left lower quadrant are usually found. Skin lesions are more frequently seen with this variant than with the common variety of ulcerative colitis (see Chapter Eight).

Macroscopic Observations in Toxic Megacolon

The colon is dilated in virtually all cases; however, the extent of the dilatation is variable (Figs. 5-47, 5-48, 5-49, and 5-50). Occasionally, the entire length of the bowel will be dilated; however, more frequently the dilatation will be limited to the region proximal to the splenic flexure. The diameter of the bowel may be increased up to 10 cm. The second major feature noted on external examination is marked vascular congestion, especially in the area of dilatation. The serosa is usually dull, cloudy, and opaque, and the bowel wall is thin and friable. In less than a third of the cases, evidence of perforation with perirectal abscess or peritonitis may be found. In still others, adhesions between the bowel and other viscera may also be noted. These are characterized by some degree of acute inflammation in the involved areas with enlargement of the adjacent lymph nodes and a

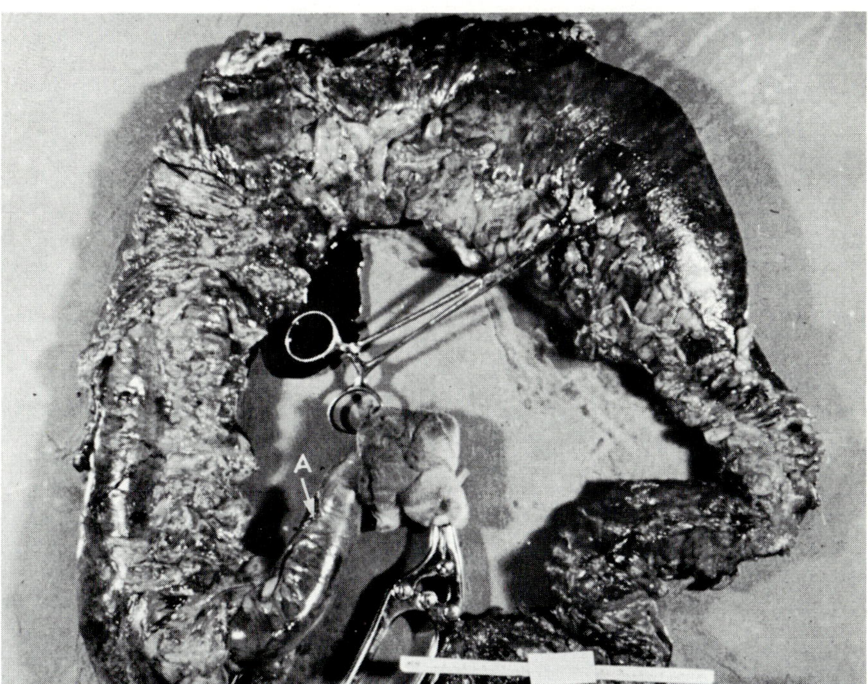

Figure 5–47 Unincised colon and terminal ileum (A) characteristic of the "acute toxic megacolon" of severe ulcerative colitis. In contrast to the usually unremarkable external appearance of ulcerative colitis, this variant reveals a massively dilated, congested, and friable external surface. In this patient, ulcerative colitis had not been previously diagnosed, and the lesion probably represents an abrupt onset.

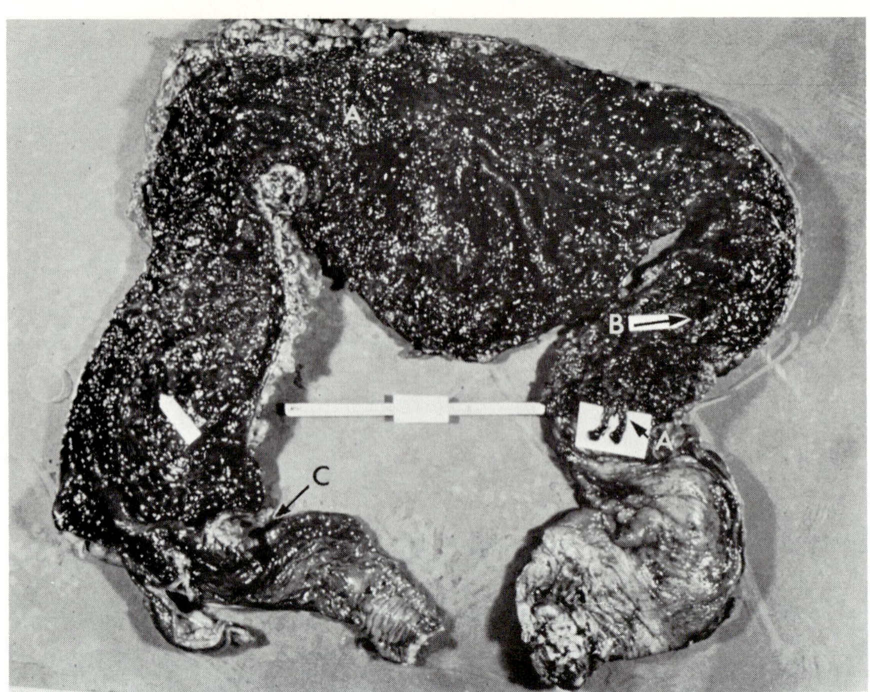

Figure 5–48 Incised specimen shown in Figure 5-47. Massively, severely inflamed mucosa reveals extensive shredding (A) and possible perforation (B). "Backwash" changes in the terminal ileum are also found (C).

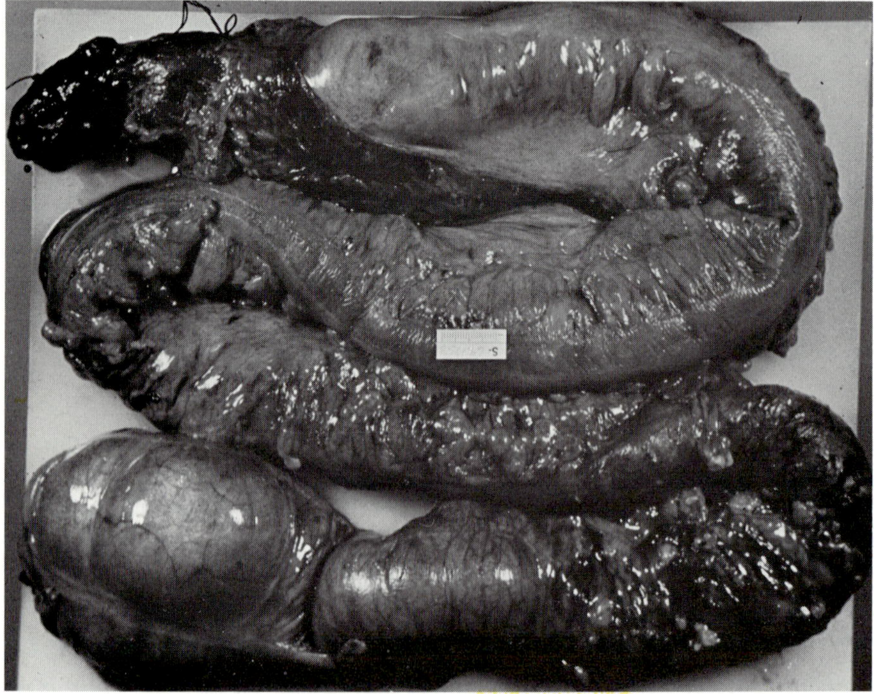

Figure 5–49 Toxic megacolon variant of ulcerative colitis revealing serosal vascular congestion and extensive dilatation of the colon.

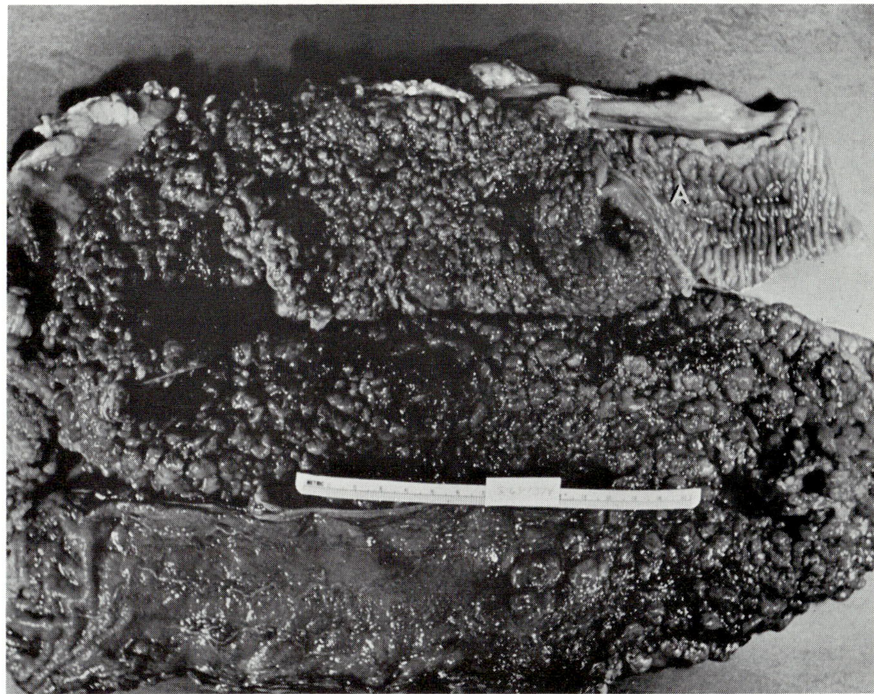

Figure 5–50   Same specimen shown in Figure 5–49 has been incised to reveal the mucosal surface. Diffuse extensive punctate ulcerations are seen in all regions except the terminal ileum (A). Pseudopolypoid appearance of the remaining mucosa is seen. This patient had long-standing ulcerative colitis and a severe acute exacerbation.

fibrin or fibrinous exudate. Because of the extreme friability of the bowel wall, the surgeon occasionally will perforate the bowel in the process of excision. Such defects may be noted on external examination.

Upon opening the bowel along its anterior long axis, one observes that the site of maximum mucosal involvement may not coincide with the site of maximum dilatation and may frequently be distal to it. The site of maximum disease in the mucosa most frequently is in the sigmoid or pelvic region of the colon; but the descending and transverse colon are often, though somewhat less frequently, involved, with the ascending colon and cecum less severely involved in about half the cases. Commonly the extension of the lesion into the ileum or even the distal jejunum may be noted. Deep ulceration through the mucosa and submucosa may involve broad areas of the surface or, more frequently, show a tendency to overlie the tenia coli, producing a linear ulcer that may be many centimeters in length. The intervening mucosa is usually edematous and may have superficial ulcers.

Microscopic Features of Toxic Megacolon

The constant microscopic feature is the deep ulceration of the colonic mucosa and submucosa, often extending into and even beyond the muscular coat. Patches of surviving mucosa may be edematous, infiltrated with lymphocytes, plasma cells, eosinophils, and polymorphs; indeed, all the features of the common type of ulcerative colitis are seen with the additional feature that the ulcers penetrate deeply rather than remaining superficial. Crypt abscesses are frequently seen, but because of the extensive erosion of the mucosa, many samples of the colon may not reveal them.

Another feature of variance from the usual form of ulcerative colitis is the existence of evidence of a vasculitis in the larger vessels of the colonic wall. This consists of swelling and irregularity of the vascular endothelium and the presence of inflammatory cells, principally polymorphs, within the muscular coat of the vessels in the submucosa muscularis and subserosa. The inflammatory lesion will often be overlaid by a thrombus within the lumen, which will reveal varying degrees of organization. In spite of the extensive mucosal necrosis and the deep penetration of the ulcers with erosion sometimes extending into the muscularis, scant if any evidence of fibrosis is seen.

Because of the high mortality with toxic megacolon, the pathologist often encounters this lesion as part of an autopsy rather than as a surgical specimen. In addition to the colonic changes already mentioned, the prosector will find localized or diffuse peritonitis, if perforation was a feature of the colonic lesion. In the absence of perforation, a rather copious amount of free clear fluid will be found in the peritoneal cavity. Severe fatty change of the liver is frequently seen, and evidence of metastatic abscesses with or without bronchopneumonia may be found. Pulmonary embolism is also frequently found in these cases. In addition the general features of dehydration and malnutrition may be present if the relapse has persisted for weeks or months.

SEGMENTAL ULCERATIVE COLITIS

Analysis and evaluation of clinical reports pertaining to segmental lesions in the colon have been made difficult by the confusion in terminology. Terms such as segmental colitis, regional colitis, regional segmental colitis, right-sided colitis, and regional ileocolitis have been applied. To clarify the problem, I have discarded all reports lacking histologic confirmation of the lesion and have included only those studies in which histopathologic examination demonstrates both grossly and microscopically the ulcerative colitis type of inflammation. Therefore, I define segmental colitis as ulcerative colitis limited to a segment of the colon, often beginning in the right half of the colon and only later extending to the more distal sigmoid and rectal segments. Granulomatous colitis, as a colonic expression of regional enteritis (also referred to by some as Crohn's disease of the colon) is discussed in the chapters on regional enteritis. The clinical entity described by Brooke and Cooke as a distinct variety of enterocolitis has been excluded.[28] Whether the histopathology of the clinical entity they describe is similar to regional enteritis or ulcerative colitis or both, or presents some other histopathologic picture, remains in doubt because only 2 of the 16 patients they originally recorded had pathologic study. Others have been unable to find similar cases in their large series of colonic inflammations. The inadequate definition of the pathologic basis for the entity leaves its existence as a separate entity in doubt.

The histopathologic features of segmental ulcerative colitis are comparable to those described previously for more general colonic involvement of ulcerative colitis, and represent a variation in the distribution and extent of the lesion. The incidence of segmental ulcerative colitis, as Table 5-1 demonstrates, is approximately 5 to 10 per cent of all colonic inflammatory lesions. This is based on study of three large series of inflammatory lesions of the colon. Considering the number of cases of segmental colitis as a percentage of all cases of nonspecific colitis, one finds a varying incidence from 1 to 17 per cent. In their large series, Kurt and Brown reported that segmental colitis represented approximately 1 per cent of their ulcerative colitis patients.[37] Their study includes those cases of ulcerative colitis that had had minimal generalized lesions that were cared for medically and did not

TABLE 5–1   Segmental Colitis Incidence

Year Reported	First Author	Location	Total Cases	Segmental Cases
All Types of Colitis				
1947	Crohn[29]	New York	600	48 (8%)
1955	Manning[41]	Boston	708	25 (3.5%)
1947	Bargen[40]	Rochester	299	18 (6.1%)
Ulcerative Colitis				
1959	Kurt[37]	Cleveland	1000	9 (1%) Cases with ileal involvement excluded
1960	Watkinson[31]	London	114	15 (13.1%) Cases with ileal lesion included
1956	Bockus[39]	Philadelphia	125	21 (17%) Some cases of ileal lesions included
1962	Cushing[38]	Washington D.C.	174	11 (6.3%) Slight "backwash" ileal lesion included

require surgical intervention. Also they excluded all cases that had ileal lesions, such as "backwash" ileitis. The report of Watkinson and that of Bockus mention 13 and 17 per cent segmental lesions, respectively.[31, 39] However, they included cases that had evidence of ileal lesions, and their material was largely surgically derived. One may assume that many of the minimal cases managed medically were excluded from their purview. Cushing and McCune included cases that had some slight "backwash" involvement of the ileum, but clearly did not have the regional enteritis type of lesion.[38] It should also be noted that it has been reported that approximately 75 per cent of the cases of segmental colitis have some degree of ileal involvement; thus, one may expect that less than 10 per cent of cases of ulcerative colitis are restricted to segmental involvement. Kurt and Brown also excluded all lesions that had some degree of rectal involvement.

The gross pathologic features of segmental colitis are comparable to those described for general ulcerative colitis with the exception that the observations are limited to a segment of colon and confined to the right colon in more than half the cases. A variable amount of transverse and left colon may be involved in approximately 30 to 40 per cent of cases and a retrograde or "backwash" ileitis may occur also in a comparable percentage. The sigmoid colon may occasionally be somewhat involved, but in no case is the rectum affected. Thus, the gross lesion represents an ulcerative colitis originating in the right colon and extending a variable distance proximally and distally. Often

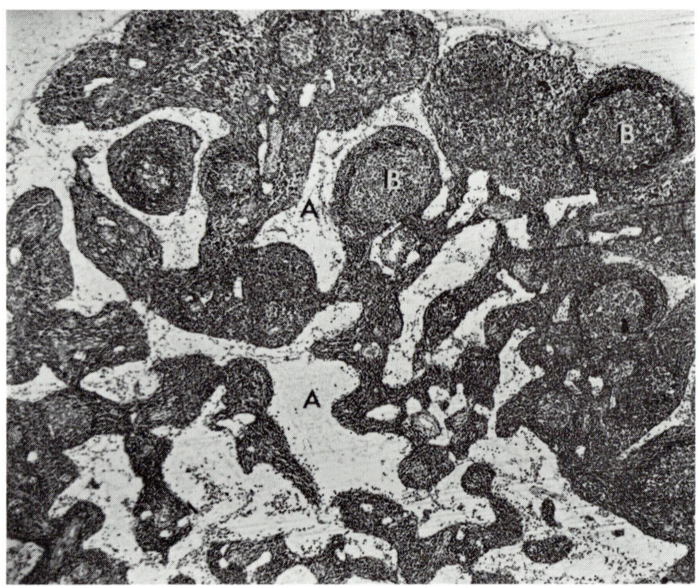

Figure 5–51   Colonic lymph node from a region with ulcerative colitis. Extensive sinusoidal congestion is seen (A) and some prominent germinal follicles (B). ×4.

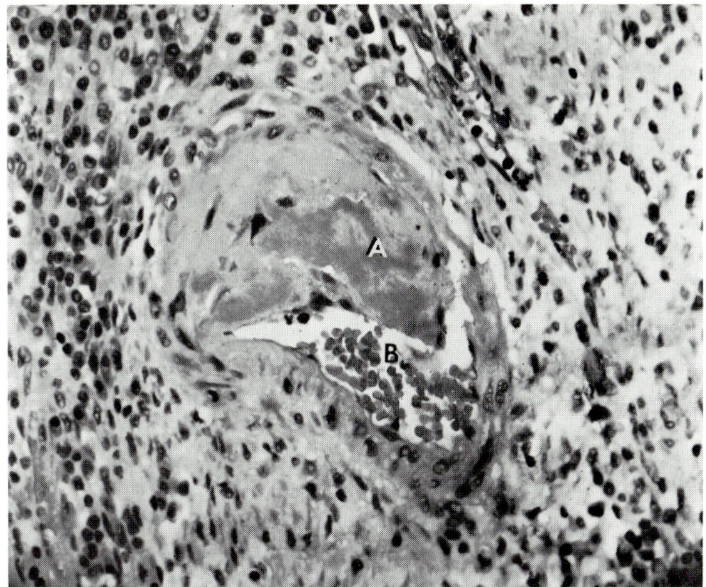

Figure 5-52 Organized thrombus (A) and recanalization (B) in a blood vessel in the vicinity of ulcerative colitis lesions. ×64.

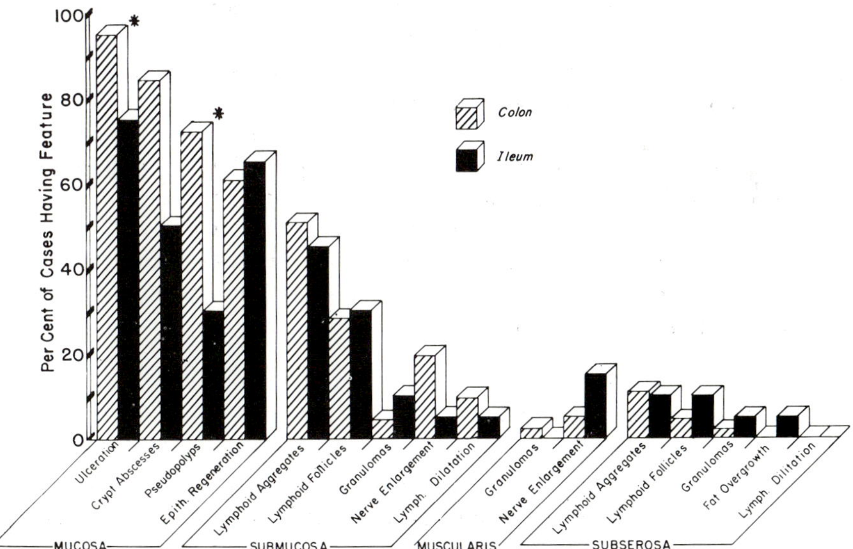

Figure 5-53 Frequency of occurrence of various histologic features in ulcerative colitis of the colon and ileum. Note that the majority of the changes are in the mucosa and that the pattern of the disease is similar in both sites. The asterisks indicate statistically significant differences in the frequency of occurrence (χ^2 3.84: $_2p$ 0.05: Yate's adjustment for continuity as necessary). (Courtesy of S. L. Saltzstein and B. F. Rosenberg, Amer. J. Clin. Path. *40*:610–623, © 1963, and The Williams & Wilkins Co. Baltimore, Md.)

the external examination of the serosa grossly does not reveal the presence of changes except for occasional slight vascular congestion. Palpation reveals some edematous induration and, upon examination of the mucosa, ulcerations of the ulcerative colitis type are observed. Microscopically the superficial erosions, crypt abscesses, and intense lymphocyte and plasma cell infiltration are seen in the involved segments, which tend to fade out into the normal colonic tissue of the noninvolved segment. A sharp border is usually not recognizable. There is a recognized tendency for segmental colitis to spread distally and proximally, as these studies have amply documented.[29, 30] Secondary types of intestinal tract lesions such as perianal disease, pseudopolyposis, stricture, and perforation and the risk of cancerous development do not appear to differ significantly in frequency from the more distal types of ulcerative colitis. Crohn observed that 22 of 77 patients with segmental colitis had perianal complications, whereas Neuman and co-workers had 22 per cent of their 201 patients with this complication. Watkinson, Thompson and Goligher observed six perianal complications in 15 patients.[31] Pseudopolyposis or the tendency to form inflammatory polypoid hyperplasias of the colonic mucosa occurs in approximately 31 per cent of cases. The formation of fibrous scars and strictures and late long-standing disease also occurs in approximately 30 per cent of the cases, though actual obstruction occurs very infrequently. Perforation of the colon occurs in about 6 per cent of cases. Reports on the incidence of carcinoma and segmental colitis are conflicting. Those of Crohn and Neuman did not reveal any cases that developed carcinoma in the affected bowel, whereas Manning and co-workers observed this change in approximately 6 per cent of their cases.[29, 30, 41] If the inflammatory lesion represents an incitement to precancerous change, one might expect that if the lesion only affected a small portion of the bowel surface, it would carry a smaller risk of carcinoma than if the entire colon were involved as is frequently the case in generalized ulcerative colitis. The systemic complications of arthritis, cutaneous lesions, and liver disease are dealt with in the discussion of secondary lesions.

ULCERATIVE PROCTITIS

Ulcerative proctitis is ulcerative colitis with a distribution limited to the rectum. This diagnosis is about one-twentieth as frequent as ulcerative colitis. Sigmoidoscopic findings are usually indistinguishable from ulcerative colitis, but less extensive. Biopsy specimens are also indistinguishable. Of the patients with ulcerative proctitis, in less than 3 per cent will it evolve into more extensive lesions of the more proximal part of the colon. As a more localized and milder form of ulcerative colitis, its prognosis is better. The gross and microscopic findings are identical with the more extensive form of the disease except for their limited distribution and severity and need not be described further here.

References

1. Dukes, C. E.: The surgical pathology of ulcerative colitis. Ann. Roy. Coll. Surg. Eng. *14*:389–400, 1954.
2. Lumb, G.: Pathology of ulcerative colitis. Gastroenterology *40*:290–298, 1961.
3a. Truelove, S. C., Horler, A. R., and Richards, W. C.: Serial biopsy in ulcerative colitis. Brit. Med. J. *4956*:1590–1593, 1955.
3b. Truelove, R.: Biopsy studies in ulcerative colitis. Brit. Med. J. *4979*:1315–1318, 1956.
4. Lumb, G.: Rectal biopsy in ulcerative colitis. Gastroenterologia (Basel) *86*:650-655, 1956.
5. Lumb, G.: Rectal biopsy in ulcerative colitis. Dis. Colon Rectum *1*:37-43, 1958.
6. Goldgraber, M. B., Kirsner, J. B., and Palmer, W. C.: The histopathology of chronic ulcerative colitis and its pathogenic implications. Gastroenterology *38*:596-604, 1960.
7. Warren, S., and Sommers, S. C.: Pathogenesis of ulcerative colitis. Amer. J. Path. *25*:657-674, 1949.
8. Lumb, G., and Protheroe, R. H.: The early lesions in ulcerative colitis. Gastroenterology *33*:457-474, 1957.
9. Buie, L. S., Sr.: Gross and microscopic criteria for the diagnosis of thrombo-ulcerative colitis. Dis. Colon Rectum *1*:209-214, 1958.
10. Counsell, B.: Lesions of the ileum associated with ulcerative colitis. Brit. J. Surg. *44*:276-290, 1956.
11. Dukes, C. E., and Lockhart-Mummery, H. E.: Practical points in the pathology and surgical treatment of ulcerative colitis: A critical review. Brit. J. Surg. *45*:25-36, 1957.
12. Allen, M. S., Jr.: Hamartomatous inverted polyps of the rectum. Cancer, *19*:257-265, 1966.
13. Gonzales-Licea, A., and Yardley, J. H.: Nature of the tissue reaction in ulcerative colitis. Light and electron microscopic findings. Gastroenterology *51*:825-840, 1966.
14. Bassler, A.: Intramural abscess of the colon wall in chronic ulcerative colitis. Amer. J. Gastroent. *21*:200-204, 1954.
15. Jacobson, M. A., and Kirsner, J. B.: The basement membrane of the epithelium of the colon and rectum in ulcerative colitis and other diseases. Gastroenterology *30*:279-285, 1956.
16. Watson, A. J., and Roy, A. D.: Paneth cells in the large intestine in ulcerative colitis. J. Path. Bact. *80*:309-316, 1960.
17. Patterson, J. C., and Watson, S. H.: Paneth cell metaplasia in ulcerative colitis. Amer. J. Path. *38*:243-249, 1961.
18. McAuley, R. L., and Sommers, S. C.: Mast cells in nonspecific ulcerative colitis. Amer. J. Dig. Dis. *6*:233-236, 1961.
19. Storsteen, K. A., Kernohan, J. W., and Bargen, J. A.: The myenteric plexus in chronic ulcerative colitis. Surg. Gynec. Obstet. *97*:335-343, 1953.
20. Greco, V., Lauro, G., Fabbrini, A., and Torsoli, A.: Histochemistry of the colonic epithelial mucins in normal subjects and in patients with ulcerative colitis. A qualitative and histometric investigation. Gut *8*:491-496, 1967.
21. Hellstrom, H. R., and Fischer, E. R.: Estimation of mucosal mucin as an aid in the differentiation of Crohn's disease of the colon and chronic ulcerative colitis. Amer. J. Clin. Path. *48*:259-268, 1967.
22. Hradsky, M., Langr, F., Nerad, V., and Skaonic, V.: Alterations of the histological and histochemical pattern in ulcerative colitis biopsy specimens. Amer. J. Proctol. *18*:392-398, 1967.
23. Lunderquist, A., and Lunderquist, A.: Angiography in ulcerative colitis. Amer. J. Roentgen. *99*:18-23, 1967.

24. McConnell, F., Hanelin, J., and Robbins, L. L.: Plain film diagnosis of fulminating ulcerative colitis. Radiology *71*:674-682, 1958.

25. McInerney, G. T., Sauer, W. G., Baggenstoss, A. H., and Hodgson, J. R.: Fulminating ulcerative colitis with marked colonic dilation: A clinicopathologic study. Gastroenterology *42*:244-257, 1962.

26. Rankin, J. G., Goulston, S. J., Bonen, R. W., and Morrow, A. W.: Fulminant ulcerative colitis. Quart. J. Med. *29*:375-390, 1960.

27. Sampson, P. A., and Walker, F. C.: Dilatation of the colon in ulcerative colitis. Brit. Med. J. *5260*:1119-1132, 1961.

28. Brooke, B. N., and Cooke, W. T.: Non-specific enterocolitis. Quart. J. Med. *24*:1-22, 1955.

29. Crohn, B. B., Gerlock, J. H., and Yarnis, H.: Right-sided (regional) colitis. J.A.M.A. *134*:334-338, 1947.

30. Neuman, H. W., Bargen, J. A., and Judd, E. S., Jr.: A clinical study of 201 cases of regional (segmental) colitis. Surg. Gynec. Obstet. *99*:563-571, 1954.

31. Watkinson, G., Thompson, H., and Goligher, J. C.: Right-sided or segmental ulcerative colitis. Brit. J. Surg. *47*:337–351, 1960.

32. Jankey, N., and Price, L. A.: Small intestine histochemical and histological changes in ulcerative colitis. Gut *10*:267–269, 1969.

33. Binder, V.: Histochemical studies of the colonic mucosa in ulcerative colitis and other colonic diseases. Scand. J. Gastroent. *3*:611-621, 1968.

34. Lewin, K.: Histochemical observations on Paneth cells. J. Anat. *105*:171-176, 1969.

35. Goulston, S. J., and McGovern, U. J.: The nature of benign strictures in ulcerative colitis. New Eng. J. Med. *281*:290-295, 1969.

36. Jalan, K. N., Sireus, W., Card, W. I., Falconer, C. W. A., Bruce, J., Crean, G. P., McManus, J. P. A., Small, W. P., and Smith, A. N.: An experience of ulcerative colitis. I. Toxic dilation in 55 cases. Gastroenterology *57*:68-82, 1969.

37. Kurt, E. J., and Brown, C. H.: Segmental ulcerative colitis, classification; report of nine unusual cases. Amer. J. Gastroent. *31*:419-431, 1959.

38. Cushing, W. J., and McCune, W. S.: Segmental ulcerative colitis. Amer. J. Surg. *103*:27-34, 1962.

39. Bockus, H. L., Roth, J. L. A., Buchman, E., Kalser, M., Staub, W. R., Finkelstein, A., and Valdes-Dapena, A.: Life history of non-specific ulcerative colitis: Relation of prognosis to anatomical and clinical varieties. Gastroenterologia (Basel) *86*:549-581, 1956.

40. Bargen, J. A.: Management of ulcerative colitis. Postgrad. Med. *2*:167-177, 1947.

41. Manning, J. H., Warren, T. R., and Adi, A. S.: Segmental colitis, results of surgery. New Eng. J. Med. *252*:850-883, 1955.

42. Söltoft, J.: Immunoglobulin-containing cells in normal jejunal mucosa and in ulcerative colitis and regional enteritis. Scand. J. Gastroent. *4*:353–360, 1969.

43. Spencer, R. G., Huizenga, K. A., Hammer, C. S., and Shorter, R. G.: Further studies on the kinetics of rectal epithelium in normal subjects and patients with ulcerative colitis or granulomatous colitis. Dis. Colon Rectum *12*:406–408, 1969.

Chapter Six

Enterocolitis To Be Differentiated from Regional Enteritis and Ulcerative Colitis

The central thesis of this monograph is to view regional enteritis and ulcerative colitis from the vantage point of pathologic process. In keeping with this, it is important to devote some attention to other inflammatory processes of the intestinal tract and to compare them with the two primary diseases under consideration, emphasizing the major features of the differential pathologic diagnosis. Therefore, regional enteritis and ulcerative colitis are not dealt with per se in this chapter.

GENERAL FEATURES

There are three cardinal features of intestinal inflammations that must be emphasized at the outset. The first is that most intestinal inflammatory processes can involve more or less both the large and small intestines. Many, as is pointed out later, are primarily situated in the small intestine and secondarily or occasionally involve the large intestine; with others the reverse may be true. The overlap in involvement is sufficient, however, to make it of primary importance that one consider the process irrespective of which segment is involved, because in a particular entity the histopathologic appearance of the lesion is usually comparable in either site. The second cardinal feature of intestinal inflammations is that the extent of the pathologic changes correlates very poorly with the extent of the clinical signs and symptoms. A most outstanding example of this is human cholera (*Vibrio comma* infection). The patient may have massive diarrhea of rice water-like stools and extensive fluid and electrolyte depletion, and may suffer collapse or death; yet modern studies of the pathology of the lesion reveal no anatomic changes, but rather a reversal of the fluid and electrolyte transport across the intestinal epithelium. Similar though less startling disassociation of the signs and symptoms and the extent of pathologic process is seen with most intestinal inflammations. Conversely, there are many instances in which the pathologic lesions of the intestinal tract are massive, but the patient may have virtually no signs or symptoms.

The third cardinal feature is that, with few exceptions, the etiologic agents of intestinal inflammations can produce a spectrum of changes varying from a mild mucorrhea to massive necrosis (gangrene). Whereas some agents tend to produce principally a mucorrhea, others predominantly produce changes at the other end of the spectrum. Therefore, on the basis of gross and microscopic findings alone, it often is impossible to decipher the etiologic agent. One must view the clinical and other laboratory evidence and deduce a presumptive etiologic agent. This has led to considerable confusion, as the presumptive cause may be in error. Whether the process is viewed in an early or late phase also affects one's presumption.

Before describing the spectrum of lesions, it is necessary to define the terms "membranous" and "pseudomembranous." In current usage they are synonymous, referring to the membrane-like material coating the mucosa. To be accurate, the term pseudomembranous should be used, because in no respect is this a true biologic membrane. It consists of a swollen red mucosa with petechial hemorrhages or, occasionally, pinpoint ulcers. The mucosal surface is coated with a variable mixture of fibrin, necrotic debris principally derived from the cellular components of the mucosa, and inflammatory infiltrates, principally polymorphs (Figs. 6-1, 6-2, 6-3, and 6-4). In the past, pathologists devoted considerable effort to dividing the pseudomembranes into two types, "croupous" and "diphtheritic." The former referred to a pseudomembrane that was composed almost entirely of a coating of fibrin that could be easily stripped off the surface of the epithelium (Fig. 6-2). Diphtheritic referred to a pseudomembrane that had in addition to the fibrinous exudate, extensive necrosis of the mucosa, inflammatory cell infiltrate, and associated relatively small areas of ulceration. The close intertwining of the fibrinous exudate and coagulative necrosis of the mucosa resulted in a tough, adherent membrane that on transection resembled a thickened mucosa (Fig. 6-4). It is now clear that the different features of the pseudomembranes represent different stages of the same process and give no clue to the etiologic agent. The characteristics of pseudomembranes refer to the stage or severity of the process rather than to the causative agent, though some agents are more prone to produce one type than the other. Another gross feature of the pseudomembrane is that it tends to be relatively diffuse, and the term is not usually applied to the necrotic debris found in focal ulcers.

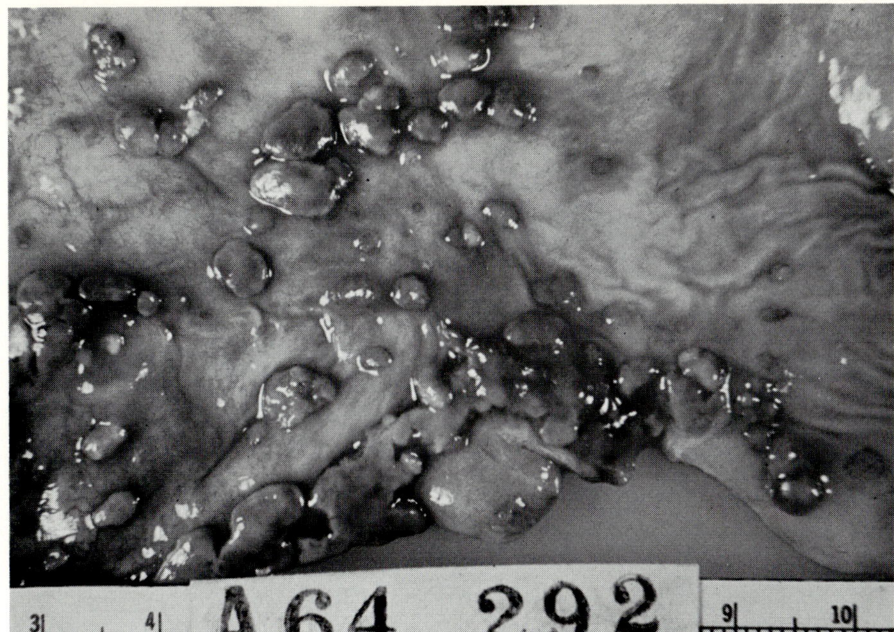

Figure 6–1 Pseudomembranous colitis. This close-up view of a portion of the colon reveals numerous round button-like zones of pseudomembrane projecting from the mucosal surface. This autopsy specimen is from a 50 year old woman who died of renal failure following generalized peritonitis and a prolonged period of hypotension.

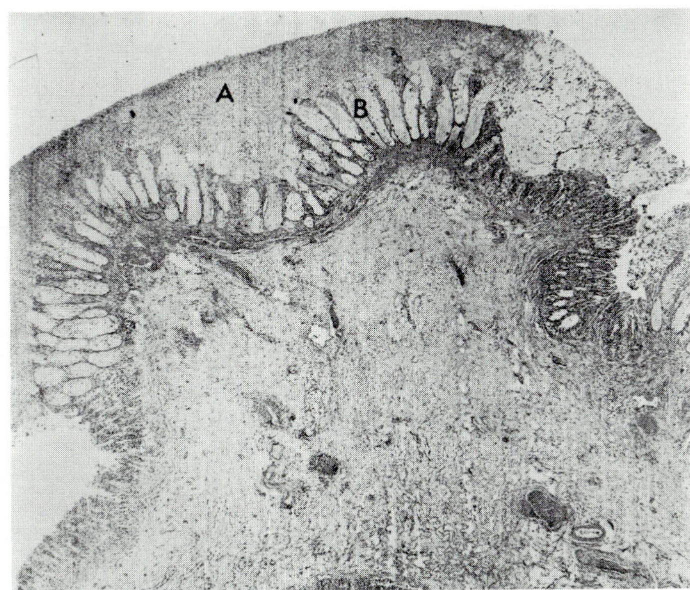

Figure 6–2 Microscopic view of one of the pseudomembranous lesions shown in Figure 6–1. The pseudomembrane (A) is firmly attached to the mucosal surface and crypts of mucus-distended glands (B). Necrosis involves the surface aspect of the mucosa only, and the pseudomembrane consists of a mixture of mucus, fibrin, and necrotic debris. Compare this "croupous" type with the more advanced lesion shown in Figure 6–4. ×16.

157

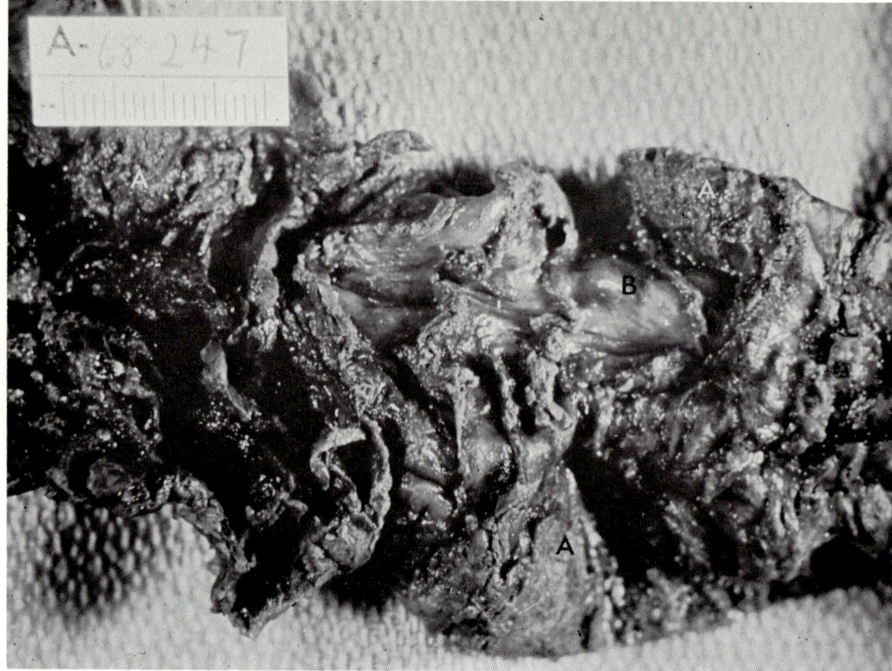

Figure 6-3 Pseudomembranous colitis, severe. Sheets of granular, irregular pseudomembrane (A) are firmly attached to the mucosa and have a friable texture. A small portion of uninvolved mucosa is seen (B). This autopsy specimen is from a 49 year old woman. The anatomic diagnosis was similar to that of the case shown in Figure 6-1.

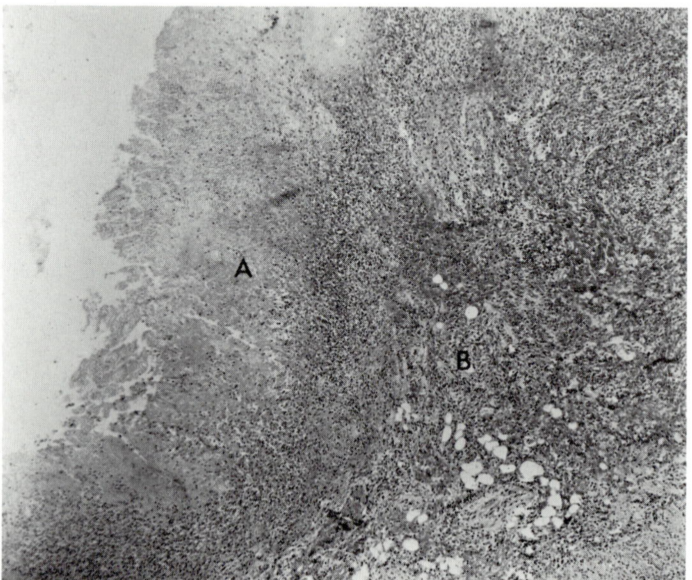

Figure 6-4 Low-power photomicrograph of the lesion shown in Figure 6-3. In this lesion, more extensive than that in Figures 6-1 and 6-2, the entire mucosa is necrotic. The cellular debris is intermixed with large amounts of dense fibrin forming a pseudomembrane (A), of the "diphtheritic" type. Numerous inflammatory cells are seen beneath it in the submucosa (B). ×34.

158

ACUTE LESIONS

Cholera

Studies on the pathogenesis of human cholera in recent years have markedly changed the prevailing conception of the disease produced by *Vibrio comma* infection. These advances have been largely due to the development of an experimental model. Injection of choleragen, a relatively pure extract of the cholera vibrio organism, into isolated loops of newborn rabbit ileum produces a syndrome indistinguishable from human cholera.[1] The model has been exploited by Norris and co-workers to provide a better understanding of the disease process.[2-4] The original concept that the human vibrio produced diarrhea by causing epithelial denudation of the intestinal mucosa resulting in fluid loss is clearly wrong. The light and electron microscopic studies of this

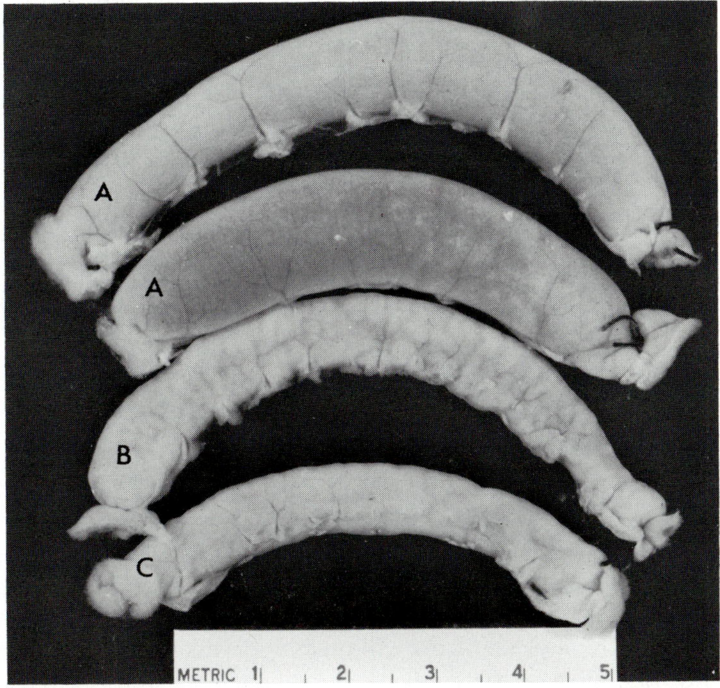

Figure 6-5   Gross specimen of four ileal loops removed from rabbits six hours after instillation of choleragen. One hour prior to sacrifice vascular markers were given intravenously. Two choleraic loops (A) are moderately distended by fluid resembling rice water stool. Control loops (B) and (C) are empty. B received 1 ml. physiologic saline, and C was left empty at laparotomy. There was no extravasation of the dye markers in ileal wall or effluent. (Courtesy of H. T. Norris, and G. Majno, Amer. J. Path. *53*:263-279, 1968, and Harper & Row, Publishers.)

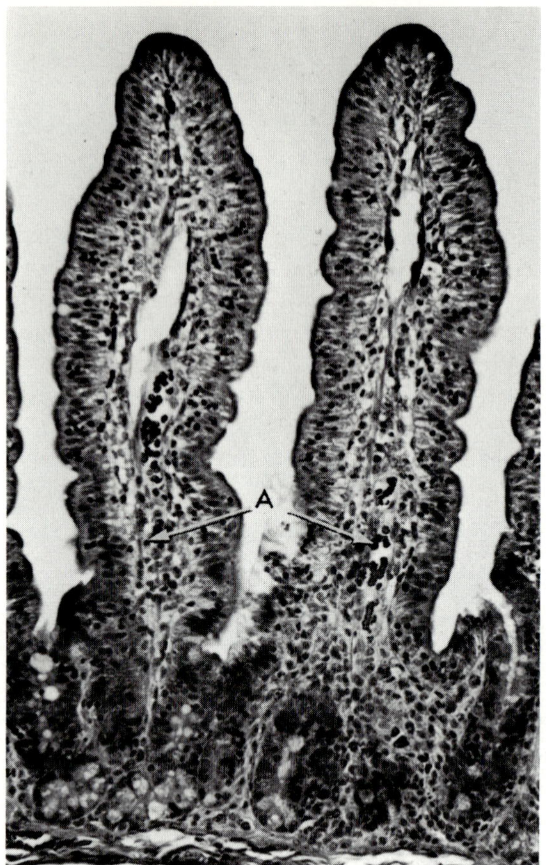

Figure 6-6   Photomicrographs of intestinal mucosa from loops similar to those labeled A in Figure 6-5. The epithelium is completely intact. The villous vasculature (A) is congested, and the central lacteal is dilated. Mucus is decreased in the epithelial cells, otherwise the epithelium is unremarkable. ×200. (Courtesy of H. T. Norris et al., J. Infect. Dis. *117:*193–196, 1967, and the University of Chicago Press.)

group have shown that choleragen did not produce epithelial cell or vascular endothelial morphologic changes, inflammatory cell infiltrate, mesenchymal tissue structural changes, or altered vascular permeability (Figs. 6-5, 6-6, and 6-7). The only demonstrable morphologic changes were minimal hyperemia of the villous blood vessels, increased mucorrhea, and dilatation of the central villous lacteals. Therefore, cholera is a disease at the end of a spectrum of intestinal lesions characterized by minimal morphologic change but maximal clinical signs and symptoms. The cholera vibrio appears to produce its effect by causing the intestinal epithelium to secrete excessive amounts of its usual product through a cellular physiologic mechanism currently being investigated.[4]

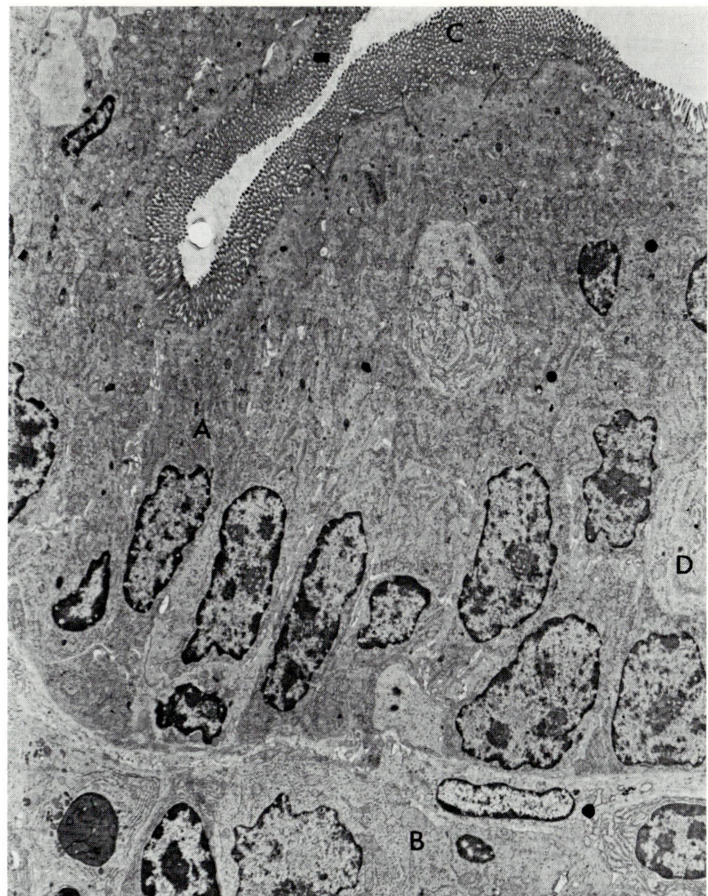

Figure 6–7　Low-power electron microscopic view of an intestinal villus from a choleraic ileal loop, demonstrating the junction between epithelium (A) and underlying lamina propria (B). No discontinuity is present between individual epithelial cells or between the epithelium and the lamina propria. Microvilli (C), and a Paneth cell (D) are shown. ×4,500. (Courtesy H. T. Norris and G. Majno, Amer. J. Path. *53*:263–279. 1968, and Harper & Row, Publishers.)

Nonspecific Acute Inflammations

Resulting from a variety of etiologic agents, the pathologic changes in nonspecific inflammations may range from mucorrhea (catarrhal enteritis) to pseudomembrane formation or, less commonly, ulcerative lesions. When the lesion is principally mucorrheal, the mucosa is grossly red, swollen, hyperemic, and may be covered with circumscribed foci of excessive amounts of mucus. The deeper layers of the bowel wall may be essentially normal. Microscopically one may see only the vascular features of inflammation characterized by hyperemia, edema, and possible exudation of erythrocytes, but no other evidence of inflammatory cell infiltrate. Older studies placed some emphasis on the existence of epithelial cell desquamation; however, recent studies of more carefully fixed material indicate that desquamation is not a feature of the lesion. Hyperplasia of lymphoid tissue in the affected region may be present, though nonspecific in nature, characterized by an increased production of lymphocytes and enlarged germinal centers in the lymphoid follicles. Basophilic inclusions may be seen in some of the histiocytes of the germinal centers. Necrosis of the germinal centers may sometimes occur in very severe cases, usually in relationship to the punctate ulcers of the epithelium.

The cause of acute mucorrhea can be any of a broad spectrum of etiologic agents. With some patients it appears to be a consequence of a psychoneurosis and, when it principally involves the colon, is termed mucous colitis. In other individuals, particularly if it involves the small intestine, it may be secondary to acute alcoholism and is termed acute enteritis. Viral infections have been suspected in cases of so-called "summer diarrhea," whereas in other instances this may be secondary to ingestion of food tainted with staphylococcal toxins. This is particularly seen in warmer climates among persons eating in institutions where foods containing dairy products and eggs are not appropriately stored. When it occurs in infants, newborn or premature, the disease may be life-threatening.

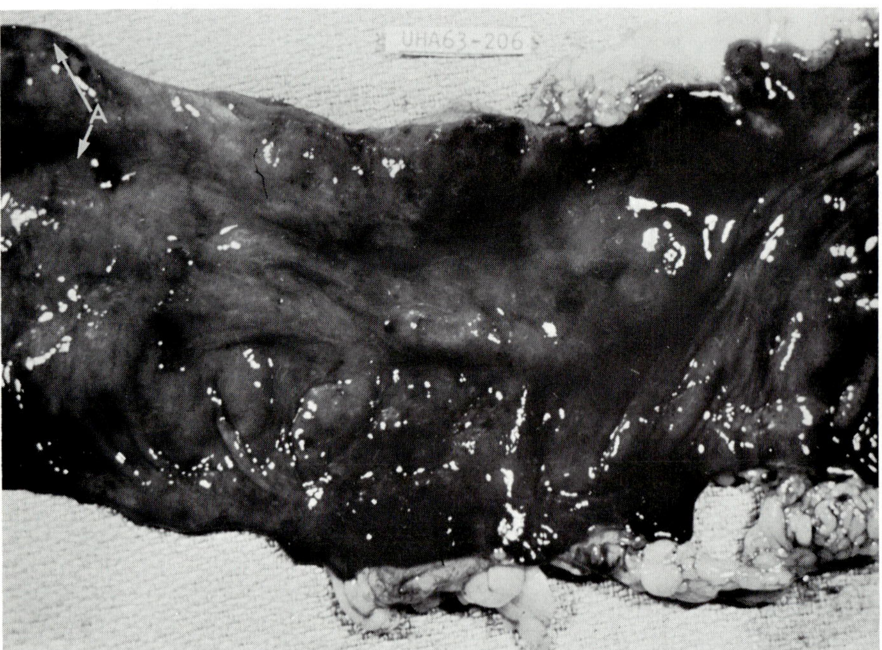

Figure 6–8 Close-up view of the intestinal mucosa at autopsy in a case of severe acute gastroenterocolitis most likely secondary to intensive oral and intravenous antibiotic therapy, though a brief period of hypotension occurred before death. Extensive vascular congestion petechiae and ecchymoses are diffusely present in the intestinal mucosa. Small irregular superficial patches of ulceration are seen (A).

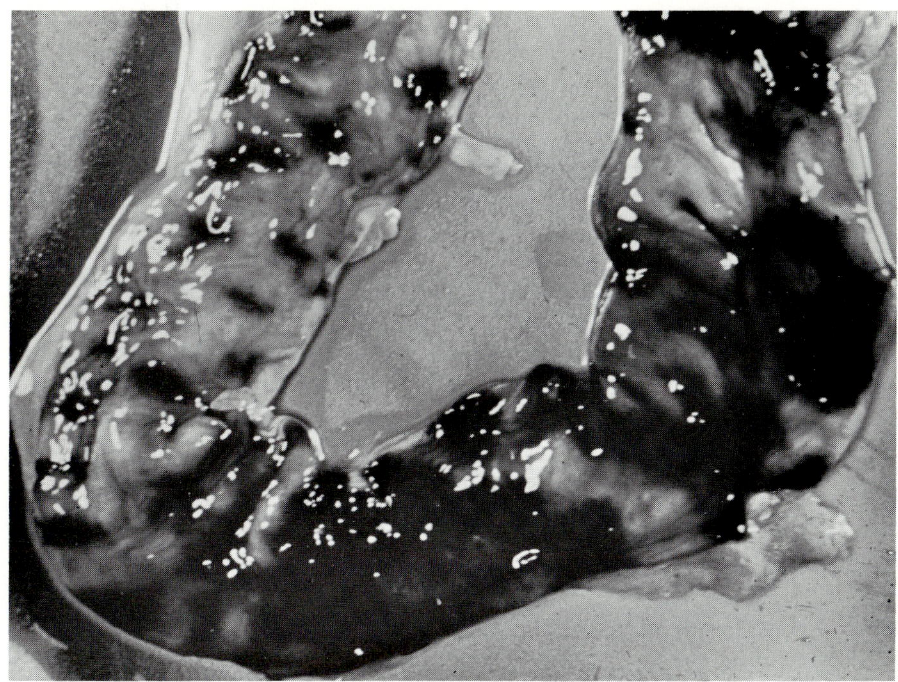

Figure 6–9   Close-up view of the intestinal mucosa at autopsy from another case of acute enterocolitis most likely secondary to intensive antibiotic therapy. Numerous random patchy mucosal ulcers are shown. Congestion and extravasation of blood are seen in the surrounding tissue. Staphylococci were the overwhelmingly predominant organism in immediate postmortem cultures of the intestinal contents.

Acute mucorrheic changes, as already noted, may be the initial phase of the pathogenesis of a more severe type of infection. Bacteria principally of the *Streptococcus, Staphylococcus, Pseudomonas, Shigella, Salmonella,* and *Proteus* groups of organisms have often been isolated from stools of individuals with acute, nonspecific changes. Antibiotic enterocolitis is an increasingly common intestinal inflammation (Figs. 6–8 and 6–9). In recent years use of antibiotics has been found to upset the normal balance of bacterial flora in the intestinal tract, resulting in a disproportionate overgrowth of some, usually *Staphylococcus, Pseudomonas,* or *Proteus.* The imbalance of organisms in the intestinal tract may lead to an acute inflammatory response ranging from a transient mucorrhea to a severe and possibly life-threatening pseudomembranous enterocolitis.

Food Poisoning

Poisoning by the toxin of *Clostridium botulinum* is a most serious intestinal problem with a high risk of mortality, but it causes little if any local intestinal inflammatory change. *C. botulinum* produces one of the most toxic chemicals known, but autopsy studies of individuals who have died from this intoxication reveal surprisingly minimal anatomic change. The entire intestinal tract may be hyperemic with little if any necrosis or other cytopathologic alteration. The mechanism of action appears to be through the autonomic nervous system and its control of muscular and vascular activity in the intestinal tract. As with cholera, referred to previously, the anatomic lesions are surprisingly minimal for these life-threatening diseases. However, in each the mechanism by which the diarrhea is produced is markedly different.

Typhoid Fever

Typhoid fever is an important predominantly ulcerative intestinal inflammation caused by *Salmonella typhi*. Though less frequently seen than in former decades, it still represents an important consideration because some features of its ulcers may be similar to the early lesions of regional enteritis. Though in its initial phases it may have in common the nonspecific intestinal inflammatory changes, very quickly the lesions become localized in the lymphoid tissue of the jejunum and ileum, the solitary follicles and the Peyer's patches. The lymphoid tissue being predominantly concentrated in the terminal portion of the small intestine, a predominantly terminal ileal location for the lesions of typhoid is the result. Though the solitary follicles are located throughout the small intestine, the Peyer's patches are principally located in the terminal portion of the ileum. The evolution of these lesions is characterized by an initial enlargement and congestion of the blood vessels in the lymphatics and secondary enlargement of the more distant lymph nodes and spleen. Bacilli may be found in the lymphoid follicles in addition to the changes of the nonspecific acute mucorrhea throughout the small intestine. The progression of the lesion is centered in the lymphoid tissue, where at first there is an enlargement or hyperplasia of the lymphoid follicles, which grossly are elevated, soft, swollen, and red. Similar kinds of changes have been observed in the earliest lesions of regional enteritis. Grossly, the Peyer's patches stand out as discrete oval structures, and in this phase may on occasion be confused with the changes seen in lymphoma or in leukemic infiltration in the intestinal lymphoid tissue.

Microscopically, the characteristic change in the lymphoid tissue is the presence of numerous large mononuclear cells scattered throughout the sinusoids of the lymph node, coupled with a blood vascular hyperemia. They have the appearance of hyperplastic monocytes or lymphocytes with a rather pronounced cytoplasm that appears reticular or foamy and may, under special bacterial stains, reveal the presence of the infective organism. When the infection is severe in these lymphoid organs, necrosis may ensue. Necrosis at first appears within the lymphoid tissue, but subsequently may extend to the overlying lamina propria and epithelium so that the oval-shaped Peyer's patches become ulcerated lesions with the surface exposed to the lumen of the intestinal tract. When this occurs the ulceration becomes more extensive and secondary invasion of other bacteria occurs. Exudation of polymorphs, lymphocytes, plasma cells, and fibrin may produce a necrotic crust on the surface of the ulcer. One may see up to 30 or 40 ulcers (corresponding to the total number of Peyer's patches) in the terminal portion of the jejunum and ileum. With the superimposition of the acute inflammatory response, principally polymorph infiltration, on the basic typhoid lesions the recognition microscopically may become more difficult, as the proportion of typhoid mononuclear cells becomes diluted by the nonspecific cellular exudate. As the lesion evolves, an attempt to wall off the inflammation ensues so that after five to seven days the ulcerated Peyer's patches are surrounded by granulation tissue. The necrotic portion of the Peyer's patches continues to slough into the lumen of the bowel, and as the lesions are walled off by granulation tissue, the ulcers become saucer-shaped with the concavity filled with necrotic debris. Because the long axes of Peyer's patches are parallel with the long axis of the intestine, the long axes of the oval ulcers are similarly disposed, which is in contrast with other inflammatory diseases of the small intestine that do not particularly involve the Peyer's patches. After a week or more of inflammation, the reparative processes become predominant in the usual course of events. The ulcers become smaller as the granulation tissue closes the wall and its characteristic appearance with granules of punctate developing capillaries surrounded by a rather myxoid connective tissue becomes visible grossly. Epithelial regeneration ensues at the periphery, with hyperplastic, densely staining, non-mucus-secreting epithelial cells growing over the granulation tissue. The subsequent scars remain as rather flattened buttons covered with smooth epithelium, and on microscopic examination the layers of the lamina propria, muscularis mucosa, and submucosa may be bound together in dense, collagenous connective tissue. Occasionally, severe typhoid infection may lead to perforation in which the necrosis is so extensive that it penetrates through the muscular coats and through the serosa into the peritoneal cavity.

Bacillary Dysentery

This type of inflammatory lesion is principally caused by a group of rod-shaped, gram-negative organisms, *Shigella shigae, s. flexneri,* and *s. sonnei.* These are of a lower order of pathogenicity than the typhoid organisms, though the lesions they produce bear some similarities to the typhoid infection. Bacillary dysentery is more common in the tropics than in temperate zones. Like typhoid, it is principally confined in its more advanced stage to the lymphoid tissue of the intestinal tract; however, unlike typhoid, the predominant lesion tends to be in the large rather than the small intestine. Also, the initial or minimal lesion begins with a nonspecific mucorrhea and diffuse nonspecific inflammation of the bowel. As in typhoid, however, the lesions become more confined to the lymphoid tissue, producing "snail-track" ulcerations in the mucosa. In the acute phase, intense hyperemia may be seen with moderate diffuse exudation of polymorphs. Usually most of the colon as well as the distal portion of the ileum may be involved (Fig. 6–10).

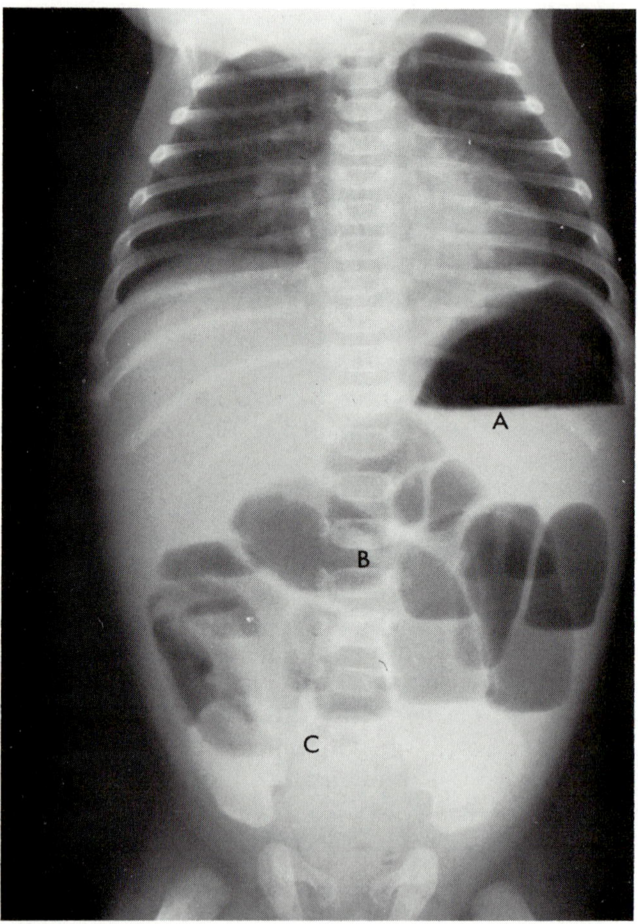

Figure 6–10   Radiograph of the abdomen of an infant with severe *Shigella sonnei* infection. The radiographic findings of paralytic ileus are demonstrated. The stomach is dilated and largely fluid filled (A). Both small and large intestine are also distended and filled with fluid (B). The probable presence of extraluminal gas (C) suggested the possibility of perforation. (Courtesy of Dr. M. M. Figley, Professor and Chairman, Department of Radiology, University of Washington School of Medicine.)

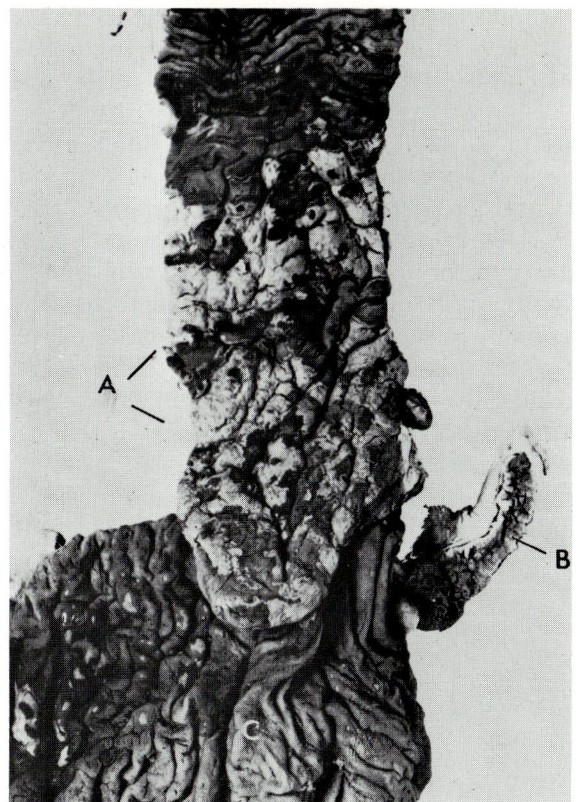

Figure 6–11   Shigellosis. The terminal ileum (A), the appendix (B), and the cecum (C) are shown. The inflammatory lesions are seen in the colon and appendix as well as the terminal ileum. Multifocal irregular, sometimes confluent, ulcers covered with necrotic debris are scattered throughout, producing a thin pseudomembrane.

Following the initial diffuse response, necrosis ensues in the lymphoid tissue of the large intestine, producing an ulcer similar to that described for typhoid. However, the involvement of the lymphoid tissue and the necrosis are seldom as severe as in the usual case of typhoid, and more frequently, especially with the less pathogenic shigella organisms (*s. flexneri* and *s. sonnei*), only the diffuse hyperemia and mild nonspecific inflammation of the mucous membrane may be involved (Fig. 6–11). In these cases, ulceration does not ensue. In the more severe cases of bacillary dysentery, however, chronic ulceration of the colon may occur and persist for a long period. These ulcers may be similar to those seen in amebic dysentery. Microscopically, one sees a mononuclear infiltrate in the lymphoid tissue as well as in the perilymphatic region that consists of enlarged macrophages of the hyperplastic type, which can on occasion, because of their size, be confused with amebas. When ulceration occurs, the process of repair is comparable to that described for typhoid. Extravasation of blood is frequently seen in the submucosa, and large zones of coagulation necrosis of the mucosa may also be present superficial to the developing granulation tissue. Secondary infection of these lesions does not occur unless ulceration eventuates.

The lesion of bacillary dysentery must be differentiated from those of ulcerative colitis and amebic dysentery (Figs. 5–41 and 5–46). The ulcers of bacillary dysentery, when present, occur on the free edges of the transverse folds of the mucous membrane and are usually distributed transversely to the long axis of the gut (Fig. 6–11). Only rarely are they serpentine in outline, with ragged edges that are undermined in a manner similar to ulcerative colitis. The bases of these ulcers are predominantly granulation tissue with a collagenogenic response, which is also in contrast to ulcerative colitis. The prevalence of the granulation tissue response, with its characteristic veil of young capillaries and a mucoid kind of connective tissue producing a saucer-shaped circumscribed button, distinguishes these ulcers from those of ulcerative colitis. Microscopically, the nonulcerated lesion differs from ulcerative colitis in centering on the lymphoid tissue and lacking crypt abscesses, but is similarly restricted to the superficial layers.

Amebic Dysentery

A third type of lesion that may resemble ulcerative colitis and must be differentiated from it is amebic dysentery. As with other dysenteries, this lesion centers in the colon, though scattered ulcers may occur in the terminal part of the ileum occasionally. The initial lesion of amebic dysentery is a minute yellow spherical elevation in the mucosa that appears as a small mucosal cyst and is the surface of a deep-lying focus of necrosis produced by the invading protozoan. Indeed, the base of this flask-shaped cyst, the surface of which is visible on the mucosal aspect, may be adjacent to or within the submucosa. These punctate lesions, the surface of which is frequently ulcerated, may be scattered throughout the large intestine. Following ulceration and the extension of the lesion laterally, it may become 2 or 3 cm. in diameter and rarely larger. The undermining of the lateral margins produces a rolled edge, and the base may be covered with a necrotic char. Occasionally the necrotic char and fibrin may be sufficiently extensive to project luminally through the relatively small opening of the ulcer. The lesions usually predominate in the cecum and tend to diminish in frequency in the more distal portions of the colon. Microscopically, the lesion centers in the lamina propria and submucosa, producing a gelatinous necrosis of the connective tissues. It is within these necrotic zones that the lesion may become secondarily invaded by bacteria, and its characteristic features be destroyed.

Though the necrosis is relatively extensive, a surprisingly scanty inflammatory cell infiltrate is present, usually lymphocytes, until the secondary invasion occurs. This is in sharp contrast with regional enteritis, which has a massive cellular infiltrate, even in the early lesion. The additional feature that distinguishes amebic dysentery from ulcerative colitis is the presence of the ameba, and the diagnosis cannot be made without its identification. Special stains may be employed to assist in this differentiation. However, even on conventional hematoxylin and eosin stains, the amebas appear as large cells of approximately 35 microns in diameter (about three to five times the diameter of an erythrocyte) (Fig. 6–12). The nucleus may be eccentrically placed. Because a characteristic feature is the ingestion of red blood cells, their presence in the cytoplasm of the ameba is one of the principal distinguishing features. However, one must be cautious to distinguish between amebas and macrophages, which may simulate them. Frequently the amebas are seen not only in the zone of necrosis at the base of the flask-shaped ulcer, but also in surrounding lymphatic and blood vessels. Indeed, thrombosis of the blood vessels may be a prominent feature at the base of the ulcers. Necrosis involving arterioles may produce foci of relatively severe hemorrhage.

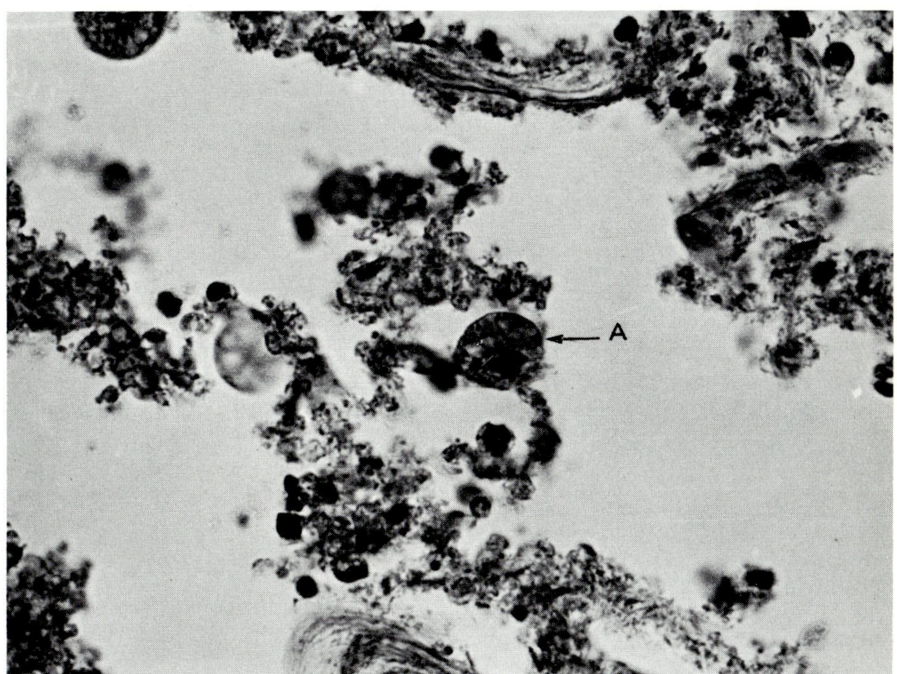

Figure 6–12 Amebic colitis. Within a submucosal abscess, necrotic debris and inflammatory cells are seen. One of many ameba (A) is shown here. ×200.

Vascular Lesions

Acute focal or diffuse ulcerations of the ileum and colon may occur as a result of vascular insufficiency. Periarteritis nodosa, which frequently obstructs arterioles and venules as they enter the intestinal wall, may produce a circumscribed ulcerated lesion in the mucosa and submucosa at the area of distribution of the involved vessel. The vascular wall inflammation and subsequent thrombosis may compromise the blood supply to multiple segments of the intestine, producing well-circumscribed ischemic ulcerations with elevated, rolled borders. Two cases have been reported in which an ulcerative colitis-like lesion occurred in relation to systemic lupus erythematosus.[5] During the past 20 years many surgeons have ligated the inferior mesenteric artery in the course of the management of carcinoma of the colon or aortic aneurysms, thus producing an ischemic lesion in the bowel as an undesired complication of the operation.[6] At first the lining of the bowel is edematous and hemorrhagic and soon ulcerates but does not have the "red velvet" appearance of ulcerative colitis. Necrosis of the mucosa ensues. It is friable, and petechial hemorrhages occur. With repair the ulcer is replaced by collagen-rich scar tissue that ultimately contracts, producing a stricture.

Morson has extensively studied the pathologic appearance of acute ischemic colitis in adults.[7] He observed that usually the two salient gross features of the external surface of the large intestine are dilatation of the colon and a thickened, friable wall. The mucosa may be extensively denuded in patches, or the extent of the lesion may be circumscribed. Unlike ulcerative colitis it may be sharply segmental in distribution. Vascular congestion with or without demonstrable thrombosis may be prominent. Microscopically, broad areas of necrosis may be seen associated with extensive capillary congestion, extravasation of blood, and intravascular thrombosis. The necrosis may extend into the muscularis. These features of the acute lesion are essentially the same as those seen with infarction of the small intestine.

At later stages, varying amounts of reparative change may be present. Capillary and fibroblast-rich granulation tissue may be seen at the edges of the necrotic zone that eventually produces fibrous scars and stricture. It is quite easy to distinguish both the early and late lesions from those of ulcerative colitis and regional enteritis in the colon.

Recently a series of investigations of necrotizing enterocolitis, probably ischemia caused, in the newborn have been reported from the University of Washington.[8, 9] The clinical and pathologic features of neonatal necrotizing enterocolitis were studied in 21 surgically treated cases and in 13 autopsies of premature infants who died as a consequence of the respiratory distress syndrome. In most instances the colonic lesion was rapidly progressive and led to free perforation, sepsis, shock, and death unless operated upon. The lesions were located predominantly in the lower ileum, cecum, and ascending colon. The earliest lesions were marked broadening of the mucosal villi because of severe capillary and venule congestion. The interstitium was infiltrated with mononuclear cells. Hemorrhage into the lamina propria was accompanied by sloughing of the epithelium (Figs. 6-13, 6-14, and 6-15). The denuded areas were covered with fibrin, necrotic debris, and inflammatory cells. No vasculitis or thrombosis was found. Though final proof of a hypoxic etiology is lacking, the presumptive evidence is overwhelming. In the autopsy study, pulmonary immaturity was seen in all cases.[9] Those infants who had pulmonary hyaline membranes had died within three days of delivery, whereas those who died later did not have demonstrable membranes.

A diffuse membranous inflammatory response may occur in the colon or terminal intestinal tract as a consequence of restriction of the blood supply from a variety of causes. Hypotension may lead to a coagulation necrosis of the mucosa with subsequent acute inflammatory response, and repair may lead to a diffuse membranous change with the gross microscopic features just described.

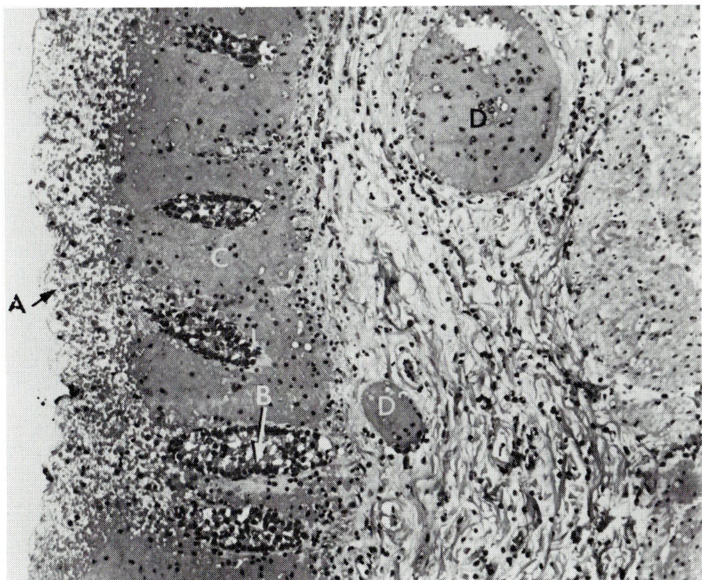

Figure 6-13 Neonatal necrotizing enterocolitis. Intestinal lumen is to the left. The necrotic mucosa (A) has only a few remaining epithelial cells in the crypts (B). The lamina propria is extensively suffused with erythrocytes (C), capillary congestion is seen (D). ×45. (Courtesy of V. E. Goldenberg, Associate Professor of Pathology, University of Washington School of Medicine.)

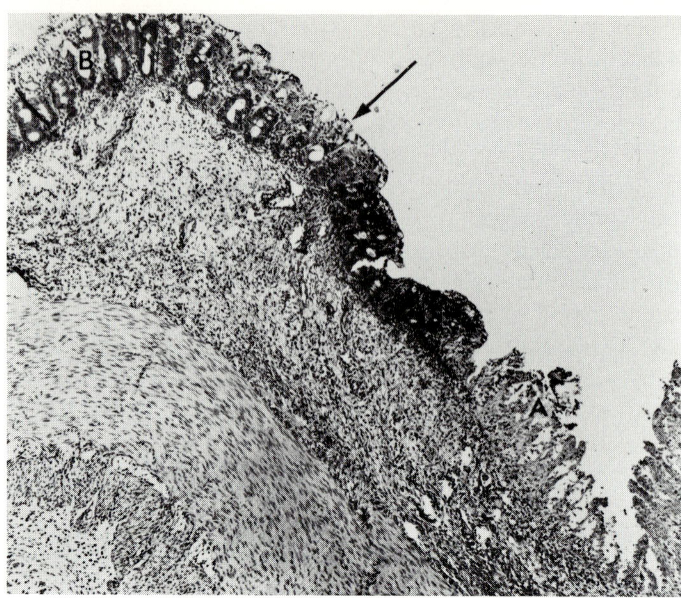

Figure 6–14   Neonatal necrotizing enterocolitis. Another region from the same specimen shown in Figure 6-13. This view is taken from the junction of the necrotizing (A) and the uninvolved (B) colon. The narrow zone of transition (arrow) is shown as well as the superficial distribution of the necrosis. ×45.

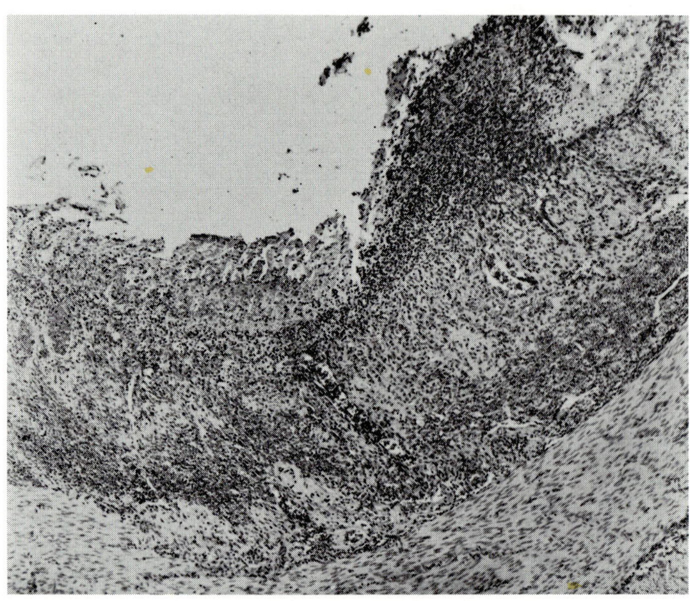

Figure 6–15   Neonatal necrotizing enterocolitis. Another region from the same specimen shown in Figures 6-13 and 6-14. Mucosal erosion and subjacent inflammatory infiltration are noted. ×45.

GRANULOMATOUS LESIONS

Ileocecal Tuberculosis

Indeed a rarity in the United States at present, ileocecal tuberculosis is, however, occasionally seen in Europe. This is in sharp contrast to the situation a century ago when, in 1875, Wilks and Moxon, in their *Lectures on Pathological Anatomy* on "Tubercular Disease and Ulceration of the Intestine," stated, "This is perhaps the commonest form of disease to which the intestine is liable."[10]

The portal of entry into the body of tubercle bacilli does not alter the sequence of events in the intestinal tract. When the primary lesion is in the intestine, the chances are two to one that the bacilli are of the bovine type and were acquired by ingesting contaminated milk. Without pulmonary lesions, the intestinal lesion is virtually certain to be of the bovine type. Of the 30 per cent of cases that involve the intestine that are not of the bovine type, almost all are the product of a miliary spread from pulmonic lesions to the intestines in far-advanced cases. The primary lesion is an ulcer that is usually solitary and quite small. It is usually in the small intestine, principally the terminal ileum, probably related to the concentration of lymphoid tissue at this site. This predilection for the terminal ileum usually represents secondary or miliary spread of tuberculosis from a primary site elsewhere in the body, whereas the primary bovine intestinal tuberculosis may be found in equal distribution from the duodenum to the ileocecal valve, and, less commonly, in the large intestine. The initial complex represents a primary ulcer, rarely seen in pathologic specimens now, and its related primary lymphoidal structure, whether it be a solitary follicle, Peyer's patch, or adjacent small group of mesenteric nodes (Fig. 6-16). Any one or a group of these lymphoid structures may undergo enlargement with the production of the primary complex of a tuberculoma composed of histiocytes, epithelioid cells, Langerhans' giant cells, and a few lymphocytes that soon undergo caseation necrosis in a manner identical with primary pulmonary tuberculosis. In actual experience, except in specialized institutions, one seldom sees the primary ulcerated lesion on the mucosa of the intestine. One may, however, find the lymphoid tissue involvement and with careful search find the site of a healed ulcer in the mucosa overlying the lymphoid tissue. The scar may be very small and inconspicuous and easily overlooked.

With healing of the primary complex in the abdominal lesion, no further extension of the disease may become evident, which is the usual course of events. Indeed, at the autopsy table one frequently finds calcified clusters of lymph nodes associated with the small intestine, which presumably are the tombstone of a previous tuberculous infec-

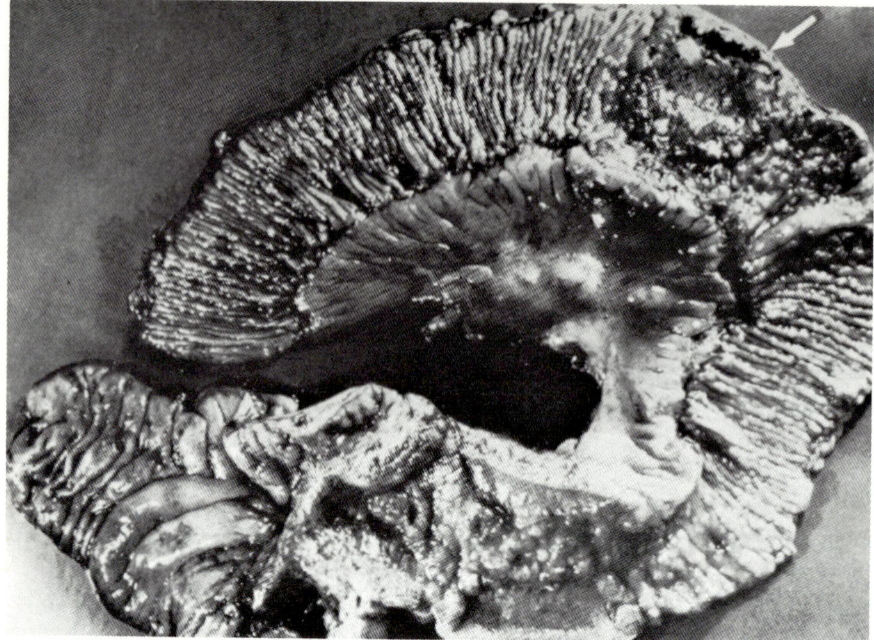

Figure 6–16   Primary tuberculous ileitis. An excavated circumferential ulcer of tuberculosis is shown (arrow). Necrosis, a characteristic of tuberculosis, has produced the saucer-shaped excavation. The granulomatous response has produced a thickened wall, which can be seen at this ulcer and at the larger more distal one. Enlarged lymph nodes project outward from the mesentery. (Courtesy of H. L. Bockus, Amer. J. Med. *27:*509, 1959, and Reuben H. Donnelley Co., New York.)

tion, though one must bear in mind the possibility of mycotic and other types of infections that can also produce calcified lymph nodes. Rarely, the primary lesion may progress to a more extensive ulcerative lesion, in which multiple ulcers of the mucosa of the small and large intestines may be found, which may become chronic and encircle the bowel, producing a cicatrizing stricture. This hypertrophic form of lesion is usually found in the ileocecal region, and may produce a tumor-like mass. More commonly, if the host does not constrain the infectious process, the tuberculoma may extend to the mesenteric lymph nodes and beyond, and rarely produce a tuberculous peritonitis. In this instance the peritoneum may be studded with innumerable tuberculous granulomas.

Sarcoidosis

Sarcoidosis, involving the intestinal lymph nodes, is a third type of granulomatous lesion resembling both ileocecal tuberculosis and regional enteritis. The histologic appearance of the granulomas may be identical with those of tuberculosis or regional enteritis when viewed macroscopically. However, distinction between the lesions may be made both by using stains for acid-fast bacilli and, clinically, the Kveim test. In addition, coagulation necrosis is not a feature of sarcoidosis, whereas it is a characteristic feature of virtually all tuberculous granulomas. A further distinguishing point is that sarcoidosis is rarely if ever limited to the intestinal tract and will characteristically involve extraintestinal tissues. Considering the differential diagnosis between various granulomatous lesions that may affect the small intestine in regional enteritis, one must not overlook the increasingly frequent possibility of fungal infections involving the intestine as the etiologic factor.

Mycotic Infections

Mycotic disease processes such as actinomycosis, histoplasmosis, and coccidioidomycosis may indeed be more frequent causes of small intestinal granulomas than either tuberculosis or sarcoidosis. In an extensive study of granulomas it was found that, excluding oral infections, 70 per cent of *Actinomyces bovis* infections in man involve the ileocecal area.[11] Twenty-five per cent of all actinomycotic lesions occur in this area. Grossly these lesions are separate or confluent hard nodules of granulomatous tissue that on transection reveal central necrosis and pus. Within the pus may sometimes be found the characteristic "sulfur granules," colonies of branching mycelial threads that microscopically have club-shaped ends. Distinguishing microscopic features of these granulomas are central necrosis, colonies of the *Actinomyces*, and intense polymorph infiltrate surrounding the abscesses.

Parasitic Infestations

Among the less common causes of chronic ulcerated lesions in the large or small intestine are helminths. Parasitic infestations of the intestinal tract may be extensive without producing significant anatomic changes in the bowel wall. However, on occasion *Schistosoma* will produce a dysentery coupled with ulceration of the large intestine. These ulcers are few in number, circumscribed, and chronic in nature with an intense fibrosis at their base. The embryonic *Ascaris* as it burrows through the wall of the small intestine to enter the bloodstream may produce ulceration. More commonly, the pinworm *Enterobius vermicularis* is found. This exceedingly common infestation occurs in the upper part of the large intestine, especially the cecum, but may also involve the appendix and terminal ileum. The mature worm at these sites, though usually residing within the lumen of the intestine, may occasionally penetrate the mucosa to produce a cyst in the submucosa, causing chronic inflammatory response with ulceration. Some evidence suggests that approximately 2 per cent of acute appendicitis is caused by these worms.

NEOPLASTIC DISEASES

Membranous enterocolitis is now occasionally seen in patients with advanced neoplastic disease who are under treatment with anticancer drugs. In some instances, the colitis is associated with the invasion of fungi, which can be easily demonstrated in histologic sections. Patients suffering from neoplastic disease of the lymphoma-leukemia group, with special involvement of the intestinal lymphoid structures, may present both the clinical and pathologic appearances of enteritis. The enlarged lymph nodes may simulate the lesions of typhoid fever.

References

1. Benyajati, C.: Experimental cholera in humans. Brit. Med. J. *1:*140-142, 1966.
2. Norris, H. T., Schultz, S. G., Curran, P. F., and Finkelstein, R. A.: Active sodium transport across rabbit ileum in experimental cholera induced by choleragen. J. Infect. Dis. *117:*193-196, 1967.
3. Norris, H. T., and Majno, G.: On the role of the ileal epithelium in pathogenesis of experimental cholera. Amer. J. Path. *53:*263-279, 1968.
4. Norris, H. T., Curran, P. F., and Schultz, S. G.: Modification of intestinal secretion in experimental cholera. J. Infect. Dis. *119:*117-125, 1969.
5. Brown, C. H., Haserick, J. R., and Shirey, E. K.: Chronic ulcerative colitis with systemic lupus erythematosus. Cleveland Clin. Quart. *23:*43-46, 1956.
6. Bernstein, W. C., and Bernstein, E. F.: Ischemic ulcerative colitis following inferior mesenteric arterial ligation. Dis. Colon Rectum *6:*54-61, 1963.
7. Morson, B. C.: Histopathology of ischemic enterocolitis. Proc. Roy. Soc. Med. *59:*889-890, 1966.
8. Stevenson, J. K., Graham, C. B., Oliver, T. K., Jr., and Goldenberg, E. E.: Neonatal necrotizing enterocolitis. A report of twenty-one cases with fourteen survivors. Amer. J. Surg. *118:*260-272, 1969.
9. Hopkins, G. B., Gould, V. E., Stevenson, J. K., and Oliver, T. K., Jr.: Necrotizing enterocolitis in premature infants. A clinical and pathologic evaluation of autopsy material. Amer. J. Dis. Child. *120:*229-232, 1970.
10. Wilks, S., and Moxon, W.: Lectures on Pathological Anatomy. 2nd Ed. London, J. and A. Churchill Ltd., 1875, p. 414.
11. Palumbo, L. T.: Nonspecific granuloma. J. Iowa Med. Soc. *38:*6-9, 1948.

Chapter Seven

Extraintestinal Lesions of Regional Enteritis

The intestinal pathology of regional enteritis has attracted much attention from descriptive morphologists. Relatively few reports are available regarding the secondary intestinal and nonintestinal lesions. Collection of necropsy data has been scant, perhaps because regional enteritis in the acute phase is not a common cause of death and postmortem examinations have been scattered and not accumulative. The major study of the secondary lesions, as revealed by autopsy, reviewed all the pathologic anatomic material at the Mayo Clinic for the period of 1923 to 1954.[1] Selected on the basis of clinical history and histologic examination for the characteristic small bowel, mesentery, and lymph node lesions of regional enteritis, 39 cases formed the basis of the report. Of these, 27 were males and 12 were females. Age at the time of death ranged from 14 to 65 years with an average of 54 years. Duration of symptoms prior to death ranged from six months to 19 years with an average duration of 5 years. Generalized peritonitis was the immediate cause of death of approximately half the patients, whereas the remainder died as a consequence of pneumonia, congestive heart failure, uremia, adrenal infarction, and sepsis. Thirty-six per cent of the patients had fistulous tracts, of which 21 per cent were internal, 10 per cent external, and 5 per cent both internal and external. In all the patients reported, the primary pathologic process involved the terminal ileum, there was jejunal involvement as well in five patients. One patient had a primary lesion in the duodenum and stomach. Thirty-eight per cent of these patients also had the primary regional enteritis pathologic process extending to the colon, principally in the cecum and ascending colonic areas. Two cases also had lesions in the colon that were compatible with concurrent ulcerative colitis. The findings that follow are primarily derived from this study, but data from other less extensive studies are referred to as well.

LIVER LESIONS

The liver was more frequently involved by pathologic changes than any other organ in the study by Chapin and co-workers.[1] Fatty change was the most common finding and was present in approximately 51 per cent of their cases. In an attempt to grade the severity of the fatty change, from minimal to severe, the majority was recorded as moderate to severe. Focal necrosis was the next most common lesion of the liver, being found in 36 per cent of the autopsies. It consisted of small scattered foci of necrosis of liver cells throughout the liver lobules. In most of these there was an accompanying acute inflammatory cell infiltrate consisting principally of polymorphs, though a few had principally lymphocytic and histiocytic infiltrates. In 36 per cent of the cases leukocytic infiltration of the periportal areas occurred and consisted principally of lymphocytes. Three of the cases had histopathologic features of portal cirrhosis, with characteristic fibrosis and nodular regeneration. Large granulomas of the type seen in the primary intestinal lesions of regional enteritis were found in four autopsies. These were negative for acid-fast organisms.

What is the significance of these liver lesions? Though perhaps not seen as frequently as in ulcerative colitis, the fatty changes in the liver in about half the cases, focal necrosis in approximately a third, and cirrhosis in three, suggest that either a dietary nutritional deficiency or a toxic product absorbed from the intestine may be involved in some long-standing cases. Those that were found to have fatty change and focal necrosis had no prior evidence of functional impairment as demonstrated by liver function tests. The existence of peritonitis could not be related to the changes because it was present in as many patients without peritonitis as it was in those with peritonitis. Rappaport found seven cases of fatty liver in 17 autopsies from the Armed Forces Institute of Pathology.[31] Others have reported the necropsy findings of seven regional enteritis cases from a series of 112 patients reviewed.[2] They found hepatic amyloidosis in one, congestion and fatty infiltration in four, and biliary cirrhosis in two cases. Monto reported the liver findings in four autopsy cases of regional enteritis, one of which had a clinical history of icterus.[3] Three of the four livers showed fatty change to varying degrees with some portal cirrhosis and periportal inflammatory cell infiltrate.

In contrast to the prevalence of fatty change and cirrhosis in the necropsy liver specimens, Kleckner performed liver needle biopsies on 20 consecutive patients with regional enteritis.[4] In all but three of these patients the disease was confined exclusively to the ileum; in two of the three the disease involved the entire small intestine and in the other, the duodenum as well. Fourteen of the cases had the diagnosis confirmed by abdominal surgery. In none was there clinical or laboratory evidence of hepatic disease. In 17 of the 20 patients no evidence of hepatic lesions was found in the biopsy specimens. The average duration of symptoms in the 17 cases was approximately three years. In three patients (two with intestinal lesions restricted to the ileum and one whose disease involved the entire small intestine), the liver biopsies disclosed fatty infiltration; in only one was it regarded as moderately severe. The duration of symptoms in the three cases averaged four years. The author contrasted the sparsity of hepatic disease associated with regional enteritis with its frequency in ulcerative colitis. In his own series of 32 patients with ulcerative colitis, 9 had various grades of fatty infiltration of the liver demonstrated by needle biopsy.

A second type of liver lesion associated with regional enteritis that is of particular pathogenetic significance is the presence within the liver of granulomas of the type commonly seen in the ileum. Warren and Sommers, in their study of 120 cases of regional enteritis, observed 2 with one or more granulomas in the liver.[5] Morphologically they closely resembled those seen in the intestine; a cluster of histiocytes and giant cells of the foreign body and Langerhans type was surrounded by an infiltrate of lymphocytes and plasma cells. Chapin also observed four cases with granulomas in the liver, of which one was of the characteristic type and three were described as small subcapsular healed tubercles.[1] To this Maurer, Hughes, and Folley added an unusual case of a 38 year old white man who had suffered from regional enteritis for 15 years.[6] At operation it was observed that the gallbladder and biliary tract were normal. Scattered throughout the liver were focal granulomas consisting of epithelioid cells and giant cells without areas of necrosis, most of them rimmed by lymphocytes and plasma cells. Histologic preparations to demonstrate fungi or acid-fast organisms were negative. Rappaport found one hepatic granuloma in the 140 cases he reviewed from the Veterans' Administration and the Armed Forces Institute of Pathology.[31] Comfort and co-workers also observed one case of liver granuloma in their series.[7] The data are insufficient to calculate the incidence of liver granulomas in regional enteritis. One may anticipate that it would approximate 5 to 10 per cent of regional enteritis cases if adequate liver samples were examined.

Liver abscess as a secondary lesion of regional enteritis is surprising because of its rarity. One case is reported of a 43 year old white man with known regional enteritis who was admitted with the chief complaint of fever, shaking chills, and severe sweating.[8] At operation a large abscess cavity was found in the right lobe of his liver, and a total of 500 ml. of pus was evacuated. This was the only case of pylephlebitis and liver abscess secondary to regional ileitis in the extensive experience at a large New York hospital. The authors reviewed the literature for suppurative pylephlebitis since 1940 and found 79 cases. Theirs was the eightieth. Seventy per cent were caused by appendiceal inflammation, and the remainder by a wide variety of inflammatory diseases of the intestinal tract, such as diverticulitis, ulcerative colitis, perforated carcinoma, pancreatitis, perforated duodenal ulcer, typhoid fever, pyosalpinx, omphalitis, and schistosomiasis and by procedures such as hemorrhoidectomy. It is curious that acute appendicitis coupled with perforation and periappendiceal abscess represents the most frequent cause of pylephlebitis, whereas its association with regional enteritis is so rare. More recently, case reports have added three more examples of liver abscesses complicating regional enteritis.[9, 10]

Sclerosing cholangitis occurs rarely as a sequel to regional enteritis but is frequently associated with ulcerative colitis. In an extensive correlative study it was found that 7 of 20 consecutive cases of sclerosing cholangitis were secondary to regional enteritis or ulcerative colitis, 6 of them the latter.[11] The cause of the cholangitis remains unknown; however, it occurs with sufficient frequency with ulcerative lesions of the small and large intestines to suggest the diagnosis. Indeed, ulcerative colitis was the second most common cause of sclerosing cholangitis. A case of sclerosing cholangitis occurring 11 years after the onset of regional enteritis has been recorded.[12]

PANCREATIC LESIONS

The pancreatic lesions are of two types. In 15 cases (38 per cent) Chapin and co-workers found interlobular and periductal fibrosis to a moderate degree.[1] It was severe in only one patient who also had an associated cholecystitis. A second prominent pancreatic lesion was acinar dilatation that consisted of expansion of the individual pancreatic acini; an acidophilic material was present in the cyst-like lumen in 31 per cent of the patients. Though the pathogenetic mechanism remains unknown, it has been shown experimentally that dilatation of pancreatic acini is an accompaniment of nutritional derangement due to a variety of causes, as well as to uremia.

MISCELLANEOUS LESIONS AT AUTOPSY

Thrombosis of the portal vein was seen in four cases by Chapin.[1] These also had an associated acute infarction of the liver. Focal cortical necrosis of the adrenal glands was found in six patients, and thrombosis of the adrenal vessels was noted in three. Thrombosis represents a major problem in regional enteritis; eight (21 per cent) of the patients in this series had thrombotic problems. Only half of these had associated peritonitis; thus, no correlation with the peritonitis was evident. One patient had bilateral thrombosis of the central adrenal veins with bilateral infarction. Congestion of the spleen was noted in approximately half the cases. The heart and lungs were carefully examined for granulomatous lesions of the Boeck's sarcoid type; however, none were found. Mild nonspecific changes in the kidney, consisting of an endothelial proliferation in the glomeruli, were seen in approximately a third of the cases and proximal tubular degeneration and necrosis in about a third. These changes are nonspecific and are associated with many types of acute and chronic inflammatory processes. Other findings in the study by Chapin and co-workers include one case with severe pyoderma gangrenosum and two with generalized secondary amyloidosis of the kidneys, adrenals, and liver. Prior to death, 23 patients had an anemia varying from moderate to severe. Macrocytosis was frequently seen.

SKIN LESIONS

The existence of skin manifestations as an associated feature of regional enteritis has been long known.[13] A case was reported of regional enteritis with granulomatous involvement of the perianal area of the perineum that also had granulomatous involvement of the skin of the groin. Another case report described perianal ulceration, ulcers of the groin, and one beneath the right breast in a 70 year old woman with regional enteritis.[15] Biopsy of the skin lesion showed the characteristic granulomas and chronic inflammation of regional enteritis.

Extensive study of the dermatologic manifestations of regional enteritis has recently been reported by McCallum and Kinmont.[16] They reviewed 138 cases of regional enteritis, the records of which were submitted to them by physicians in the Nottingham and Derby regions of England. Of the 138 cases studied, 44 per cent were found to have skin lesions. These they dividied into two categories: (1) Those that were direct extensions of the disease process in having the characteristic granulomatous histologic picture and (2) two types of vascular reactions of the skin. Of the 60 skin manifestations in their first group, perianal ulceration, ischiorectal abscesses, and fistula-in-ano accounted for 25. Ulcerations or fistulas or both on the anterior abdominal wall and related to operative procedures in the treatment of regional enteritis accounted for 28. Involvement of the skin of the groin and submammary region was found in 2 and granulomas of the buttocks were found in 1. Thus, the overwhelming proportion of skin manifestations of regional enteritis in this study was essentially in association with lesions of the gastrointestinal tract.

Of the vascular skin reaction group in the same study, one case of erythema nodosum and one of pyoderma gangrenosum were recorded.[16] A case of pyoderma gangrenosum in a 19 year old girl with regional enteritis has been reported.[17] The patient presented with erythematous tender nodules on both lower limbs; one of them progressed to form a small discharging ulcer that healed in about six weeks with local therapy. Six months later an ulcer formed on the left calf, beginning again as a number of small erythematous nodules that became confluent and necrotic. The biopsy examination of the ulcer edge showed a slit-like abscess with deeply undermined edges. Most of the lesion was located deep in the dermis. At the center of the ulcer was a zone of purulent inflammation surrounded by an area of giant cells. No active arteritis was seen, and cultures of the biopsy specimen failed to reveal acid-fast bacilli or other pathogen. These ulcers healed under local treatment. One year later, regional enteritis was diagnosed, and surgical excision of the terminal 30 cm. of ileum and 61 cm. of small intestine proximal to it, as well as the cecum and a portion of the ascending colon, was performed. An abscess was present in the mass of adherent small bowel loops, and two fistulous tracts were present within this mass. One month following discharge from the hospital, steroids were discontinued; one week later there was a recurrence of the skin lesion on the posterior aspect of the left calf, which increased rapidly in size until it became soft, raised, and red with a deep central ulceration. Over the subsequent two months increasing numbers of these skin lesions appeared in the vicinity.

Erythema nodosum is a more frequent accompaniment of regional enteritis than pyoderma gangrenosum. Van Patter described five cases of the former and one of the latter in 600 patients with regional enteritis.[18] Crohn and Yarnis reported seven cases of erythema nodosum in a series of 542 patients with regional enteritis, but did not record pyoderma gangrenosum.[19] Perry and Brunsting also described a case of pyoderma gangrenosum in association with regional enteritis.[20] One may estimate that 1 to 5 per cent of regional enteritis patients will have erythema nodosum or pyoderma gangrenosum.

JOINT LESIONS

Though the autopsy studies of Chapin et al. and of Rappaport do not mention joint lesions, probably because it is not customary to investigate the joints in autopsies, arthritis is now a well-recognized feature of regional enteritis, though certainly not as prevalent as it is in ulcerative colitis.[1, 31] The joint lesions are principally of two types: migratory polyarthritis and ankylosing spondylitis. Histologic verification of the former in regional enteritis is wanting, therefore only some brief clinical comments are included here. Ford and Vallis recorded the clinical course of arthritis associated with ulcerative colitis and regional enteritis.[21] They reported only four patients with regional enteritis who ranged in age from 30 to 47. One presented with a chronic polyarthritis involving most joints of the body that lasted for five years and subsided slowly after bowel resection. X-rays revealed a chronic active residual arthritis in the right wrist. Another patient had polyarthritis of the right knee and left elbow on two occasions within three months without residual changes. Another patient had two attacks of subacute peripheral arthritis with no residual at this site; however, x-rays revealed a blurring of the sacroiliac joints. Their fourth patient developed ankylosing spondylitis without peripheral joint disease with a residual of moderate rigidity of the spine.

Acheson clearly established the association between ankylosing spondylitis and regional enteritis.[22] He obtained data on 2,320 male patients, discharged from 174 Veterans' Administration hospitals with a diagnosis of regional enteritis or ulcerative colitis during 1956 and 1957. A total of 54 cases of ankylosing spondylitis was found in this group. The minimum evidence required for the diagnosis of ankylosing spondylitis was radiologic demonstration of bilateral disease of the sacroiliac joints, namely, the loss of definition or regularity of the joint spaces with subchondral eburnation. For controls, information was also collected from cases of two chronic diseases with an age distribution similar to those of regional enteritis, Hodgkin's disease and multiple sclerosis.

Seventeen of a total 742 cases of regional enteritis had ankylosing spondylitis (2.3 per cent). This incidence was compared with that of ankylosing spondylitis in patients of a similar age distribution with diagnoses such as Hodgkin's disease and multiple sclerosis, all with medical and surgical discharges. The association with regional enteritis proved to be 20 times greater than with other diseases in a 25 per cent systematic sample of all patients admitted to the general medical-surgical beds of the Veterans' Administration hospitals. In 675 admissions for Hodgkin's disease, ankylosing spondylitis was not encountered. Only two instances of the disease were found in 813 cases of multiple sclerosis. Also supporting the association and militating against the bias of possible awareness of the connection of joint diseases with regional enteritis, 14 of the cases with ankylosing spondylitis had been diagnosed before the abdominal condition was diagnosed. Acheson was able to uncover two cases of ankylosing spondylitis associated with regional enteritis in the literature prior to his study. Bowen and Kirsner reviewed all types of arthritis that may occur with ulcerative colitis and regional enteritis.[23] They noted that arthritis occurred less frequently with regional enteritis, ranging from 3 to 10 per cent, in contrast with ulcerative colitis. Also, the incidence of ankylosing spondylitis in 1 to 2 per cent of regional enteritis patients was less than in ulcerative colitis, in which it ranges up to 25 per cent. Others have reported similar findings.[24]

The peripheral migratory arthritis seen with regional enteritis is characterized by a clinical picture of asymmetrical reversible inflammation of large joints, chiefly knees, hips, and ankles. Although any single joint or combination of joints may be affected, the arthritis less frequently involves the smaller joints of the hands and feet. The severity of the inflammation varies and is not always proportional to the severity of the inflammatory bowel disease, nor is it related to the age of the patient. Very frequently the joint inflammation may be so intense as to result in rupture of the joint capsule with drainage of sterile, purulent contents followed by complete repair. Cases have been reported in which regional enteritis presents as acute arthritis.[25]

AMYLOIDOSIS

In 1948, Olsan and Sussman and, in 1949, Cohen and Fishman reported what appears to be the first recognition of regional enteritis as a cause of secondary amyloidosis.[26, 27] Since then there have been relatively few cases reported. Unless pathologists have the possibility of amyloidosis in mind and utilize special procedures to reveal the deposits they will quite likely overlook many cases with moderate or slight infiltration. It is quite likely that the reports in the literature are deceptively sparse because of these oversights.

When amyloidosis is suspected a large array of tests is available to confirm its presence. When seen with hematoxylin-eosin stains it appears as an amorphous eosinophilic, waxy hyaline, extracellular substance that may occur widely distributed in the body. At the autopsy table added evidence for suspected deposits may be obtained by use of Virchow's iodine solution and dilute sulfuric acid staining procedure. A blue-purple color is presumptive evidence of an amyloid deposit, though false negatives sometimes occur with the procedure. Amyloid stains metachromatically with both crystal violet and Congo red. The unique green birefringence of the latter stain, when stained sections are viewed with polarized light, provides perhaps the most convenient and useful confirmatory test for amyloid. The Van Gieson stain, which colors amyloid a light tan, is especially useful with amyloids associated with multiple myeloma, which often are Congo red negative. Amyloids fluoresce when stained with thioflavine-T, but a wide variety of substances react similarly, and further work on the parameters of its specificity is needed. Of course, a major aid in confirming the presence of amyloids is the electron microscope, which reveals characteristic nonbranching fibrils of amyloid.[28] For general information about amyloidosis the reader is referred to a recent review by Cohen.[29]

Though amyloidosis is a frequent sequel to chronic necrotizing granulomatous diseases such as tuberculosis, it appears to be much less frequent with nonsuppurative granulomatous disease such as regional enteritis. Werther and co-workers reviewed all autopsies of patients who died as a result of regional enteritis at a New York hospital over a 20 year period.[30] Of the 17 cases autopsied, 4 had amyloidosis. Chapin's compilation of autopsies, referred to earlier, had two instances of amyloidosis in 39 autopsies of patients who died with regional enteritis. I have been able to find 14 case reports in the literature, which are summarized in Table 7-1. Study of these cases reveals that the distribution of amyloids was predominantly of the secondary type with principal involvement of the adrenals, kidneys, liver, and spleen. Blood vessel walls throughout various internal organs were also very frequently infiltrated. The presence of amyloids did not correlate well with the clinical features of the disease. The age range was variable from 20 to 70, and the duration of regional enteritis symptoms was 4 to 25 years. Chronic suppuration and fistulas were absent in many of the cases. About half the patients died as a result of adrenal or renal failure due to amyloid infiltration of these organs.

Other extraintestinal sequelae of regional enteritis occur in special circumstances. Children and adolescents who incur the disease are often retarded in growth and development. In adults and children alike, bone marrow and peripheral blood changes characteristic of the

TABLE 7–1   Amyloidosis and Regional Enteritis

First Author	Year	No. of Cases	Duration of Symptoms (Years)	Severity of R.E.	Distribution of Amyloid	
					Severe	*Moderate*
Olson[26]	1948	1	10	(not recorded)	Spleen Kidneys Adrenals	Thyroid Heart
Cohen[27]	1949	1	14	1+	Adrenals Kidneys Blood vessels	Bone marrow Spleen Pancreas Urogenital tract
Hirst[32]	1953	1	4	(not recorded)	Adrenals Kidney Liver Blood vessels	Spleen
Chapin[1]	1956	2		(not recorded)	Kidneys Adrenals Liver	
Werther[30]	1960	4	8	(not recorded)	Adrenals Kidneys Blood vessels	Spleen Liver Bone marrow
			10	(not recorded)	Adrenals Kidneys Spleen Blood vessels	Heart Endometrium Skin Thyroid Gastrointestinal tract Pancreas
			4	(not recorded)	Spleen	
			10	(not recorded)	Spleen	Liver Kidneys
Briggs[33]	1961	1	(not recorded)		(not described)	
Palmer[2]	1963	1	(not recorded)		(not described)	
Ogg[34]	1965	2	11	2+	Kidney	(limited autopsies)
			25	4+	Renal Liver	
Weisiger[35]	1966	1	18	4+	Intestine Spleen Kidneys Adrenals	Liver Heart Pancreas Blood vessels

microcytic hypochromic anemia may occur. The bone marrow may be hyperplastic in response to blood loss from intestinal bleeding into the lumen with consequent depletion of iron stores. In other cases the anemia may be macrocytic hyperchromic with a megaloblastic bone marrow, presumably a result of the defective absorption of hematopoietic factors.

References

1. Chapin, L. E., Scudamore, H. H., Baggenstoss, A. H., and Bargen, J. A.: Regional enteritis: Associated visceral changes. Gastroenterology *30*:404–415, 1956.
2. Palmer, W. L., Kirsner, J. B., Goldgraber, M. B., and Fuentes, S. S.: Disease of the liver in regional enteritis. Amer. J. Med. Sci. *246*:663–672, 1963.
3. Monto, A. S.: The liver in ulcerative disease of the intestinal tract: Functional and anatomic changes. Ann. Intern. Med. *50*:1385–1394, 1959.
4. Kleckner, M. S., Jr.: The liver in regional enteritis. Gastroenterology *30*:416–420, 1956.
5. Warren, S., and Sommers, S. C.: Cicatrizing enteritis (regional enteritis) as a pathological entity: analysis of 120 cases. Amer. J. Path. *24*:475–501, 1948.
6. Maurer, L. H., Hughes, R. W., Folley, J. H., and Mosenthal, W. T.: Granulomatous hepatitis associated with regional enteritis. Gastroenterology *53*:301–305, 1967.
7. Comfort, M. W., Weber, H. M., Baggenstoss, A. H., and Kielly, W. F.: Nonspecific granulomatous inflammation of the stomach and duodenum; its relation to regional enteritis. Amer. J. Med. Sci. *220*:616–632, 1950.
8. Lerman, B., Garlock, J. H., and Janowitz, H. D.: Suppurative pylephlebitis with multiple liver abscesses complicating regional ileitis. Ann. Surg. *155*:441–448, 1962.
9. Sparberg, M., Gottschalk, A., and Kirsner, J. B.: Liver abscess complication regional enteritis: Report of two cases. Gastroenterology *49*:548–551, 1965.
10. Taylor, F. W.: Regional enteritis complicated by pylephlebitis and multiple liver abscesses. Amer. J. Med. *7*:838–840, 1949.
11. Smith, M. P., and Loe, R. H.: Sclerosing cholangitis, review of recent case reports and associated diseases and four new cases. Amer. J. Surg. *110*:239–246, 1965.
12. Atkinson, A. J., and Carroll, W. W.: Sclerosing cholangitis. Association with regional enteritis. J.A.M.A. *188*:183–184, 1964.
13. Berger, S. S.: Regional enteritis. Amer. J. Gastroent. *26*:81–99, 1956.
14. Scott, O. L. S.: Granuloma of the groins and perineum secondary to chronic proctocolitis. Proc. Roy Soc. Med. *54*:1019, 1961.
15. Parks, A. G., Morson, B. C., and Pegum, J. S.: Crohn's disease with cutaneous involvement. Proc. Roy. Soc. Med. *58*:241–242, 1965.
16. McCallum, D. I., and Kinmont, P. D. C.: Dermatological manifestations of Crohn's disease. Brit. J. Derm. *80*:1–8, 1968.
17. Stathers, G. M., Abbott, L. G., and McGuiness, A. E.: Pyoderma gangrenosum in association with regional enteritis. Arch. Derm. (Chicago) *95*:375–380, 1967.
18. Van Patter, W. N., Bargen, J. A., Dockerty, M. B., Feldman, W. H., Mayo, C. W., and Waugh, J. M.: Regional enteritis. Gastroenterology *26*:347–450, 1954.
19. Crohn, B. B., and Yarnis, H.: Regional ileitis. 2nd Ed. New York, Grune and Stratton, 1958.
20. Perry, H. O., and Brunsting, L. A.: Pyoderma gangrenosum. A clinical study of nineteen cases. Arch. Derm. (Chicago) *75*:380–386, 1957.
21. Ford, D. K., and Vallis, D. G.: The clinical course of arthritis associated with ulcerative colitis and regional ileitis. Arthritis Rheum. *2*:526–536, 1959.
22. Acheson, E. D.: An association between ulcerative colitis, regional enteritis, and ankylosing spondylitis. Quart. J. Med. *29*:489–499, 1960.
23. Bowen, G. E., and Kirsner, J. B.: The arthritis of ulcerative colitis and regional enteritis ("intestinal arthritis"). Med. Clin. N. Amer. *49*:17–32, 1965.

24. Stewart, J. S., and Ansell, B. M.: Ankylosing spondylitis associated with regional enteritis. Gastroenterology *45*:265-268, 1963.
25. Austad, W. R., Thompson, G. R., and Joseph, R. R.: Regional enteritis presenting as acute arthritis. Mich. Med. *67*:324-329, 1968.
26. Olsan, E. S., and Sussman, M. L.: Nonspecific enterocolitis. Amer. J. Roentgen. *60*:471-478, 1948.
27. Cohen, H., and Fishman, A. P.: Regional enteritis and amyloidosis. Gastroenterology *12*:502-508, 1949.
28. Cohen, A. S., Frensdorff, A., Lamprecht, S., and Calkins, E.: A study of the fine structure of the amyloid associated with familial Mediterranean fever. Amer. J. Path. *41*:567-578, 1962.
29. Cohen, A. S.: Amyloidosis. New Eng. J. Med. *277*:522-530, 574-583, and 628-638, 1967.
30. Werther, J. L., Schapira, A., Rubenstein, O., and Janowitz, H. D.: Amyloidosis in regional enteritis. A report of five cases. Amer. J. Med. *29*:416-423, 1960.
31. Rappaport, H., Burgoyne, F. H., and Smetana, H. F.: Pathology of regional enteritis. Milit. Surg. *109*:463-502, 1951.
32. Hirst, A. E., Jr., and Munson, R.: Amyloidosis from regional ileitis with multiple fistulae and abscesses. Med. Arts Sci. *7*:9-12, 1953.
33. Briggs, G. W.: Amyloidosis. Ann. Intern. Med. *55*:943-947, 1961.
34. Ogg, C. S.: Regional enteritis associated with amyloidosis. Postgrad. Med. J. *41*:185-186, 1965.
35. Weisiger, B. B., and Lan, C. W.: Massivie hemorrhage in amyloidosis secondary to regional ileitis. Southern Med. J. *59*:776-784, 1966.

Chapter Eight

Extraintestinal Lesions of Ulcerative Colitis

As with regional enteritis, some types of skin, liver, and joint lesions frequently occur in association with ulcerative colitis. Whether these are an integral part of the host response to an etiologic agent in parallel with the intestinal lesions, or whether they are secondary ("in series") to the intestinal, remains unproved. Therefore, I have selected the noncommital term "extraintestinal" rather than "secondary." I have avoided the clinical term "complications" because of its breadth. In common usage "complications" may include multiple primary and secondary responses to an agent as well as untoward side effects and inadequacies of therapy and the patient's unique reaction thereto. To describe these latter responses would be to write a textbook of pathology. I have limited this chapter to consideration of those lesions that have a reasonable likelihood of being an integral part of the primary process. In some instances, these extraintestinal lesions precede or are concomitant with the apparent onset of the intestinal manifestations.

LIVER LESIONS

Biopsy and autopsy examination of the liver have revealed three general patterns of liver lesions: fatty change and periportal cirrhosis of Laennec's type, pericholangitis, and carcinoma of the bile duct type. The existence of fatty change and cirrhosis associated with chronic ulcerative colitis has been recognized for many years, from necropsy studies, laboratory data, biopsy examination, and clinical observations. Logan reported that in 10 of 13 cases of ulcerative colitis in which he performed the autopsy, there was fatty infiltration of the liver and in 1 there was also cirrhosis.[1] The fatty change was more prominent in the peripheral portions of the lobule, but might extend to involve the entire liver lobule. Occasionally it tended to be focal in distribution, but generally it was diffuse and comparable in appearance to the so-called alimentary fatty change. Grossly, the liver might be enlarged and yellow, weigh up to 5 kg., and have rounded borders. Microscopically, vacuoles of fat-staining material were present in the cytoplasm of the hepatic cells. The vacuoles were of variable size and number in the cytoplasm of various cells and from case to case. Occasionally, enlarged distorted liver cells containing fat were ruptured, producing fatty cysts. The liver was otherwise unremarkable.

Three types of cirrhosis have been described in relationship to ulcerative colitis.[2] Several authors describe cases with varying degrees of a periportal (Laennec's) cirrhosis. Grossly, the liver may be normal or small in size, and a fine to rough nodular pattern may be seen on the surface. Coexistence of fatty change and the cirrhosis has not been observed in the cases reported. Microscopically the principal change is an increase in collagenous connective tissue extending from the periportal areas from lobule to lobule, dividing each into multiple compartments (Figs. 8-1 and 8-8). The fibrous strands may subdivide the liver lobule into several portions, some of which lack central veins. Foci of liver cell regeneration can be seen in some lobules and in others

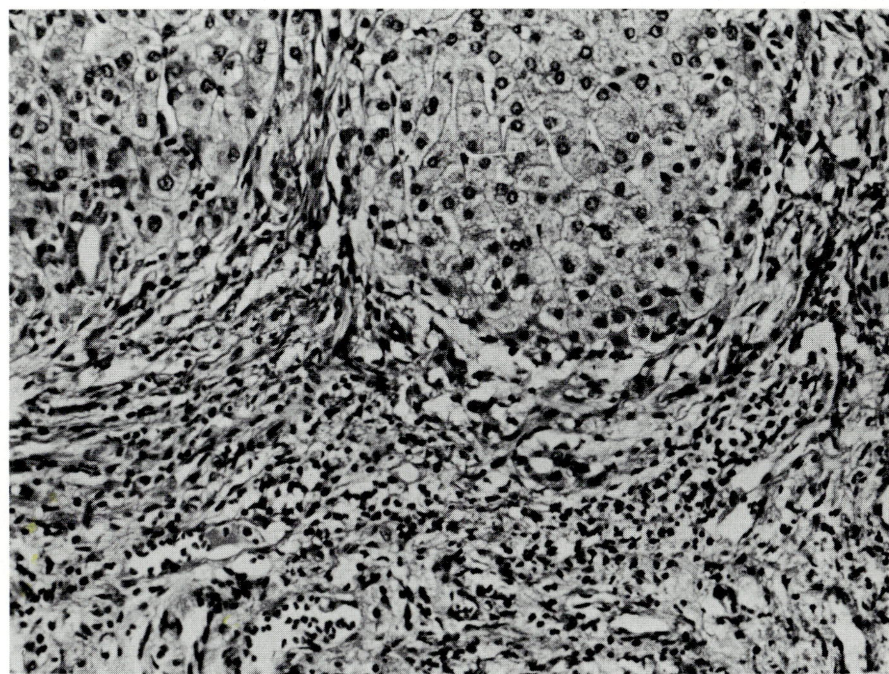

Figure 8–1 Liver biopsy specimen from a patient who had many years of ulcerative colitis. Fatty change is not present. Periportal cirrhosis with extensive lymphocyte and plasma cell infiltrate is shown. ×50.

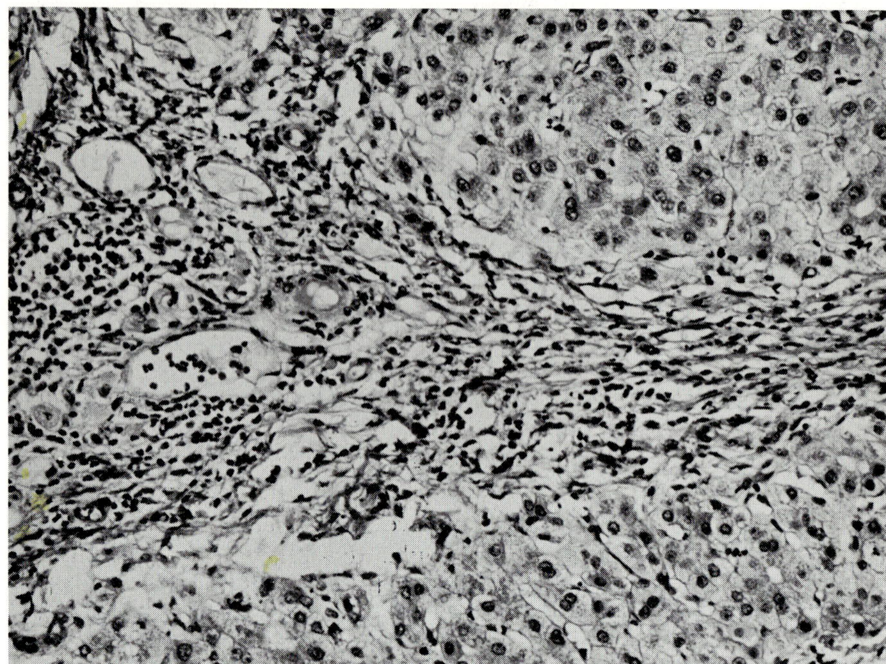

Figure 8–2   Liver biopsy specimen. Another region of the same specimen shown in Figure 8–1. All the lesions had similar periportal changes. ×50.

microfoci of necrosis are present. The remaining blood vessels are compressed and distorted by the fibrous scars. Many cases tend to have less fibrous tissue than is commonly seen with alcoholic cirrhosis, and the extent of lymphocytic infiltration, which is frequently extensive in alcoholic cirrhosis, is not a prominent feature of cirrhosis associated with ulcerative colitis. Similarly, Mallory bodies have not been described in this type of cirrhosis. Bargen, in his extensive study of 693 cases of chronic ulcerative colitis, reported the incidence of various complications associated with the disease.[3] This clinical study was done before the extensive use of needle biopsies, and its histologic work-up was therefore limited; the author encountered only 2 cases of cirrhosis. Another group studied 150 unselected cases of ulcerative colitis and found no clinical evidence of liver disease.[4] In 27 of them an autopsy was later performed; no more liver change than that seen with other chronic disease was found. In another study, 5 cases of cirrhosis in 151 patients with ulcerative colitis were reported.[5]

A more recent study reported necropsy observations of 91 cases of chronic ulcerative colitis.[6] In about half (47) there was moderate to severe fatty change, and cirrhosis was observed in 3 cases. Warren and Sommers in their report of 120 surgical cases of chronic ulcerative colitis and 60 necropsy cases found fatty change in the liver of 33 of 60 necropsies and portal cirrhosis in 3.[33] Needle biopsies in 26 cases of ulcerative colitis revealed 5 without histologic evidence of hepatic change and 9 with varying degrees of fatty infiltration.[7] Chronic pericholangitis was found in 3 cases, without other concurrent liver lesions, and in 3 others there was also an associated bile stasis. Patches of necrosis were observed in 1 case and cirrhosis was present in 6. In these latter cases there was no accompaniment of fat infiltration. Nodular regeneration and distortion of the histologic architecture by fibrosis and destruction of hepatic cells were the criteria used for cirrhosis. These investigators correlated their histologic findings with the clinical and laboratory evidence and with hepatic dysfunction. The cases were chosen on the basis of clinical and laboratory evidence of hepatic disease. In one report, 11 of 17 cases of chronic ulcerative colitis studied at autopsy had hepatic histopathologic changes, cirrhosis was present in 2, and fatty change in the remainder.[8]

The significance of these liver changes has been intensely disputed (Table 8-1). The presence of fatty change in the liver at autopsy, particularly when associated with long-drawn-out debilitating disease could, in part, indicate a terminal or agonal change. Perhaps the best evidence that there is an increased association of fatty change of the liver and cirrhosis with ulcerative colitis has been provided by Jones and by Kimmelstiel.[6, 9] Jones compared the frequency and extent of fatty infiltration of the liver in the chronic ulcerative colitis group reported earlier with that in two control groups, one consisting of 90 consecutive necropsies (excluding infants and children) and a second consisting of 57 patients with peritonitis. The latter group was selected because peritonitis was often a terminal complication of ulcerative colitis. He found that, whereas ulcerative colitis patients had 15 per

TABLE 8-1   Frequency of Fatty Change and Cirrhosis of Liver in Ulcerative Colitis

First Author	Year	Source of Cases	U.C. Total Cases	Moderate to Severe Liver Fatty Change	Liver Cirrhosis (all types)
Autopsied Cases					
Logan[1]	1919	Seattle	13	10	1
Pollard[8]	1948		17	9	2
Warren[10]	1949	Boston	60	33	3
Jones[6]	1951	Mayo	91	47	3
Kimmelstiel[9]	1952	A.F.I.P.	93	14	8
Monto[11]	1959	New York	100	40	8
Biopsied Cases (Clinical evidence of liver lesions)					
Kleckner[7]	1952	Minnesota	26	9	6
Anthonisen[12]	1966	Denmark	55	—	0
Parker[13]	1954	London	39	14	1
Olhagen[14]	1958	Stockholm	674	?	10 (1.5%)

cent moderate and 35 per cent severe fatty infiltration, the control groups ranged between 2 and 4 per cent. A mild fatty infiltration was approximately equal in each group. In a similar study, Kimmelstiel and co-workers found 29 per cent of their ulcerative colitis cases had degenerative liver lesions, whereas 1,000 cases in the control series had only 11.5 per cent.[9] Noteworthy in this study was the observation that the incidence of cirrhosis in ulcerative colitis was only 1 per cent and in the control series 2.3 per cent. Inflammatory liver lesions consisting of interlobular hepatitis and foci of inflammation similarly were much more frequent in ulcerative colitis than in the control series. They found 15 per cent of the ulcerative colitis patients had inflammatory liver lesions, whereas only 2 per cent of the control series had this type of change.

The cause or causes of the liver lesions just mentioned is also disputed. Fatty change of the liver has been shown to be caused by nutritional, metabolic (endocrine), toxic chemical, bacterial, anoxic factors, and so on. Each of these has been proposed as a cause for the fatty change in the liver seen with ulcerative colitis. Unlike regional enteritis patients, ulcerative colitis patients are prone to loss of blood into the fecal stream, and anemia is a prominent problem. The frequent administration of blood transfusions to ulcerative colitis patients exposes them to a greater risk of serum hepatitis and thus the greater risk of developing fatty change and cirrhosis in the liver. It has also been postulated that the absorption of toxic products from the colon into the portal stream, thus to be delivered to the liver, may accentuate liver cell injury and promote fatty change and cirrhosis. These postulated toxic products present features of either bacterial toxins or chemical toxic substances derived from the necrotic mucosal tissue or a combination of these. Also nutritional imbalance associated with long debilitation, loss of blood, and anemia may precipitate a hypoproteinemia and contribute to the liver change. Frequently the fatty change is transient in nature, as are the alterations in liver function tests. The cause of the liver cirrhosis seen in some ulcerative colitis patients remains unknown. Less frequently, hepatic cell necrosis, pericholangitis and bile duct hyperplasia, and rarely a case of bile duct carcinoma have been reported in association with ulcerative colitis.

Though numerous studies have been carried out to associate liver lesions with ulcerative colitis and with various clinical findings, histopathologic descriptions are relatively sparse. Kimmelstiel analyzed the histopathology of the liver lesions in his study, noted that the fatty change tended to be prominent at the periphery of the lobules and that evidence of central lobular congestion was absent.[9] This fatty change was frequently associated with evidence of regeneration characterized by enlarged atypical and hyperchromatic nuclei and liver cells at the periphery of the lobule. He could not find a correlation between the course or duration of the colitis and the presence of this change. Focal necrosis was seen in several of his cases, and in some it was rather extensive. Acute inflammatory cell infiltrates consisting principally of polymorphs appeared around the foci of necrosis in some; however, the degree of inflammatory changes varied, and in some there was no infiltrate whatsoever. Numerous bile pigmented macrophages could be found within and surrounding areas of necrosis frequently, and partially disintegrated liver cells loaded with bile pigment could also be seen. The architecture of the liver in general was preserved, but the foci of necrosis were confluent. They were sharply delineated in cases of cirrhosis. The lobular architecture was obscured, and central veins could only occasionally be found. There was a marked predominantly periportal fatty change, and in some lobules there was marked fibrosis around central veins. The periportal spaces had insignificant amounts of round cell infiltration and no fibrosis. The cirrhosis was centrolobular. Kimmelstiel also found, in some cases, small foci of inflammation that occurred anywhere within the lobule or in the periportal tissues and consisted of small patches of polymorph infiltrate. Though in Kimmelstiel's cases the fibrosis was centrolobular, the majority of reports indicate a periportal fibrosis. Monto observed the liver changes in 100 autopsy cases.[11] Though he found that fatty change was prominent, he did not describe its location. Ten of his cases had some degree of fibrosis or bile duct proliferation or both. Periportal inflammatory infiltrates and foci of necrosis were seen, often in association with bile duct proliferation and some degree of periportal fibrosis. He did not regard any of his cases as representative of characteristic Laennec's cirrhosis.

In the absence of a specific quantitative measurement of fatty change it is difficult to compare the incidence of fatty change in the various articles. In one report of seven autopsied cases of cirrhosis, three that had histologic features of Laennec's or portal cirrhosis were patients who had denied alcoholism.[15] Four patients exhibited a histopathologic pattern of postnecrotic or toxic cirrhosis. Their age at death ranged from 14 to 52 years, and the mode of death was either hepatic coma or bleeding esophageal varices. The duration of their ulcerative colitis from clinical diagnosis to death ranged from 3 to 15 years, and in all but one the colitis was severe. Four had healed ulcerative colitis lesions at the time of death. Parker and Kendall observed the predominantly peripheral lobular distribution of fatty change in the liver, confirming the observation of Kimmelstiel.[13] Their biopsy tissue did not reveal the presence of a periportal or pericholangiolar inflammatory cell infiltration. Their only case of cirrhosis was in a patient who also developed carcinoma of the extrahepatic bile ducts and a secondary suppurative cholangitis. The cirrhosis appeared biliary in type. In four of their cases there appeared to be foci of slight fibrous thickening in occasional portal tracts, but in none was there linkage of adjacent tracts disrupting the architectural pattern of the liver. Five of their cases had focal zones of necrosis, irregularly distributed, principally in the central lobular areas. One case of severe amyloidosis was found, ·and in two there were organized thrombi in the hepatic vein. They concluded that the incidence of cirrhosis was not materially greater than in the general population. Olhagen studied all the cases at the Karolinska Sjukhuset from 1940 to 1956 in which ulcerative colitis and liver cirrhosis coexisted.[14] He found 10 in 674 cases of ulcerative colitis. This represented 4 per cent of all the liver cirrhosis seen at that institution for the period. In 8 of the 10 cases there were signs of liver cirrhosis present either at the time of the diagnosis of ulcerative colitis or preceding it, or occurring so early in the course of the colonic disorder that the condition could not have been the cause of the cirrhosis, which raised the possibility of portal blood stasis as an etiologic factor in ulcerative colitis.

Perhaps the most significant, though infrequent, hepatopathologic conditions in ulcerative colitis patients are pericholangitis and bile duct carcinoma. In the reports of fatty change and portal cirrhosis just reviewed, I included mention of bile duct lesions reported in the several studies. Intrahepatic cholestasis is the most common hepatic clinical finding in ulcerative colitis. In a review of 25 cases of sclerosing cholangitis, Smith and Loe found 6 to have had ulcerative colitis also and 1 to have had regional enteritis.[16] Many of the other patients had diseases such as retroperitoneal fibrosis, retropleural fibrosis, and Riedel's struma of the thyroid, diseases commonly considered to be autoimmune in nature.[17] This raises interesting possibilities regarding the pathogenetic mechanism of ulcerative colitis, at least in some instances. Since Kleckner's study of three cases of pericholangitis, numerous other cases have been reported.[16, 18–22]

The already noted report by Parker and Kendall included one case of biliary cirrhosis with bile duct carcinoma. In a study of 441 patients with ulcerative colitis, three cases of bile duct carcinoma were found.[23] The occurrence of active cholangitis with subsequent biliary cirrhosis and, in some cases, bile duct carcinoma in some patients with ulcerative colitis requires further study. There are insufficient reports to indicate the frequency of biliary tract disease in ulcerative colitis. In one recent series of 1,474 patients with ulcerative colitis, sclerosing cholangitis was found in 12. A recent report by Ham lists eight cases from the medical literature and adds two more, one intrahepatic and one in the gallbladder.[24] Cholangiosclerosis was present in both.

The histopathologic appearance consists of a marked proliferation of bile ducts, an increase in connective tissue, principally in the periportal areas, intensely infiltrated with acute and chronic inflammatory cells, principally polymorphs and lymphocytes (Figs. 8-3, 8-4, 8-5, and 8-6). Mild degrees of this change have been reported many times in the livers of ulcerative colitis patients. More severe degrees leading to an extension of the fibrous scars from lobule to lobule and pro-

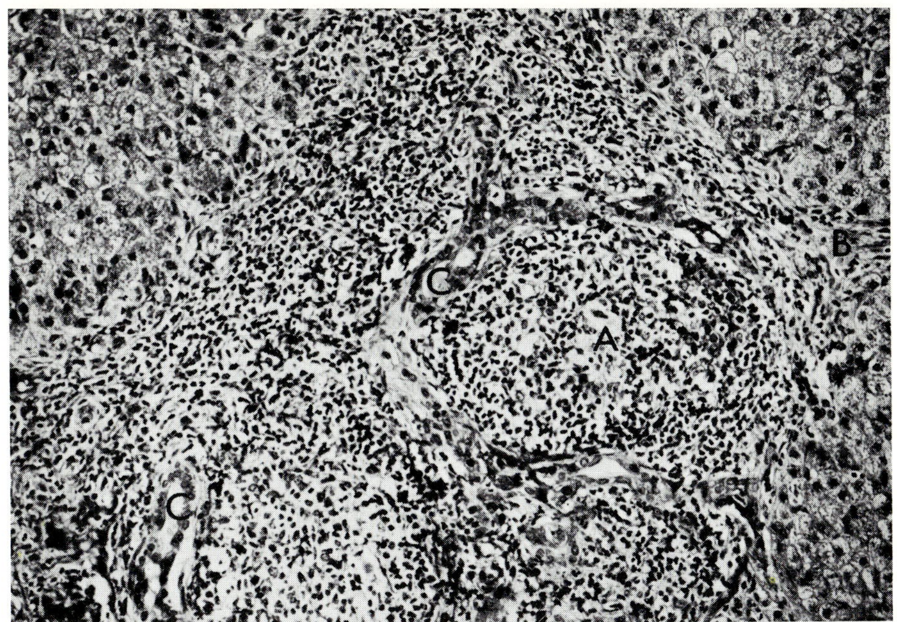

Figure 8-3 Liver biopsy specimen from an adolescent child with active ulcerative colitis. Extensive pericholangitis, seen in the surrounding bile ducts, consists of approximately equal proportions of immature lymphocytes and histiocytes (A). Scant fatty change or necrosis was found in the liver lobules, and in this region scant fibrosis in the periportal areas (B). Bile ducts are shown (C). ×50.

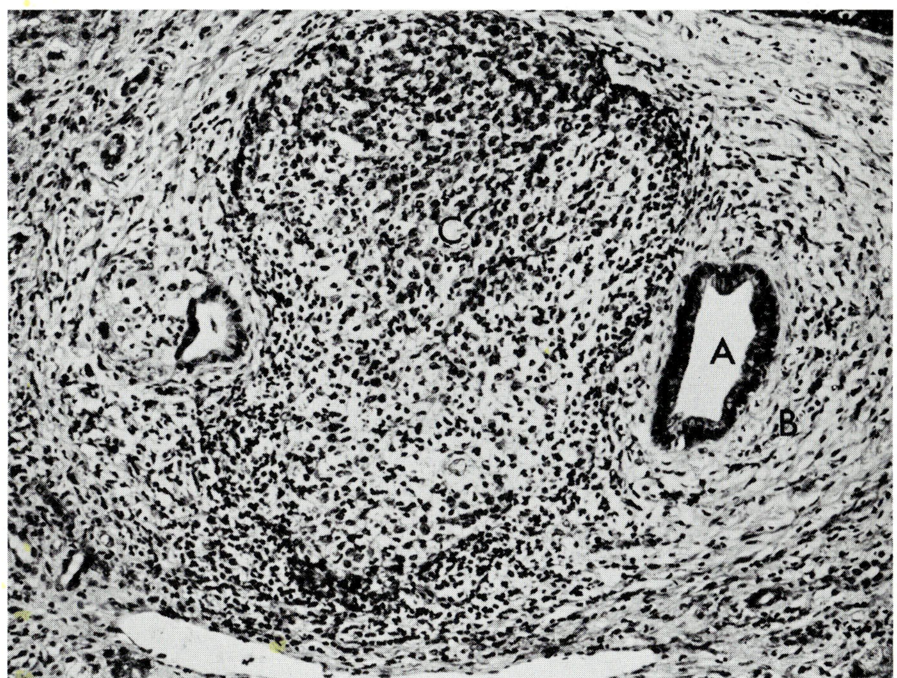

Figure 8-4 Liver biopsy specimen from the intrahepatic biliary tract of the same patient. A relatively large branch of the bile duct (A) is surrounded by an "onion skin" arrangement of rather cellular connective tissue (B). A patch of lymphocytes and histiocytes (C) is situated between two branches of the bile duct. ×50.

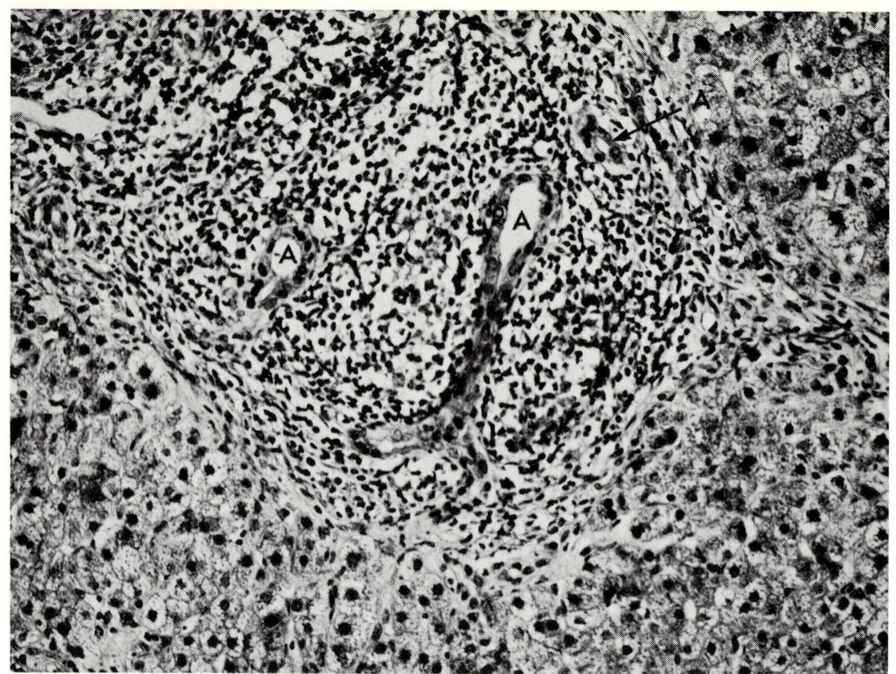

Figure 8-5 Liver biopsy specimen. A periportal zone revealing three branches of the bile duct (A) surrounded by many immature lymphocytes and plasma cells. Regressive changes are not seen in the liver cells. ×50.

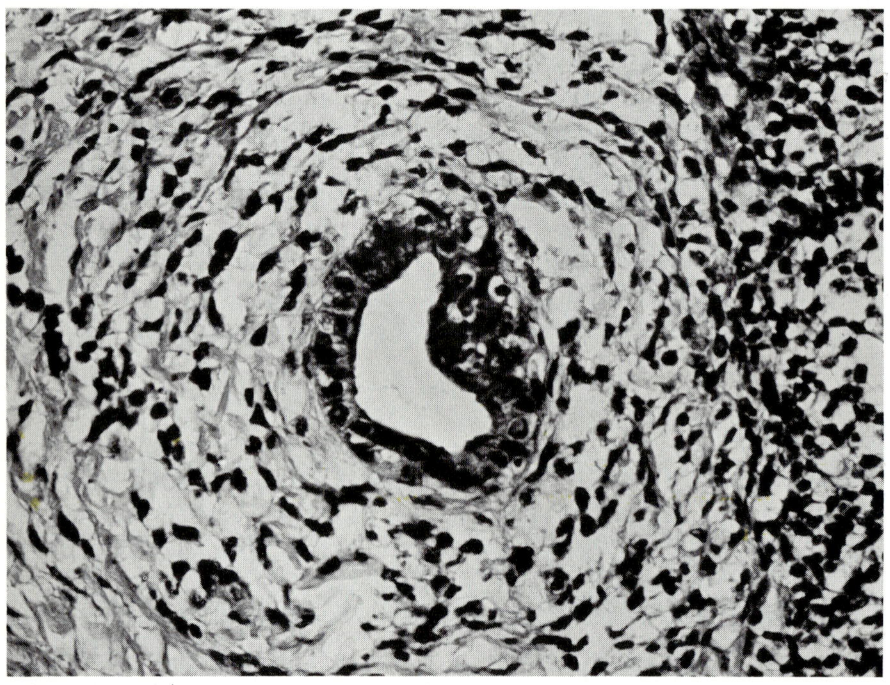

Figure 8-6 Liver biopsy specimen revealing pericholangitis. ×100.

ducing cirrhosis, bile stasis, and bile lakes have also been reported. Still other authors have emphasized the appearance of cirrhosis, in some of their patients, that resembles the postnecrotic cirrhosis of viral hepatitis. This sometimes consists of foci of necrosis or hepatic cells scattered throughout the lobules; in more extensive cases, large areas of necrotic liver substance, scattered bile duct proliferation, lymphocytes, and mononuclear cells have been described. However, no descriptions of the so-called Councilman body has been presented. Grossly, with this type of cirrhosis the liver is enlarged, with large nodules that are coarse and irregular in size and shape.

In summary, the relationship of fatty liver to ulcerative colitis appears well established, though whether the cause is nutritional or toxic remains unknown. The correlation of liver cirrhosis with ulcerative colitis remains doubtful. There was no clear presentation of the type of cirrhosis found; some observers reported a biliary, others a periportal, and others a central lobular cirrhosis. The total incidence of cirrhosis appears to be no higher in these patients than in the general population. Further, when one considers that the cirrhosis described follows no consistent histopathologic pattern but in some cases resembles Laennec's cirrhosis and in others biliary cirrhosis and in still others postnecrotic cirrhosis, the association is doubtful. Several reports mention the occurrence of small foci of necrosis and acute inflammation in the liver. These cases are too sporadic and ill-defined to indicate their prevalence or significance. Because of the reported occurrence of pericholangitis, sclerosing cholangitis, and bile duct carcinoma, it behooves the pathologist to look carefully for these lesions in biopsy and autopsy specimens. The data on their frequency and time relationships to the onset of ulcerative colitis are insufficient to permit interpretation. Suffice it to say, the one moderately extensive study indicated that less than 1 per cent of ulcerative colitis patients had biliary tract lesions.

SKIN LESIONS

Numerous authors have reported the coexistence of skin lesions and ulcerative colitis (Table 8–2). Kelley has summarized many of these reports.[25, 26] Various authors report the incidence of skin lesions of all types with ulcerative colitis to vary from 2 to 34 per cent. Part of this variability is related to the thoroughness with which the lesions are sought and part to their evanescent nature and the severity and activity of the disease, which may affect the observed frequency. Judging from the reports, some authors may have eliminated some of the less commonly associated skin lesions, considering them coincidental in a patient with chronic ulcerative colitis. Kelley reviewed approximately 330 admissions to the University of Rochester Medical Center for chronic ulcerative colitis. Excluding those cases that he regarded as inade-

TABLE 8–2   Cutaneous Lesions Associated with Chronic Ulcerative Colitis*

Author and Location	Year	No. Cases of Chronic Ulcerative Colitis	No. Cases with Cutaneous Lesions	Per cent
Bargen[3] (Mayo Clinic, Rochester, Minn.)	1929	693	17	2.5
Hurst[27] (New Lodge Clinic, England)	1935	40	1	2.5
Ricketts and Palmer[28] (Billings Hospital, Chicago, Ill.)	1946	206	22	10.7
Warren and Sommers[10] (Deaconess Hospital, Boston, Mass.)	1949	180	16	9
Rice-Oxley and Trulove[29] (Radcliffe Infirmary, Oxford, Eng.)	1950	129	12	9.3
Brown et al.[30] (Montefiore Hospital, New York, N.Y.)	1951	147	17	11.6
Samitz and Greenberg[31] (Graduate Hospital, Philadelphia, Pa.)	1951	189	65	34
Banks et al.[32] (Beth Israel Hospital, Boston, Mass.)	1957	245	31	12.6
Bacon[33] (Temple University Medical Center, Philadelphia, Pa.)	1958	317	7	2.2
Hightower, et al.[34] (Scott and White Clinic, Temple, Tex.)	1958	220	13	6

*Courtesy of M. L. Kelley: Amer. J. Dig. Dis. 7:255–272, 1962, and Harper and Row, Publishers, New York.

quately documented for the primary lesion, he selected 119 patients, 55 men, 57 women, and 3 boys and 4 girls under the age of 12 for his study. As Tables 8-3 and 8-4 demonstrate, the most frequently observed skin lesion was erythema nodosum. It would seem to be more frequent in females than in males. This lesion occurred in each case concomitant with activity of the inflammatory process in the intestine and subsided with its remission. Though the occurrence of the erythema nodosum lesion was associated with the activity of the colitis, it was not apparently related to the extent, duration, and severity of the disease. Grossly, the erythema nodosum lesion was tender, warm, and had raised nodules that usually underwent slow involution with decreased activity of colitis that did not ulcerate. In some patients the lesions became flocculent, and ulceration developed. Erythema multiforme developed in three of Kelley's patients, and a variety of papular and pustular eruptions occurred in seven. He regarded these to be principally related to bacterial infection. In some, numerous furuncles developed, whereas in others a few localized large abscesses were present. These he regarded as being probably secondary to debilitation due to the primary process of metastatic abscesses caused by bacteremia from the inflamed bowel. He did not have any patients who had the degree of necrotic skin ulceration that could be termed pyoderma gangrenosum as many others have reported to be associated with

TABLE 8–3   Skin Manifestations Among 119 Patients with Chronic Ulcerative Colitis*

Condition	No. of Patients†	F	M
Erythema nodosum	12 (21 bouts)	9	3
Erythema multiforme	3 (4 bouts)	2	1
Papular-pustular dermatitis	7	5	2
Aphthous stomatitis	6	5	1
Neurodermatitis (eczema)	4	2	2
Herpes zoster	2	1	1
Nonspecific maculopapular eruption	2	1	1
Sacral decubitus	1	1	—
Abscess base of scrotum	1	—	1
Bleeding gums	1	—	1
Clubbing of fingers	5	3	2
Total	44	29	15

*Courtesy of M. L. Kelley: Amer. J. Dig. Dis. 7:255–272, 1962; and Harper and Row, Publishers, New York.

†At Strong Memorial and Rochester Municipal Hospitals.

TABLE 8–4   Erythema Nodosum in Patients with Chronic Ulcerative Colitis*

Author and Location	Year	No. Patients	Cases of Erythema Nodosum
Jackman and Bargen[35] (Mayo Clinic, Rochester, Minn.)	1940	871 (776 adults, 95 children)	9 adults, 1 child
Elitzak and Widerman[36] (Mount Sinai Hospital, New York, N.Y.)	1941	23 children	3
Rice-Oxley and Truelove[29] (Radcliffe Infirmary, Oxford, England)	1950	129	4
Samitz and Greenberg[31] (Graduate Hospital, Philadelphia, Pa.)	1951	189	8
Rowe and Rowe[37] (Oakland, Calif.)	1954	138	4
Foster and Brick[38] (Georgetown University Hospital, Washington, D.C.)	1954	37	7
Kelley[25] (Strong Memorial Hospital, Rochester, N.Y.)	1954	71	6
Totals		1458	33

*Courtesy of M. L. Kelley and V. W. Logan. Gastroenterology 31:285–295, 1956, and Williams & Wilkins Co., Baltimore.

ulcerative colitis. Another more recent report has presented essentially similar data.[39]

Whether some of the skin lesions are an integral part of the inflammatory process in the patient or are secondarily related to treatment remains unknown. There is no clear association of the occurrence of skin lesions with the utilization of drugs or other forms of therapy. The well-documented fact that the occurrence of the erythema nodosum lesion correlates with the activity of the bowel lesion strongly suggests an integral relationship between them.

The pathologic findings in erythema nodosum consist of the gross presence of tender red nodules that are raised slightly above the level of the skin. These are frequently seen on the shins, vary from 1 to 5 or 6 cm. in diameter, and are usually limited to the anterior surface of the legs. They may, however, occur anywhere on the body. They usually do not break down, but involute gradually within a few weeks. Occasionally they may persist longer, and new lesions may appear while others are involuting. Microscopically the changes are principally located in the upper levels of the subcutaneous tissue (Figs. 8–7, 8–8, and 8–9). The dermis has a slight amount of perivascular infiltration of chronic inflammatory cells, predominantly lymphocytes. In the upper

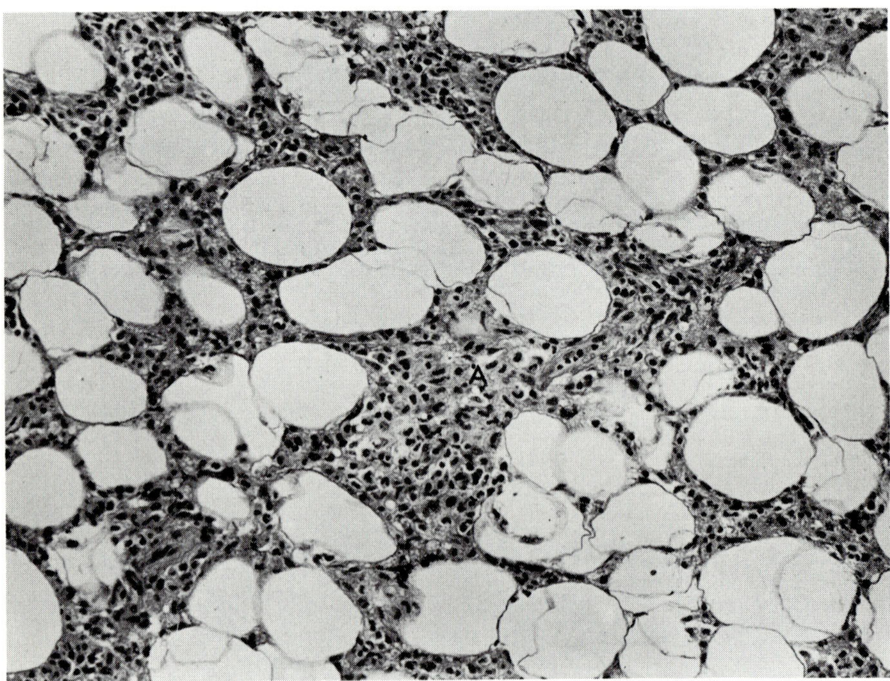

Figure 8–7   Erythema nodosum. The infiltration of the subcutaneous fat shown here produces grossly red, elevated, tender nodules that are often multiple and appear on the anterior surface of the legs. The cellular infiltrate (A) consists of polymorphs and lymphocytes. ×50.

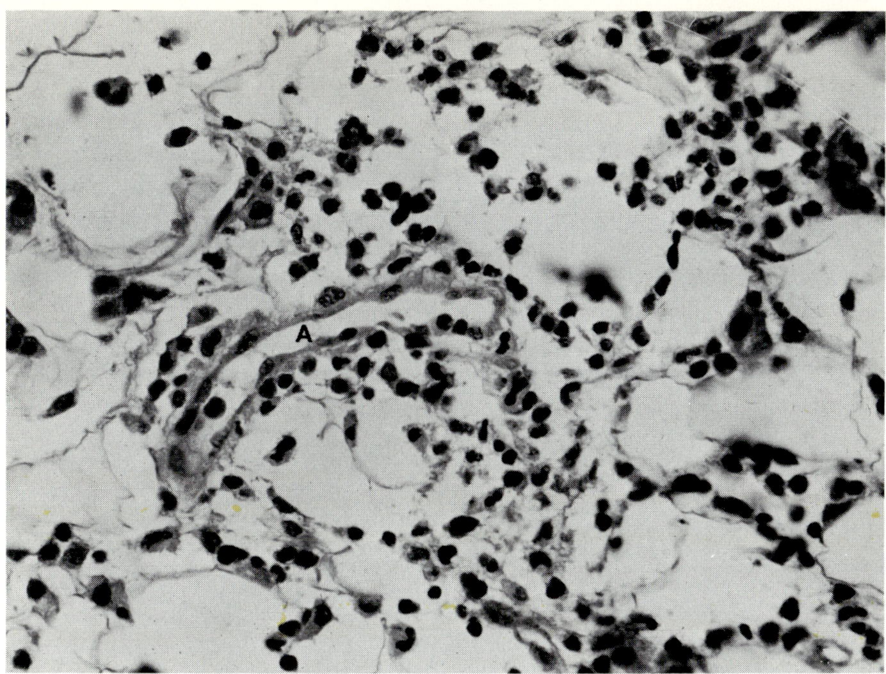

Figure 8-8 Erythema nodosum. A capillary (A) in the subcutaneous fat is closely cuffed by lymphocytes and polymorphs. ×100.

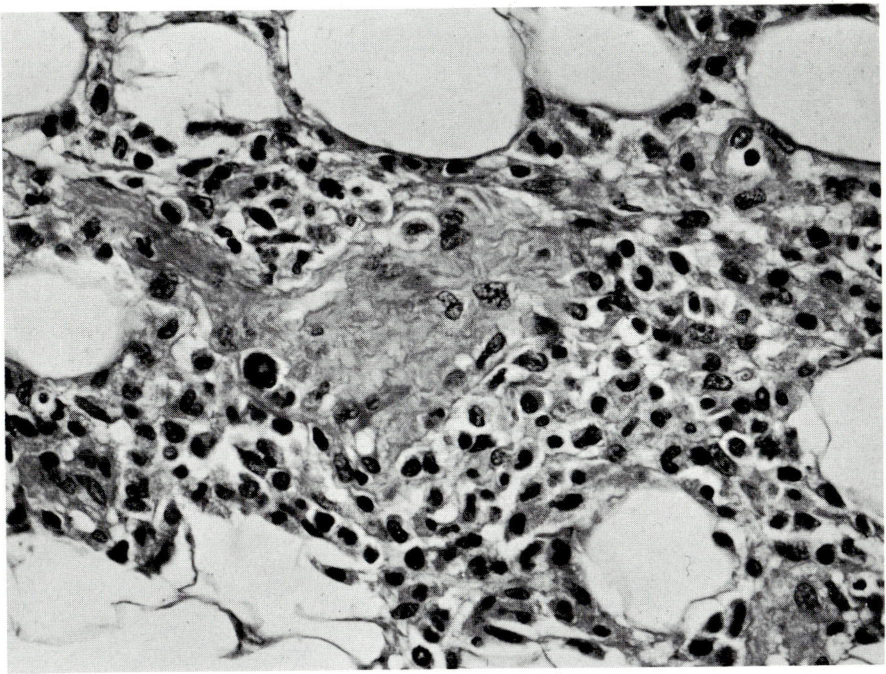

Figure 8-9 Erythema nodosum. Subcutaneous fat revealing the cellular infiltrate within the septa. ×100.

portion of the subcutaneous tissue, a scattered infiltrate consists mainly of neutrophils and lymphocytes. Some histiocytes and occasionally eosinophils are present, but plasma cells are rarely found. In later stages the inflammatory cellular infiltrate may involve the fatty tissue surrounding sweat glands; it is moderate in quantity and multifocal in distribution. Abscess formation in most instances does not occur, nor does necrosis. The lesions are frequently associated with veins, but the vascular wall itself may not show recognizable change, except in the endothelium, though occasionally the inflammatory infiltrate may extend into its outer layers (Fig. 8–10). In advanced cases, giant cells, an epithelioid type of histiocytes, may be located centrally in the lesion or form palisade arrangements around a central cleft. The giant cells are principally of the foreign body type, and in older lesions the polymorphs are fewer in number and the relative preponderance of chronic inflammatory cells, principally lymphocytes, may be noted. Also, increased fibrosis may be present, characterized by increased collagen fibers.

Pyoderma gangrenosum represents a catch-all for a variety of histologic appearances of infected skin lesions that begin as abscesses that subsequently ulcerate and spread to adjacent areas of the skin. Grossly, the advancing borders tend to be red to purple, elevated, and

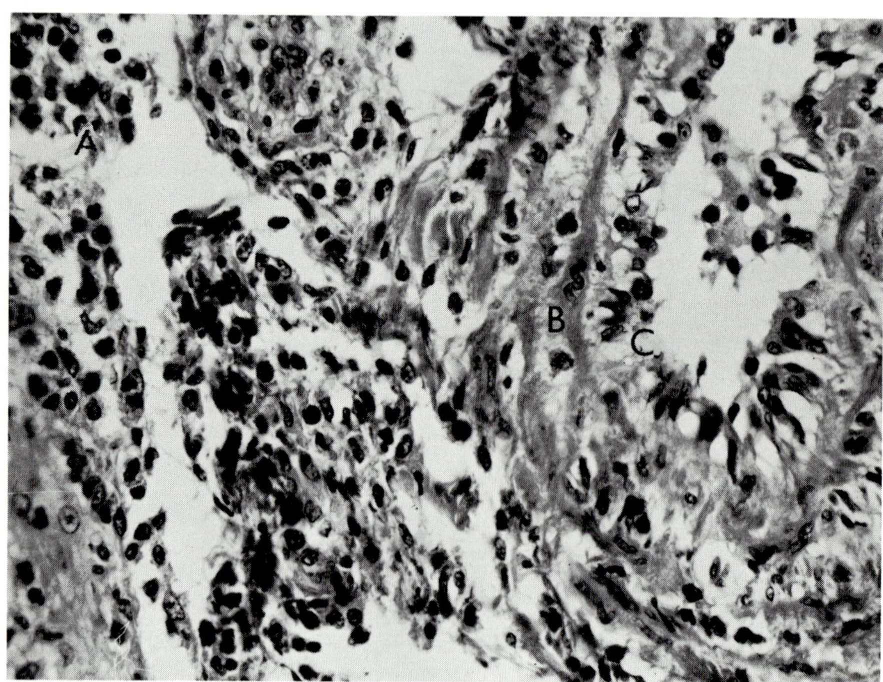

Figure 8–10   Erythema nodosum. Subcutaneous fat infiltrated with lymphocytes and polymorphs (A) in the vicinity of an arteriole (B). The endothelium of the arteriole (C) has swollen vacuolated cells. ×100.

undermined and rolled. The pathogenesis of this lesion and its etiology are unknown, whether it represents primarily a septic abscess or whether it is related to an immune reaction of the skin (Figs. 8–11 and 8–12). Microscopically the lesions are nonspecific in appearance, characterized by necrosis and acute inflammation involving the dermis and upper layers of the subcutaneous tissue (Fig. 8–13). In more long-standing cases, chronic inflammatory infiltrates may be present with lymphocytes, plasma cells, histiocytes, and fibroblasts predominating. Often the bed of the ulcer has increased proliferation of vascular channels of young granulation tissue, young fibroblasts, and connective tissue. An attempt at regeneration of the epithelium is seen in the proliferation at the edges of the ulcer, and relatively bizarre appearing epithelial cells may be found. When healing ensues, extensive scarification, characterized by large bundles of dense collagen fibers and fibroblasts is seen.

Aphthous stomatitis is another sequela of ulcerative colitis and is believed by some to have the same pathogenetic basis as the more common sequelae of erythema nodosum and arthritis; that is, a hyperergic reaction. Evidence for the relationship of aphthous stomatitis to ulcerative colitis has been reported.[29, 40, 41]

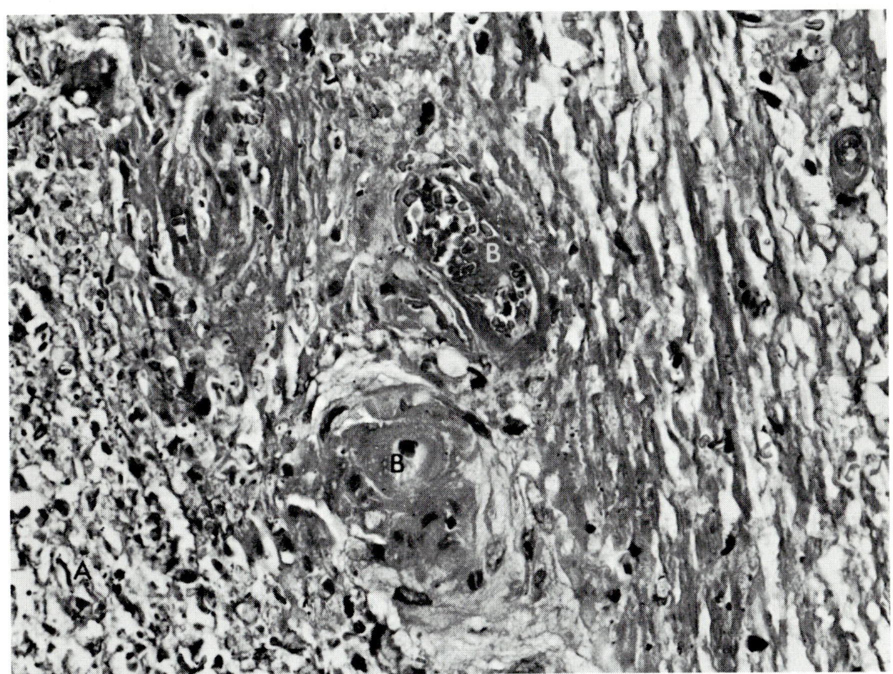

Figure 8–11 Pyoderma gangrenosum. Edge of necrosis (A) is adjacent to degenerating and necrotic blood vessels (B). ×100.

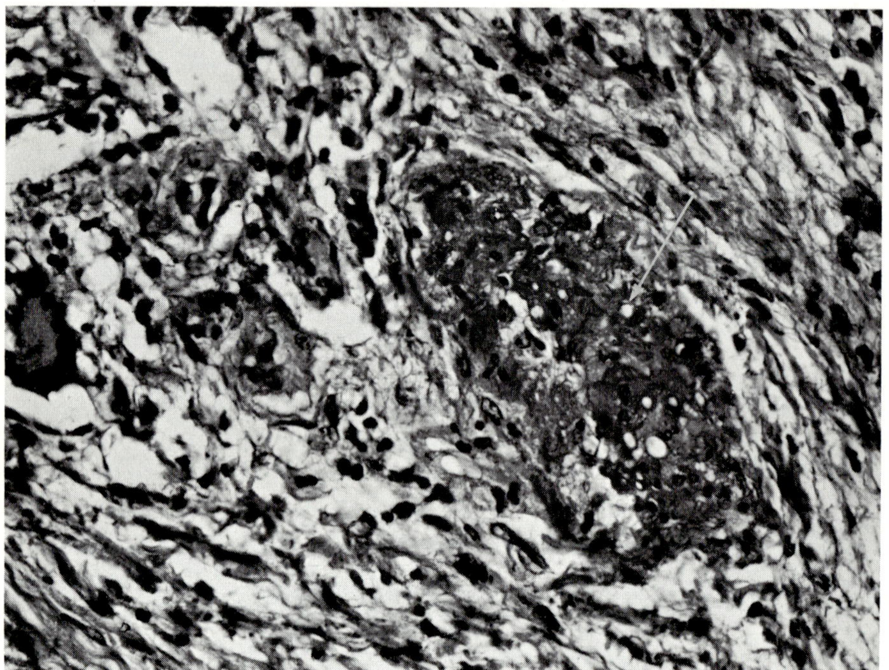

Figure 8–12   Pyoderma gangrenosum. A thrombosed necrotic vessel (arrow) is shown in the vicinity of an abscess. ×100.

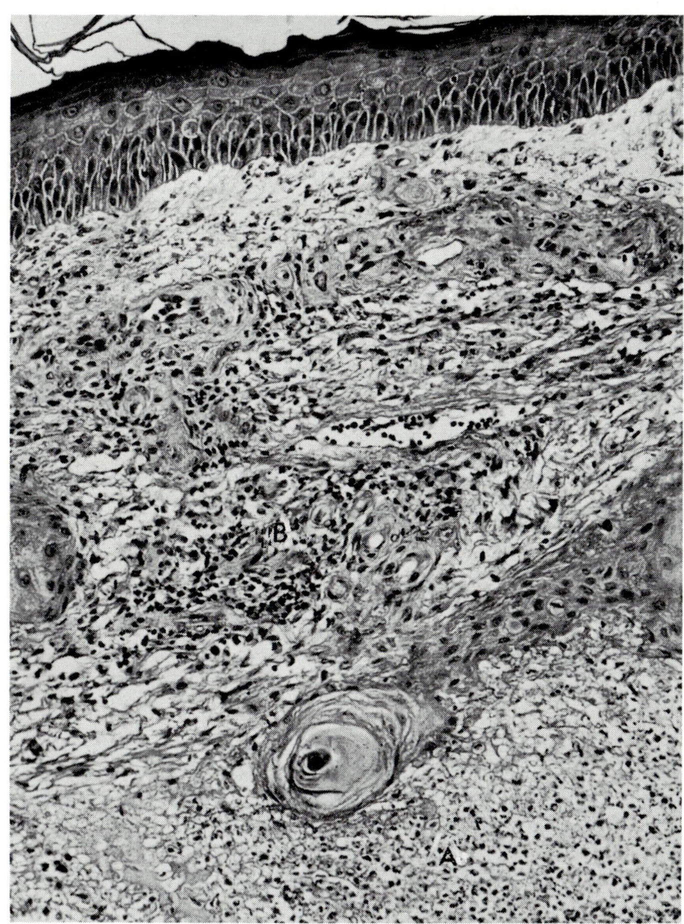

Figure 8–13 Pyoderma gangrenosum. An abscess (A) at the level of the tips of the skin appendages consists of an ill-defined region of necrosis surrounded by some polymorphs (B). The overlying stratified squamous epithelium (C) is not yet eroded. ×50.

JOINT LESIONS

Articular involvement as a sequela of chronic ulcerative colitis has long been known. Bargen called attention to the arthritis affecting peripheral joints.[3] He, as well as subsequent authors, noted that the arthritis tended to flair and subside with exacerbations and remissions of the colitis. The several reports in the literature subsequently have attempted to establish the incidence of articular manifestations, and as Table 8–5 shows, the data is somewhat variable, ranging from 8 to 17 per cent. In part this variability may be explained by the fact that different observers may have used differing criteria regarding the diagnosis of arthritis, and there may have been some hospital based selection in terms of the severity of the underlying disease.

In addition to the mild nonspecific arthralgias that are frequently encountered in ulcerative colitis, two principal specific lesions are associated: migratory polyarthritis and ankylosing spondylitis (Tables 8-6, 8-7, and 8-8). Depending on the stringency of the criteria utilized by the observer to separate the migratory nonspecific arthralgias from the more specific migratory arthritis, the recorded frequency of joint involvement can be markedly altered. Because of the more precise capacity to identify ankylosing spondylitis, the reported data by the various authors for this disease is much more consistent. Fernandez-Herlihy, in his analysis of 555 cases of chronic ulcerative colitis, found 95 with joint lesions (Table 8–5).[42] Of these, 46 had the onset of arthritis simultaneously with or before the colitis, whereas 49 had the onset of the arthritis after the colitis (Table 8-7). Almost identical results were reported in a subsequent study, 43 of 333 cases, with comparable

TABLE 8–5   Ulcerative Colitis with Arthritis (All Types)

First Author	Year of Report	Total Ulcerative Colitis	Total Arthritis	Migratory	Ankylosing Spondylitis	Other
Jankelson[50]	1942	145	15 (10%)	3		
Crohn[49]	1947	77 (segmental)	10 (13%)			
Kirsner[53]	1948	100	8 (8%)			
Brown[30]	1951	147	11 (8%)			
Neuman[48]	1954	201 (segmental)	30 (15%)			
Brooke[55]	1956	131	17 (13%)			
Bywaters[51]	1958	109	16 (15%)			
Fernandez-Herlihy[42]	1959	555	95 (17%)	33	28	18
Wright[54]	1959	108	17 (16%)			
Acheson[45]	1960	1175			23 (2%)	
Zvaifler[52]	1960	100			6	
Rotstein[43]	1963	333	34 (10%)	14	9	11

TABLE 8–6   Cutaneous Lesions in Patients with Ulcerative Colitis and Arthritis* **

Cutaneous Lesions	Patients (no.)	Peripheral Arthritis (52 patients)				Spondylitis (19 patients)			
		Total		*Synchronous with Arthritis*		*Total*		*Synchronous with Arthritis*	
		No.	*%*	*No.*	*%*	*No.*	*%*	*No.*	*%*
Erythema nodosum	13	12	23	9	17	1	5	1	5
Pyoderma gangrenosum	3	2	4	1	2	1	5	1	5
Other	5	4†	8	—	—	1‡	5	0	—
Total	21	18	35	10	19	3	15	2	10

*Various rashes thought to be due to drug reactions are not included.

†Includes one patient (Case 18) with deep ulceration of legs possibly due to pyoderma gangrenosum, one patient (Case 20) with intracutaneous nodules, one patient (Case 24) with nodules in the skin of the calf of the leg, and one patient (Case 26) with lesions typical of discoid lupus erythematosus.

‡This patient (Case 56) had urticaria synchronous with a flare-up of colitis and conjunctivitis.

**Courtesy of C. McEwen et al.: Amer. J. Med. *33*:923–941, 1962, and Reuben H. Donnelley Co., New York.

TABLE 8–7   Time Relationship Between Onset of Colitis and Arthritis*

Authors	Peripheral Arthritis					Spondylitis				
	Patients (no.)	*Colitis Onset Before or Simultaneous with Arthritis*		*Colitis Onset After Arthritis*		Patients (no.)	*Colitis Onset Before or Simultaneous with Arthritis*		*Colitis Onset After Arthritis*	
		No.	*%*	*No.*	*%*		*No.*	*%*	*No.*	*%*
Bywaters, Ansell[51]	37	30	81	7	19	0	—	—	—	—
Fernandez-Herlihy[42]	44	40	90	4	10	28	23	82	5	18
Ford, Vallis[44]	14	14	100	0	—	2	1	—	1	—
Acheson[45]	0	—	—	—	—	31	19	61	12	39
McEwen et al.[56]	52	47	90	5	10	19	14	74	5	26
Combined series	147	131	89	16	11	80	57	71	23	29

*Courtesy of C. McEwen et al.: Amer. J. Med. *33*:923–941, 1962, and Reuben H. Donnelley Co., New York.

TABLE 8–8   Simultaneous Flares of Ulcerative Colitis and Arthritis**

| | Peripheral Arthritis | | | Spondylitis | | |
| | | Patients with Simultaneous Flares | | | Patients with Simultaneous Flares | |
Authors	Patients (No.)	No.	%	Patients (No.)	No.	%
Fernandez-Herlihy[42]	30*	19	63	28	4	14
Wright, Watkinson[54]	16	14	88	0	—	—
McEwen et al.[56]	52	31†	60	19	5‡	26

*Includes 18 cases diagnosed as rheumatoid arthritis, 2 with arthritis and erythema nodosum and 10 with "acute toxic arthritis."

†In 20 of these patients, flares were always simultaneous; and in 11 they were usually or sometimes simultaneous.

‡In 4 of these patients, flares were simultaneous in all attacks and in one only at onset.

**Courtesy of C. McEwen et al.: Amer. J. Med. *33:*923–941, 1962, and Reuben H. Donnelley Co., New York.

temporal relationship between the occurrence of ulcerative colitis and arthritis. Age at onset of the disease and the sex ratio were also almost identical in these two series (Table 8-9). Several authors have studied the relative frequency of the migratory arthritis and ankylosing spondylitis in those patients with ulcerative colitis who have joint lesions (Tables 8-5 and 8-9). A rheumatoid arthritis-like lesion has been identified in about 1 to 2 per cent of the ulcerative colitis patients. The occurrence of ankylosing spondylitis in patients with ulcerative colitis is about fiftyfold above the frequency that occurs in the general population.

Ford and Vallis presented evidence to indicate that the arthritis of ulcerative colitis is a distinct clinical entity.[44] Their basis for separation was clinical observation rather than the specific morphologic nature of the joint lesions. On the basis of pathologic study of the lesions, most observers do not adhere to this view.

TABLE 8–9   Sex Distribution in Patients with Arthritis and Accompanying Ulcerative Colitis*

| | Total Cases | | | | Peripheral Arthritis | | | | Spondylitis | | | |
| | | | Females | | | | Females | | | | Females | |
Authors	Cases (No.)	Males (No.)	No.	%	Cases (No.)	Males (No.)	No.	%	Cases (No.)	Males (No.)	No.	%
Bywaters, Ansell[51]	37	9	28	76	37	9	28	76	0	—	—	—
Fernandez-Herlihy[42]	72	34	38	53	44	14	30	68	28	20	8	29
Wright, Watkinson[54]	17	5	12	71	17	5	12	71	0	—	—	—
Ford, Vallis[44]	14	7	7	50	13	7	6	46	1	0	1	—
Zvaifler[52]	6	4	2	33	0	—	—	—	6	4	2	33
McEwen et al.[56]	67	36	31	46	52	23	29	56	15	13	2	13

*Courtesy of C. McEwen et al.: Amer. J. Med. *33:*923–941, 1962, and Reuben H. Donelley Co., New York.

Acheson presented conclusive evidence that the frequency of ankylosing spondylitis associated with ulcerative colitis exceeds that of the general population and that the two are related diseases.[45] He studied 45 cases of ankylosing spondylitis and 36 cases of rheumatoid arthritis, occurring among 1,175 ulcerative colitis patients discharged from Veterans' Administration hospitals from 1956 and 1957. Twenty-three or 2 per cent of these patients had ankylosing spondylitis. He too found that the onset of the spondylitis occurred synchronously with or before the onset of the colitis as frequently as it occurred after. Control series of comparable age distribution, having other chronic diseases such as Hodgkin's disease and multiple sclerosis, and paired with a comparable number of all medical and surgical discharges, revealed the presence of ankylosing spondylitis to be 20 times greater in the ulcerative colitis and regional enteritis groups than in the control groups. In a series of 33 patients with ankylosing spondylitis, 6 were found to have ulcerative colitis on subsequent investigation.[46]

Watkinson and co-workers reported on the frequency of arthritis associated with segmental colitis.[47] Of a total of 114 patients with ulcerative colitis, three of those with segmental colitis also had arthritis. Similar observations were reported by Neuman, who found that 15 per cent of 201 patients with segmental colitis had joint involvement.[48] Crohn and his co-workers reported a 13 per cent joint involvement in 77 patients with segmental colitis.[49] Thus, the frequency of joint involvement in segmental colitis appears to be comparable to that found in more distal type of ulcerative colitis.

In those few patients with ulcerative colitis and with a rheumatoid arthritis type of clinical change who have undergone biopsy, a joint lesion comparable to that of rheumatoid arthritis has been revealed. There is synovial cell hyperplasia, loss of lining cells, lymphocytic infiltrate, occasional plasma cell and polymorph infiltrate with destruction of the joint cartilage, and fibroblast proliferation in the underlying tissues, increased vascularity, and fibrin incorporation and organization. Synovial fluid cell counts range up to 11,800 cells per cubic millimeter, which are principally polymorphs; synovial fluid specific gravity is low; and the viscosity is low. Ankylosing spondylitis is essentially a variant, histopathologically, of rheumatoid arthritis that is limited to the bones of the spine, particularly the sacroiliac joint.

McEwen and co-workers extensively reviewed the arthritis accompanying ulcerative colitis (Tables 8-10, 8-11, and 8-12).[56, 57] The migatory peripheral type of arthritis occurred twice as frequently in the ankles and knees as it did in the elbow, proximal interphalangeal, wrist metacarpophalangeal, and shoulder joints. Less frequently the hip and metatarsophalangeal and toe joints were involved. Ankylosing spondylitis usually occurred in the hip, shoulder, or knee joints, accounting for approximately two thirds of the lesions of this type. The remainder occurred with decreasing frequency in the ankle, wrist, elbow, hands,

TABLE 8–10   Number of Joints Involved in Each Episode of the Peripheral Type of Arthritis*

Episodes of Arthritis	Patients (no.)	Joints Involved (no.)					
		1 to 3		4 to 5		6 or more	
		Patients					
		No.	%	No.	%	No.	%
First	52	45	87	6	11	1	2
Second	44	38	86	4	9	2	5
Third	30	24	80	3	10	3	10
Fourth and fifth	12	9	75	2	17	1	8

*Courtesy of C. McEwen et al. Amer. J. Med. *33*:923–941, 1962, and Reuben H. Donnelley Co., New York.

or toes. In more than half the cases, more than one joint was affected. About one third of the patients with peripheral migratory arthritis had concomitant skin lesions, usually erythema nodosum, whereas only 15 per cent of those with spondylitis had concurrent skin lesions (Table 8-6). McEwen reported on the pathologic features of five synovial tissue biopsies from patients with migratory peripheral arthritis. During the acute phase of joint involvement, hyperplastic and hypertrophic lining cells with mild infiltration of histiocytes and lymphocytes and rare neutrophils and plasma cells were seen. Biopsies of older

TABLE 8–11   Frequency of Involvement of Individual Peripheral Joints in Patients with Spondylitis Accompanying Ulcerative Colitis Compared with That in Ankylosing Spondylitis*

Joints	Patients in Whom Involved			
	Spondylitis Accompanying Ulcerative Colitis		Ankylosing Spondylitis	
	No. Patients	%	No. Patients	%
Hip	13	33	22	23
Shoulder	13	33	19	20
Knee	14	35	23	24
Ankle	5	13	9	9
Wrist	4	10	8	8
Elbow	3	10	4	4
Proximal interphalangeal	5	13	5	5
Metacarpophalangeal	2	5	5	5
Metatarsophalangeal	1	3	3	3
Toes	0	–	2	2
Number of patients	40		95	

*Courtesy of C. McEwen: Clin. Orthop. *57*:9–17, 1968, and J. B. Lippincott Co., Philadelphia.

TABLE 8–12 Frequency of Involvement of Individual Joints in Patients with the Peripheral Type of Arthritis Accompanying Ulcerative Colitis Compared with That in Rheumatoid Arthritis*

| | Patients in Whom Involved | | | |
| | *Peripheral Arthritis Accompanying Ulcerative Colitis* | | *Rheumatoid Arthritis* | |
Joints	*No. Patients*	*%*	*No. Patients*	*%*
Knee	40	68	68	69
Ankle	39	66	59	60
Elbow	25	42	40	41
Proximal interphalangeal (finger)	25	42	86	88
Wrist	24	41	85	87
Shoulder	18	30	23	23
Metacarpophalangeal	17	29	60	61
Hip	13	22	31	32
Metatarsophalangeal	7	12	37	38
Toes	3	5	15	16
Number of patients	59		98	

*Courtesy of C. McEwen: Clin. Orthop. 57:4–17, 1968, and J. B. Lippincott Co., Philadelphia.

lesions revealed synovitis with villus formation and mild focal hyperemia and hypertrophy of the lining cells with stratification. Many distended capillaries and thick-walled venules were seen, and a diffuse lymphocytic, histiocytic, and plasma cell infiltrate was present. The infiltrates were usually diffuse, though occasionally they were focal in distribution.

AMYLOIDOSIS

Another sequela of ulcerative colitis is systemic amyloidosis. Its frequency has not been ascertained with certainty. Since Targgart and co-workers reviewed the problem, additional cases have not been reported.[66] They reviewed the 10 available cases, including their own. The age at the time of death ranged from 27 to 48, and as with regional enteritis, the duration of known amyloidosis was quite variable, from 1 to 20 years. Six of the ten patients had chronic suppurative inflammation with or without fistula and abscess. Most of these (six of eight) had extension of the ulcerative colitis lesion to the small bowel. In five of nine patients, renal amyloidosis significantly contributed to the death of the patient.

Though the number of cases of amyloidosis associated with regional enteritis and ulcerative colitis reported is insufficient to make precise analyses, some tentative observations may be made. Involve-

TABLE 8–13   Ulcerative Colitis with Amyloidosis

Case Number	First Author	Year of Report	Duration of Colitis	Age at Death	Distribution of Amyloid
1.	Moschowitz[58]	1936	(not given)	48	Kidneys
2.	Mallory[59]	1947	6	27	Kidneys, adrenals, liver, spleen
3.	Jensen[60]	1950	12	38	Kidneys, adrenals, spleen, blood vessels
4.	Frenkel[61]	1954	6	26	Kidneys, adrenals
5.	Mandelbaum[62]	1955	10	28	Kidneys, adrenals, spleen, liver
6.	Mandelbaum[62]	1955	20	48	Kidneys, adrenals, lymph nodes, spleen, intestines
7.	Hasson[63]	1957	15	32	Kidneys, adrenals, spleen, liver
8.	Warren[64]	1959	2	28	Liver, adrenals, spleen
9.	Heptinstall[65]	1960	9	—	Kidneys
10.	Targarrt[66]	1963	21	35	Kidneys, adrenals, spleen, thyroid, blood vessels, intestine

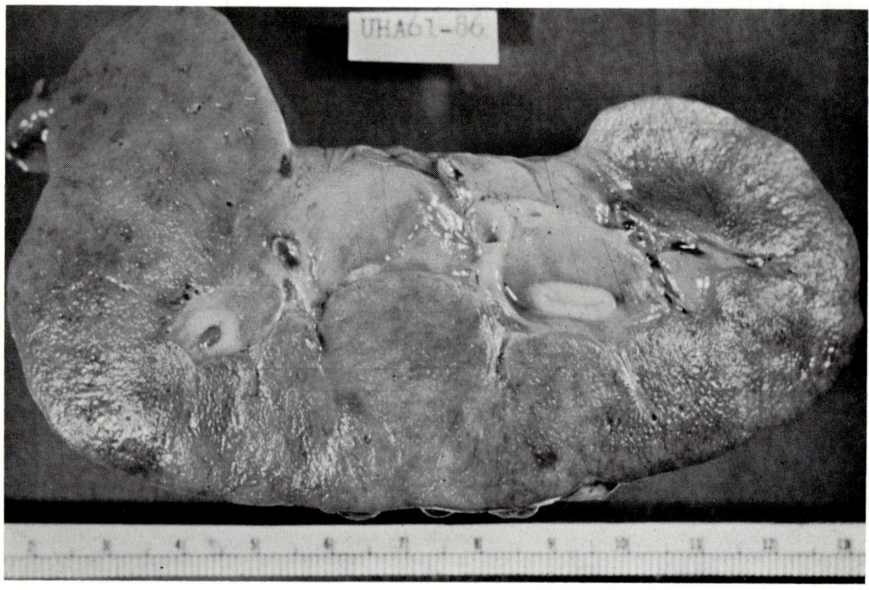

Figure 8–14   Amyloidosis of the kidney in a case of ulcerative colitis. The kidneys were moderately enlarged, pale, swollen, and firm, with a waxy appearance.

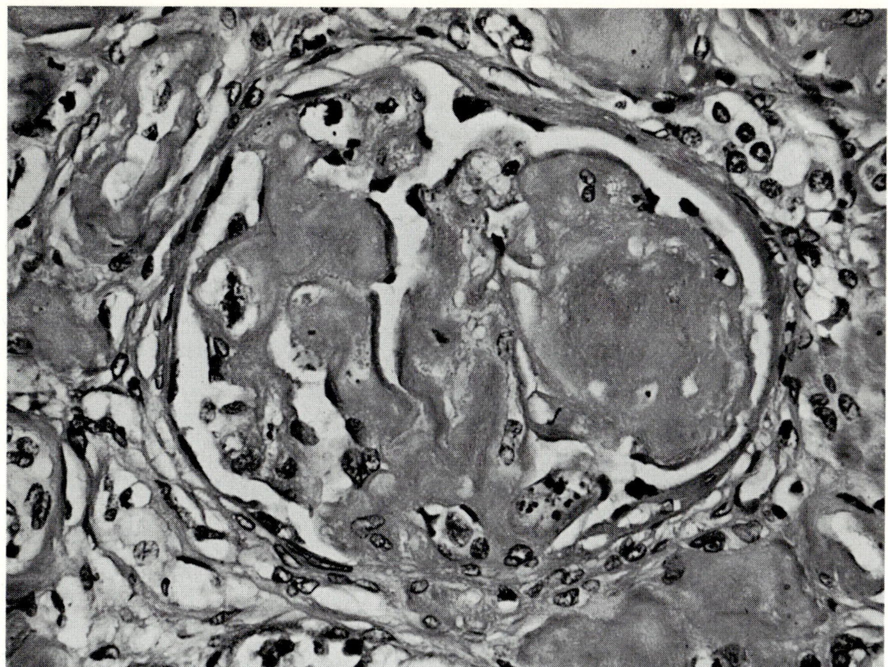

Figure 8–15 Photomicrograph of amyloidosis of the kidney in the case shown in Figure 8-14. Amyloid was extensively deposited in the glomeruli and in the tubular and vascular basement membranes. ×100.

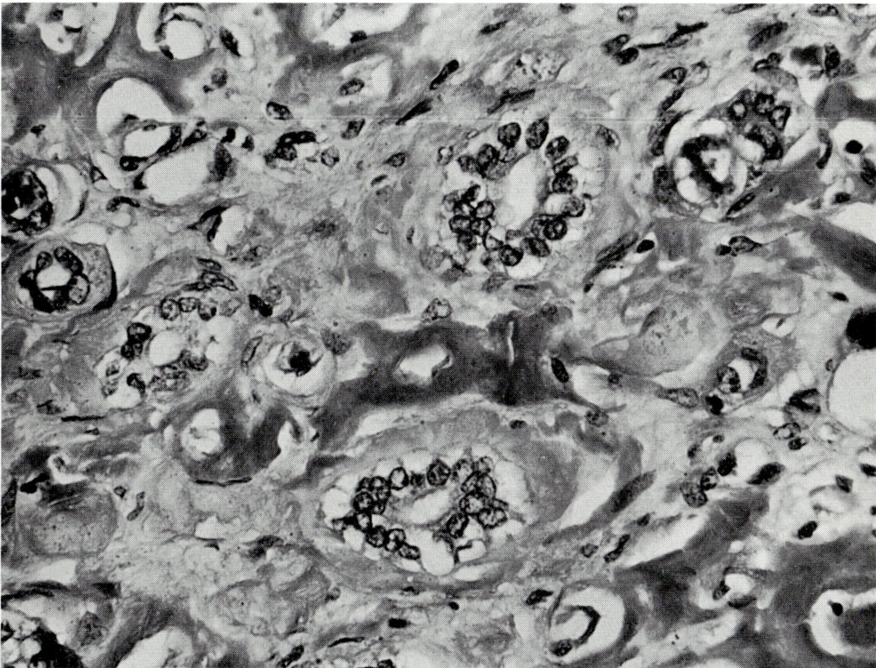

Figure 8–16 Amyloidosis of the kidney. A view of the collecting tubule region of the medulla revealing extensive deposits. ×100.

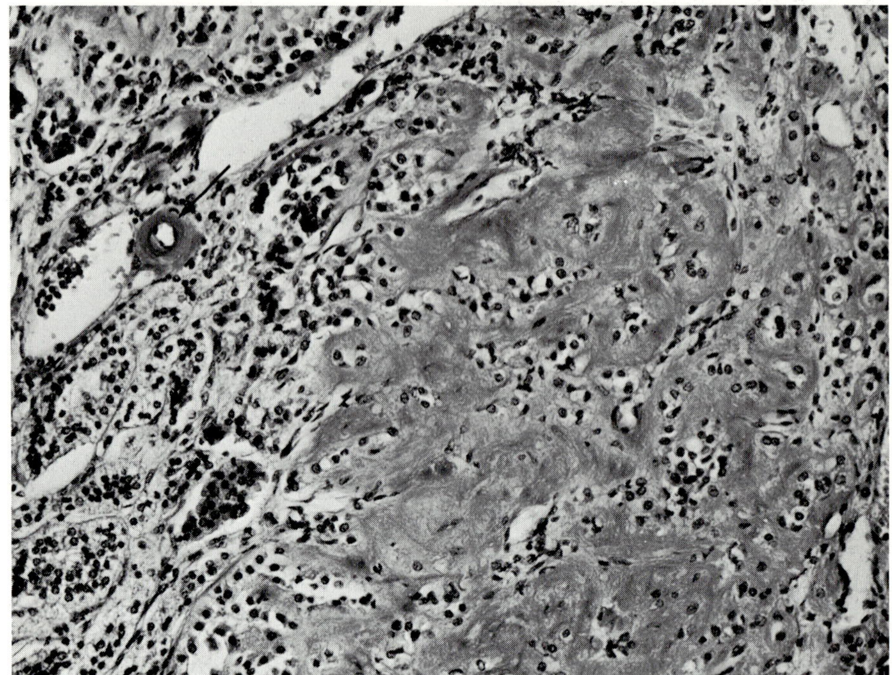

Figure 8-17   Amyloidosis of the adrenal gland from the same case shown in Figure 8-16. Deposits are seen in the wall of a blood vessel (arrow) as well as the zona fasciculata. ×100.

ment of the adrenal glands and kidneys and, to a lesser degree, the spleen, is present in most cases. This is characteristic of secondary amyloidosis. It is noteworthy that the liver involvement in both is usually minimal, though occasionally extensive. Secondary suppurative complications seem to be more prominently associated with the amyloids of ulcerative colitis than of regional enteritis. The frequency with which ileal involvement of ulcerative colitis is associated with amyloidosis leaves unanswered the question whether amyloidosis is secondary to involvement of the small intestine or whether it is a reflection of the severity of the colonic disease. The amyloidosis of regional enteritis seems less clearly associated with the suppurative process than that of ulcerative colitis. Whether it occurs more frequently with regional enteritis than with ulcerative colitis remains moot in view of the absence of incidence data on the latter. It is surprising that amyloidosis should occur so rarely in these patients with long-standing chronic inflammations.

References

1. Logan, A. A., Chronic ulcerative colitis. A review of 117 cases. Northwest Med. *18*:1-9, 1919.
2. Vinnick, E. I., and Kern, F.: Liver disease in ulcerative colitis. Arch. Intern. Med. *112*:41-49, 1963.

3. Bargen, J. A.: Complications and sequelae of chronic ulcerative colitis. Ann. Intern. Med. *3:*335-352, 1929.

4. Ross, J. R., and Swarts, J. M.: Hepatic dysfunction and cirrhosis in chronic ulcerative colitis. Gastroenterology *10:*81-95, 1948.

5. Tumen, H. J., Monaghan, J. F., and Jobb, E.: Hepatic cirrhosis as a complication of chronic ulcerative colitis. Ann. Intern. Med. *26:*542-553, 1947.

6. Jones, G. W., Baggenstoss, A. H., and Bargen, J. A.: Hepatic lesions and dysfunction associated with chronic ulcerative colitis. Amer. J. Med. Sci. *221:*279-286, 1951.

7. Kleckner, M. S., Jr., Stauffer, M. H., Bargen, J. A., and Dockerty, M. B.: Hepatic lesions in the living patient with chronic ulcerative colitis as demonstrated by needle biopsy. Gastroenterology *22:*13-33, 1952.

8. Pollard, H. M., and Block, M.: Association of hepatic insufficiency with chronic ulcerative colitis. Arch. Intern. Med. *82:*159-174, 1948.

9. Kimmelstiel, P., Large, H. L., and Verner, H. D.: Liver damage in ulcerative colitis. Amer. J. Path. *28:*259-289, 1952.

10. Warren, S., and Sommers, S. C.: Pathogenesis of ulcerative colitis. Amer. J. Path. *25:*657-674, 1949.

11. Monto, A. S.: The liver in ulcerative disease of the intestinal tract: Functional and anatomic changes. Ann. Intern. Med. *50:*1385-1394, 1959.

12. Anthonisen, P., Christoffersen, P., and Riis, P.: Liver histology in ulcerative colitis. Acta Med. Scand. *180:*551-559, 1966.

13. Parker, R. G., and Kendall, E. J.: The liver in ulcerative colitis. Brit. Med. J. *4895:*1030-1032, 1954.

14. Olhagen, L.: Ulcerative colitis in cirrhosis of the liver; report of ten cases. Acta Med. Scand. *162:*143-153, 1958.

15. Hoffbauer, F. W., McCartney, J. S., Dennis, C., and Karlson, K.: The relationship of chronic ulcerative colitis and cirrhosis. Ann. Intern. Med. *39:*267-284, 1953.

16. Smith, M. P., and Loe, R. H.: Sclerosing cholangitis, review of recent case reports and associated diseases and four new cases. Amer. J. Surg. *110:*239-246, 1965.

17. Isenberg, J. I., Goldstein, H., Korn, A. R., Ozeran, R. S., and Rosen, V.: Pulmonary vasculitis—an uncommon complication of ulcerative colitis. New Eng. J. Med. *279:*1376-1377, 1968.

18. Roberts, J. M.: Stenosing cholangitis. West. J. Surg. *63:*253-259, 1955.

19. Goldgraber, M. B., and Kirsner, J. B.: Chronic granulomatous choledochitis associated with chronic ulcerative colitis. A case report. Gastroenterology *38:*821-828, 1960.

20. Atkinson, A. J., and Carroll, W. W.: Sclerosing cholangitis. Association with regional enteritis. J.A.M.A. *188:*175-176, 1964.

21. Warren, K. W., Athanassiades, S., and Monge, J. I.: Primary sclerosing cholangitis. A study of 42 cases. Amer. J. Surg. *111:*23-38, 1966.

22. Thorpe, M. E., Scheur, P. J., and Sherlock, S.: Primary sclerosing cholangitis, the billiary tree, and ulcerative colitis. Gut *8:*435-448, 1967.

23. Rankin, J. G., Skyring, A. P., and Goulston, S. J.: Liver in ulcerative colitis: Obstructive jaundice due to bile duct carcinoma. Gut *7:*433-437, 1966.

24. Ham, J. M.: Tumors of biliary epithelium and ulcerative colitis. Ann. Surg. *168:*1088-1093, 1968.

25. Kelley, M. L., Jr., and Logan, V. W.: Erythema nodosum in association with chronic ulcerative colitis. Gastroenterology *31:*285-295, 1956.

26. Kelley, M. L., Jr.: Skin lesion associated with chronic ulcerative colitis. Amer. J. Dig. Dis. *7:*255-272, 1962.

27. Hurst, A. F.: Prognosis of ulcerative colitis. Lancet *2:*1194-1196, 1935.

28. Ricketts, W. E., and Palmer, W. L.: Complications of chronic nonspecific ulcerative colitis. Gastroenterology *7:*55-56, 1946.

29. Rice-Oxley, J. M., and Truelove, S.: Complications of ulcerative colitis. Lancet *1:*607-611, 1950.

30. Brown, M. L., Kasich, A. M., and Weingarten, B.: Complications of chronic ulcerative colitis. Amer. J. Dig. Dis. *18:*52-54, 1951.

31. Samitz, M. H., and Greenberg, M. S.: Skin lesions in association with ulcerative colitis. Gastroenterology *19:*476-479, 1951.

32. Banks, B. M., Korelitz, B. I., and Zetzel, L.: The course of nonspecific ulcerative colitis: review of twenty years experience and late results. Gastroenterology *32:*983-1012, 1957.

33. Bacon, H. E.: Ulcerative Colitis. Philadelphia, J. B. Lippincott Company, 1958.

34. Hightower, N. C., Jr., Broders, A. C., Jr., Haines, R. D., McKenney, I. F., and

Sommers, A. W.: Chronic ulcerative colitis. II. Complications. Amer. J. Dig. Dis. *3*:861-876, 1958.

35. Jackman, R. J., Bargen, J. A., and Helmholtz, H. F.: Life histories of ninety-five children with chronic ulcerative colitis. Amer. J. Dis. Child. *59*:459-467, 1940.

36. Elitzak, J., and Widerman, A. H.: Nonspecific ulcerative colitis in childhood. Amer. J. Dis. Child. *62*:115-126, 1941.

37. Rowe, A. H., and Rowe, A., Jr.: Chronic ulcerative colitis and regional enteritis; their allergic aspects. Ann. Allergy. *12*:387-402, 1954.

38. Foster, J. J., and Brick, I. B.: Erythema nodosum in ulcerative colitis. Gastroenterology *27*:417-425, 1954.

39. Johnson, M. L., and Wilson, H. T. H.: Skin lesions in ulcerative colitis. Gut *10*:255-263, 1969.

40. Lagercrantz, R.: Ulcerative colitis in children. Acta Paediat. (Suppl. 75) *37*:89-151, 1949.

41. Lagercrantz, R., Winberg, J., and Zetterstrom, R.: Extracolonic manifestations in chronic ulcerative colitis. Acta Paediat. *47*:675-687, 1958.

42. Fernandez-Herlihy, L.: The articular manifestations of chronic ulcerative colitis; an analysis of 555 cases. New Eng. J. Med. *261*:259-263, 1959.

43. Rotstein, J., Entel, I., and Zeviner, B.: Arthritis associated with ulcerative colitis. Ann. Rheum. Dis. *22*:194-197, 1963.

44. Ford, D. K., and Vallis, D. G.: The clinical course of arthritis associated with ulcerative colitis and regional ileitis. Arthritis Rheum. *2*:526-536, 1959.

45. Acheson, E. D.: An association between ulcerative colitis, regional enteritis and ankylosing spondylitis. Quart. J. Med. *29*:489-499, 1960.

46. Jayson, M. I., and Bouchier, I. A. D.: Ulcerative colitis with ankylosing spondylitis. Ann. Rheum. Dis. *27*:219-224, 1968.

47. Watkinson, G., Thompson, H., and Goligher, J. C.: Right-sided or segmental ulcerative colitis. Brit. J. Surg. *47*:337-351, 1960.

48. Neuman, H. W., Bargen, J. A., and Judd, E. S., Jr.: A clinical study of 201 cases of regional (segmental) colitis. Surg. Gynec. Obstet. *99*:563-571, 1954.

49. Crohn, B. B., Gerlock, J. H., and Yarnis, H.: Right-sided (regional) colitis. J.A.M.A. *134*:334-338, 1947.

50. Jankelson, I. R., McClure, C. W., and Sweetsir, F. N.: Chronic ulcerative colitis. II. Complication outside digestive tract. Rev. Gastroent. *9*:99-104, 1942.

51. Bywaters, E. G., and Ansell, B. M.: Arthritis associated with ulcerative colitis; a clinical and pathological study. Ann. Rheum. Dis. *17*:169-183, 1958.

52. Zvaifler, N. J., and Martel, W.: Spondylitis in chronic ulcerative colitis. Arthritis Rheum. *3*:76-87, 1960.

53. Kirsner, J. B., Palmer, W. L., Maimon, S. N., and Ricketts, W. E.: Clinical course of chronic nonspecific ulcerative colitis. J.A.M.A. *137*:922-928, 1948.

54. Wright, V., and Watkinson, G.: The arthritis of ulcerative colitis. Medicine (Balt.) *38*:243-262, 1959.

55. Brooke, B. N.: Outcome of surgery for ulcerative colitis. Lancet *2*:532-536, 1956.

56. McEwen, C., Lingg, C., and Kirsner, J. B.: Arthritis accompanying ulcerative colitis. Amer. J. Med. *33*:923-941, 1962.

57. McEwen, C.: Arthritis accompanying ulcerative colitis. Clin. Orthop. *57*:4-17, 1968.

58. Moschowitz, E.: Clinical aspects of amyloidosis. Ann. Intern. Med. *10*:73-88, 1936.

59. Mallory, T. B., Castleman, B., and Ropes, M. W.: Case records of the Massachusetts General Hospital, Case no. 33021. New Eng. J. Med. *236*:75-76, 1947.

60. Jensen, E. J., Bargen, J. A., and Baggenstoss, A. H.: Amyloidosis associated with chronic ulcerative colitis. Gastroenterology *15*:75-83, 1950.

61. Frenkel, M., and Groen, J.: Amyloidosis following adrenocorticotropic hormone therapy with report of a case. Nederl. T. Geneesk. *98*:2352, 1954.

62. Mandelbaum, I., and Bryk, D.: Idiopathic chronic ulcerative colitis and amyloidosis. J. Mount Sinai Hosp. N. Y. *22*:24-33, 1955.

63. Hasson, J., Berkman, J. I., Parker, J. G., and Rifkin, H. A.: A clinicopathologic study of chronic renal vein thrombosis in adults. Ann. Intern. Med. *47*:493-517, 1957.

64. Warren, I. A., Strygler, I., and Kobernick, S. D.: Amyloidosis secondary to chronic ulcerative colitis. Ann. Intern. Med. *51*:795-801, 1959.

65. Heptinstall, R. H., and Joekes, A. M.: Renal amyloid. A report on eleven cases proven by renal biopsy. Ann. Rheum. Dis. *19*:126-134, 1960.

66. Targgart, W. H., Trump, B. F., Lagunoff, D., and Eschbach, J.: Systemic amyloidosis and ulcerative colitis. Gastroenterology *44*:335-341, 1963.

Chapter Nine

Neoplastic Sequelae

REGIONAL ENTERITIS

I have found 21 cases in the medical literature in which carcinoma of the small or large intestine occurred within, in association with, or following the onset of the lesions of regional enteritis (Table 9-1). From the data available it is not possible to indicate with certainty whether regional enteritis predisposes the intestine to the development of carcinoma or whether it is a coincidence. Proof of the association remains wanting, though suspicion is strong that regional enteritis does predispose to the development of carcinoma. The age distribution of cases on record is relatively young, certainly considerably younger than the age of greatest prevalence of carcinomas of the intestinal tract in general. Also carcinoma of the small intestine is exceedingly rare, and the probability of coincidence with regional enteritis is remote. More than half the patients had a history of abdominal complaints suggestive of a clinical diagnosis of regional enteritis for a period of 10 years or more. Only one had a brief history of abdominal problems identifiable clinically for a week or two. In the majority of incidences the carcinoma was discovered coincidentally at the time of laparotomy for removal of the terminal ileum for regional enteritis. Though the histopathologic descriptions presented in the case reports are not in every instance complete, two cases of the pyloric type of epithelial metaplasia were identified and two others displayed an atypical hyperplasia in the vicinity of the invasive carcinoma. As indicated in a previous chapter, the prevalence of Paneth cell and pyloric gland types of metaplasia in many long-standing cases of regional enteritis is apparent. The occurrence of an increased incidence of carcinoma in this type of metaplastic epithelium would not be surprising.

Excluded from this list is the one case reported by Bersack in which clearly a carcinoma of the ileum was identified, but the presence of regional enteritis is debatable.[1] Also noteworthy are the reports by

Year	First Author	Age	Sex	Comments
1948	Warren[4]	(not given)		10 yr. of abdominal complaints; adenocarcinoma in R.E. of colon
1954	Van Patter[5]	(not given)		Carcinoma in R.E. lesion of colon
1956	Ginzburg[6]	30	M	Anaplastic carcinoma in R.E. involved jejunal segment; liver metastases
1957	Kornfeld[7]	36	F	8 yr. of R.E. adenocarcinoma distal to ligament of Treitz; metastases to liver, lymph nodes, lung, and bone
1958	Crohn[8]	(not given)		Carcinoma in R.E. lesion of colon
1958	Lear[9]	(not given)		Discovered carcinoma incidental to ileal resection for R.E.
1959	Buchanan[10]	47	M	3 yr. of R.E. adenocarcinoma in resected specimen of terminal ileum; lymph node metastases
1959	Weingarten[11]		F	21 yr. of abdominal complaints and R.E.; well-differentiated adenocarcinoma of jejunum with metastases to lymph nodes, liver, lungs, uterus, and ovaries
1960	Weingarten[11]	28	F	5 yr. of R.E.; all layers of involved ileum infiltrated with adenocarcinoma except serosa
1960	Steele[12]	38	M	14 yr. of abdominal complaints; 11 yr. of ankylosing spondylitis; anaplastic adenocarcinoma adjacent to fistula at autopsy involving all layers and extending into lymph nodes
1960	Zisk[13](Case 1)	61	F	Brief history of abdominal complaints; resection at autopsy revealed R.E. and adenocarcinoma in terminal ileum; glandular metaplasia
1960	Zisk[13] (Case 2)	62	F	20 yr. of abdominal complaints; adenocarcinoma and R.E. identified in ileum in resected specimen
1960	Almond[14]	48	F	2½ yr. of abdominal symptoms; resection revealed R.E. and adenocarcinoma of ileum
1963	Hoffert[15]	40	M	Well-differentiated adenocarcinoma in terminal ileum infiltrating to serosa and adjacent fat
1964	Berman[16]	51	M	35 yr. of abdominal cramps and diarrhea; regional enteritis and well-differentiated adenocarcinoma extending to serosa in involved ileum of resected specimen
1964	Wein[17]	48	M	20 yr. of R.E.; adenocarcinoma found in ileocecal valve of resected specimen in area of R.E. involvement
1968	Cantwell[18]	60	M	31 yr. of R.E.; carcinoma in resected ileum; metastases found at autopsy; signet ring cell type
1968	Sheil[19]	40	F	5 to 7 yr. of intermittent abdominal complaints; well-differentiated adenocarcinoma in stenotic terminal ileum
1968	Sheil[19]	50	F	11 yr. of symptoms; mucinous adenocarcinoma in rectum with R.E. lesion
1969	Tyers[20]	32	M	9½ years of abdominal complaints; pathologic diagnosis, multicentric carcinoma of jejunum arising from chronic regional enteritis
1969	Magnes[76]	71	M	14 yr. of regional enteritis before unicentric carcinoma of terminal ileum

Hughes and by Wyburn-Mason of the coincidental occurrence of a reticulum cell sarcoma of the ileum and regional enteritis.[2, 3] This occurred in a 72 year old man who had a 16 year history of abdominal complaints following trauma to the abdomen. Regional enteritis was identified in the surgically resected specimen one year after onset of abdominal symptoms. Following resection he remained largely symptom free until the terminal episode. At autopsy a tumor mass was found encircling the ileum, 35 cm. proximal to the cecum, and 37 cm. proximal to this was another tumor. The ascending colon also contained two small tumor nodules, and the mesenteric and retroperitoneal lymph nodes were similarly involved, as were the internal mammary and left supraclavicular, periaortic, and peribronchial lymph nodes. Microscopically this was identified as a reticulum cell sarcoma. The widespread involvement of the lymphoreticular system suggests the probability that the occurrence of these two diseases was coincidental.

Although the majority of carcinomas associated with regional enteritis occurred in the small intestine, a few occurred in regional enteritis lesions of the large bowel. The data are insufficient to determine whether this is proportional to the occurrence of regional enteritis in the large intestine. Most of the carcinomas (approximately three quarters) were composed of neoplastic cells that were well or moderately well differentiated. Relatively few were anaplastic. Two cases of the signet ring cell type have been recorded. Metastasis took place predominantly via the intestinal lymphatics. Distant metastases have been recorded in the liver, lungs, pancreas, adrenal glands, and ovaries. Peritoneal and omental implants were frequently observed. The prognosis was extremely poor, and rarely did a patient live for more than a year after discovery of the neoplasm.

ULCERATIVE COLITIS

During the past 20 years it has become evident that ulcerative colitis is a precancerous lesion. That is not to say that all cases of ulcerative colitis, if followed long enough, will result in carcinomatous change; however, there is a significantly greater frequency of carcinoma of the colon in individuals with ulcerative colitis than in the general population. Recognition of this fact has been tardy, and conflicting reports in the early literature have perhaps resulted from the fact that ulcerative colitis itself is not a common lesion and only a small percentage of those who have it subsequently develop carcinoma of the colon. Over the years, as reports have accumulated, their summarization has made the relationship incontrovertible. Bargen, drawing on the extensive experience of the Mayo Clinic, reported that about 2 per cent of the 693 cases he reviewed eventuated in carcinoma.[21] More recently others have summarized the reports in the literature and added their own cases to establish the causal relationship.[22a, 22b, 23] Table 9–2 is a list of the major studies on the incidence of carcinoma of the colon. I have not included the smaller reports with few cases. Excluding childhood ulcerative colitis, which is discussed separately, it is apparent from this table that the reported incidence of carcinoma in observed cases of ulcerative colitis ranges from about 1 to 14 per cent. This variability may be accounted for by the selectivity of

TABLE 9–2   Frequency of Carcinoma with Ulcerative Colitis

First Author	Year of Publication	Observed Cases of Ulcerative Colitis	Cases of Carcinoma	Percentage of Total U.C.
Bargen[21]	1929	693	15	2.1
Lynn[24]	1945	1467	25	1.9
Renshaw[25]	1945	336	2	0.59
Svartz[26]	1946	120	3	2.20
Cave[27]	1946	101	4	4.0
Ricketts[28]	1946	206	3	1.4
Cattell[29]	1947	450	9	2.0
Johnson[30]	1948	164	2	1.2
Hayes[31]	1949	451	3	0.7
Svartz[32]	1949	290	9	3.1
Kasich[33]	1949	143	7	4.9
Warren[35]	1949	180	9	5.0
Strombeck[36]	1949	54	1	1.8
Lagercrantz[37]	1949	134	1	0.7
Svartz[32]	1949	439	17	3.9
Kapel[38]	1950	143	2	1.4
Rice-Oxley[39]	1950	129	4	3.1
Sloan[40]	1950	2000	66	3.3
Lahey[41]	1950	263	18	6.7
Gleckler[42]	1950	316	12	3.8
Lyons[43]	1951	226	9	3.9
Kiefer[44]	1951	226	10	4.4
Counsell[45]	1952	63	7	11.1
Weckesser[46]	1953	118	4	3.4
MacDougall[55]	1954	126	5	3.9
Bargen[56]	1954	1564	98	6.3
Wheelock[47]	1955	319	31	8.8
Flood[48]	1956	148	1	0.67
Bacon[49]	1956	84	12	14.2
Maltby[51]	1956	81	5	6.1
Colcock[52]	1956	307	11	3.58
Hickey[53]	1956	326	19	6.0
Dukes[54]	1957	153	8	5.2
Goldgraber[22]	1958	792	22	2.8
Thorlakson[50]	1958	218	17	3.7
Slaney[57]	1959	222	18	6.7
Dawson[23]	1959	663	19	2.4
Russell[58]	1961	272	11	4.0
Total		13,987	563	3.1

referral of patients to these major hospitals and clinics and to the variable duration of follow-up. These centers tend to see only the more severe refractory cases; therefore, one may expect the actual incidence of carcinoma with ulcerative colitis to be somewhat less than reported. In a total of 13,987 observed cases of ulcerative colitis in 38 major reports, 836 carcinomas of the colon were reported for a frequency of 5.8 per cent. There appears to be no sexual preponderance, the ratio being 1:1. Sloan, Bargen, and Gage reported a female to male ratio of 0.8:1 in their series of 2,000 patients who had 66 carcinomas.[40] However, in the report of Dawson and Pryse-Davies, of 663 patients with ulcerative colitis in whom 19 carcinomas occurred, there was no specific predominance of female over male when the incidence was adjusted for the slight predominance of ulcerative colitis in females.[23]

The duration of symptoms of chronic ulcerative colitis before the occurrence of carcinoma of the colon is quite variable as Table 9-3 reveals. This not only accounts for some of the variability in the frequency of carcinoma dependent upon the duration of clinical follow-up, but is also pathologically and therapeutically significant. This table is abstracted from seven reports in the literature in which data on the duration of symptoms was available. Of these 130 cases reported, 22 per cent had ulcerative colitis symptoms for less than 10 years, whereas 47 per cent had ulcerative colitis for 10 through 19 years, and 31 per cent had symptoms for more than 20 years. The duration of symptoms prior to the onset of carcinoma in individual cases was highly variable. Many had symptoms of a year or two prior to the discovery of the carcinoma, and the maximum duration was 40 years. Though there are insufficient cases to be significant, one has the decided impression that individuals in their late teens and early twenties seem to have a shorter duration between the onset of the ulcerative colitis and the occurrence of carcinoma.

The mean age at death from carcinoma of the colon, as abstracted from the literature, is shown in Table 9-4. This was selected rather than analysis of the age at diagnosis of the carcinoma because it is more

TABLE 9–3   Duration of Ulcerative Colitis Symptoms Before Cancer

			Duration of Ulcerative Colitis (yr.)		
First Author	**Year**	**No. of Carcinomas**	*less than 10*	*10 to 19*	*20 or more*
Goldgraber[22]	1958	14	2	9	3
Thorlakson[50]	1958	8	1	3	4
Slaney[57]	1959	18	5	9	4
Dawson[23]	1959	19	4	6	9
Russell[58]	1961	22	6	15	1
White[59]	1962	17	7	5	5
Hinton[61]	1966	32	4	14	14
Total		130	29 (22%)	61 (47%)	40 (31%)

TABLE 9–4   Mean Age at Death from Cancer of Colon

First Author	Year of Report	Deaths from Carcinoma	Age in Years
Kasich[33]	1949	7	44
Counsell[45]	1952	7	45
Ascherman[62]	1953	15	32
Thorlakson[64]	1956	12	48
Tidrick[63]	1956	6	28
Goldgraber[22]	1958	14	41
Thorlakson[50]	1958	5	50
Dawson[23]	1959	13	43
Slaney[57]	1959	8	43
Russell[58]	1961	17	47
White[59]	1962	14	47
Total deaths		118	Average age 46

indicative of the biology of the neoplasm and is less subject to clinical and therapeutic variability. These data summarize the fact that death occurs at an earlier age in patients with carcinoma of the colon following ulcerative colitis than it does in patients who have carcinoma of the colon but are otherwise apparently free of colonic disease. This is further evidence that these carcinomas are biologically different from the usual colonic carcinoma and that their existence is not mere coincidence—and reinforces the evidence on their frequency.

Another distinguishing gross feature of the carcinomas associated with ulcerative colitis is that they have a different anatomic location from carcinomas of the colon in general. Table 9–5 reveals that, of 386 of these carcinomas reported by nine authors, only 45 per cent were located in the rectosigmoid region, in sharp contrast with the approximately 70 per cent reported for carcinomas of the colon in general (Table 9–6). Even if one were to include all the unclassified locations in the rectosigmoid, one would still have a significant difference. Also, the

TABLE 9–5   Anatomic Location of Carcinoma of the Colon Secondary to Ulcerative Colitis

First Author	Total Carcinomas	Cecum	Ascending Colon	Hepatic Flexure	Transverse Colon	Splenic Flexure	Descending Colon	Rectosigmoid Colon	Unclassified
Goldgraber[22]	14	1		1	3		1	8	
Slaney[57]	18		2	1	1		1	12	1
Dawson[23]	20	1	1		2		1	11	3
Rosenquist[65]	26	3		2	6	5		10	
Edling[66]	43	6	5	4	6	4	4	14	
Russell[58]	26	1	2	2	6	1	2	12	
Bargen[56]	178	17	5	3	15	7	10	70	51
Thorlakson[50, 64]	17	1	1	1	1	1	1	11	
Hinton[61]	44	1	0	2	9	4	5	23	
	386	31	16	16	49	22	25	171	55
		(8%)	(4%)	(4%)	(13%)	(6%)	(7%)	(45%)	

TABLE 9–6   Anatomic Location of Lesions in Series of Carcinoma of the Colon of all Causes*

Location	Welch and Burke 1886 cases (1962) (%)	McSwain et al. 708 cases (1962) (%)	Popper 497 cases (1952) (%)	Pittsburgh Series 280 Cases (%)
Cecum	9.5	8.6	8.3	13.6
Ascending colon	6.2	7.2	5.6	8.1
Hepatic flexure	2.0	2.5	2.5	3.6
Transverse colon	5.7	6.5	4.5	3.9
Splenic flexure	2.6	2.0	3.0	3.2
Descending colon	5.0	2.5	5.6	6.4
Rectosigmoid	68.0	68.4	70.5	60.1
Anus	1.0	2.3	—	1.1
	100.0	100.0	100.0	100.0

*Courtesy of W. C. Davis and F. C. Jackson: Ca. *18:*144, 1968, and the American Cancer Society.

frequency of carcinomas of the transverse colon associated with ulcerative colitis is almost twice that of the ordinary type, the latter occurring about 6 per cent of the time in this location. Except in the cecum, the frequency is approximately double that in other regions of the proximal colon.

The macroscopic features of carcinomas of the colon associated with ulcerative colitis are comparable to those of "ordinary" carcinomas of the colon in spite of the differences in frequency and location (Tables 9-5 and 9-6).[60] Grossly, the lesions range from exophytic (polypoid) to ulcerative and diffusely infiltrating patterns of growth. Strictures are present in approximately half, and about three quarters have evidence of metastases at the time of their discovery. Metastatic spread occurs via the lymphatics principally. Two or more separate primary carcinomas of the colon seem to occur more frequently in association with ulcerative colitis than is reported with "ordinary" carcinoma of the colon, though the data are insufficient to document this. Indeed the data on anatomic location of carcinoma of the colon is based on location of the carcinomas rather than on individual patients, because several of the reports include multiple neoplasms (Figs. 9-1 and 9-2). In some cases, because of the diffuse involvement with carcinoma, it is difficult to identify with certainty the precise site of origin. In one patient, the whole large intestine was diffusely involved by carcinomas, and careful autopsy did not reveal one particular region of primary growth.[23] This lack of precise site of origin has been reported by several observers and suggests to some that the carcinomas arise as a diffuse neoplastic change over a wide field of altered mucosa, which is in distinct contrast to the usual large intestinal carcinoma in which the edges are well defined.[22, 45] In some of the cases, the

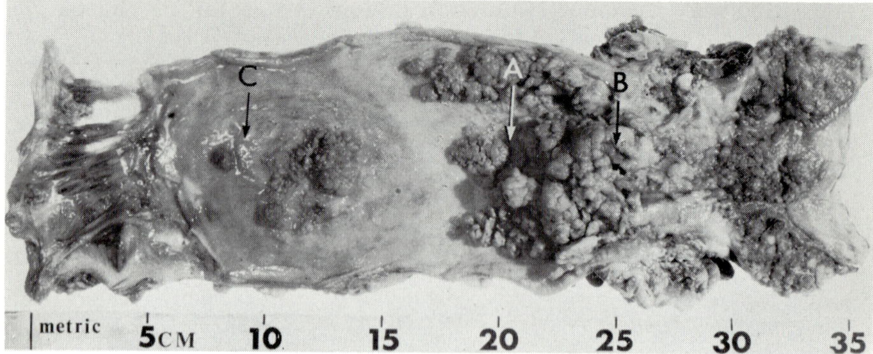

Figure 9–1   Sigmoid colon and rectum. Toward the right end of the specimen there is extensive papillary tumor that is largely benign (A), but contains a stricture due to malignancy (B) (carcinoma) about 5 cm. long. In the rectum there are smaller areas of villous overgrowth of the mucosa (C). (Courtesy of B. C. Morson and L. S. Pang, Gut *8*:423–34, 1967, and the British Medical Association.)

evidence of strictures may be noted by clinical means prior to the identification of the carcinoma. The early spread and metastasis are features frequently reported and appear to be linked with the unusually poor prognosis. In some cases, in addition to the diffuse carcinomatous involvement, there may be a locus of carcinoma at one site and adenomatous colonic polyps elsewhere (Figs. 9-2, 9-3, and 9-4). Multiple neoplasms are common in many series.[22, 34] In one study

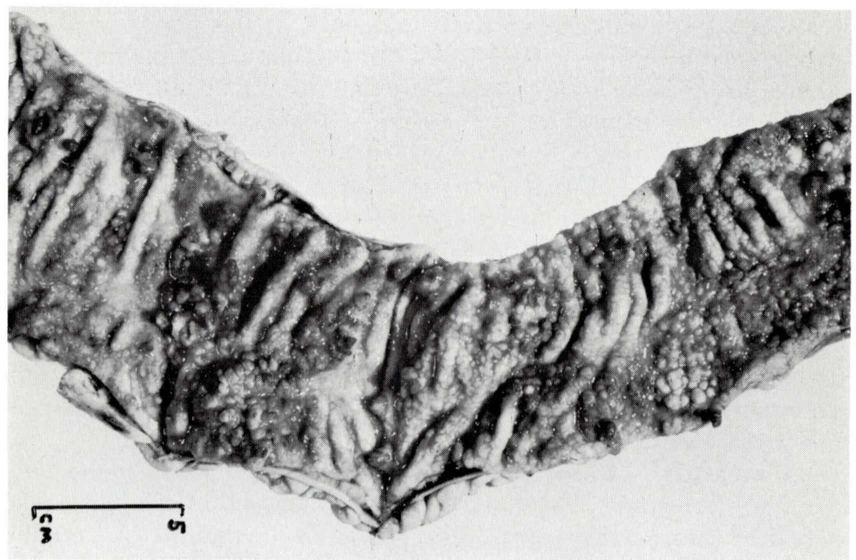

Figure 9–2   Mucosal surface of the colon from another case showing polypoid change that has a nodular and papillary surface configuration. (Courtesy of B. C. Morson and L. S. Pang, Gut *8*:423–34, 1967, and the British Medical Association.)

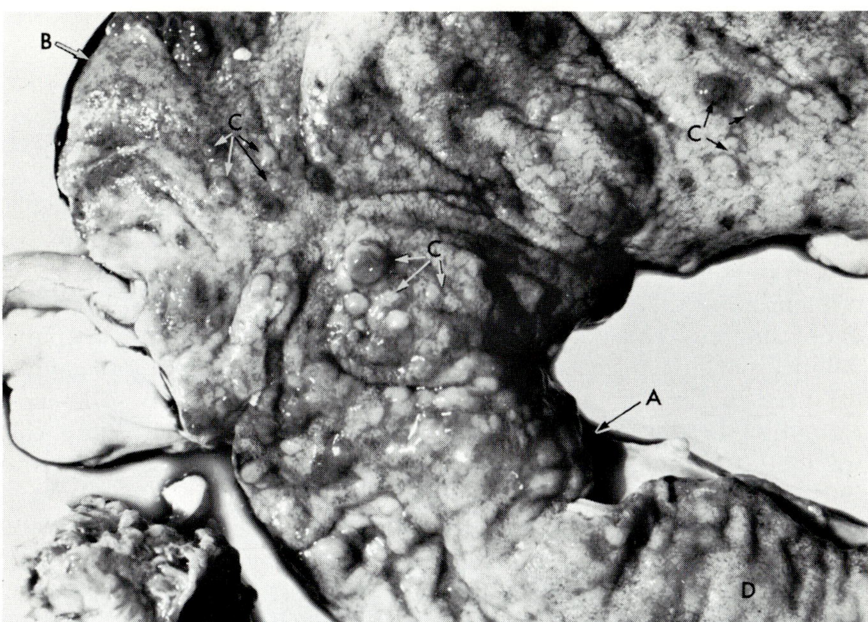

Figure 9-3 Close-up view of the terminal ileum (A) and cecum (B) from a patient with ulcerative colitis and secondary polypoid hyperplasia (C). The latter change involves the terminal centimeter or two of the ileum. Uninvolved ileal mucosa is seen at (D).

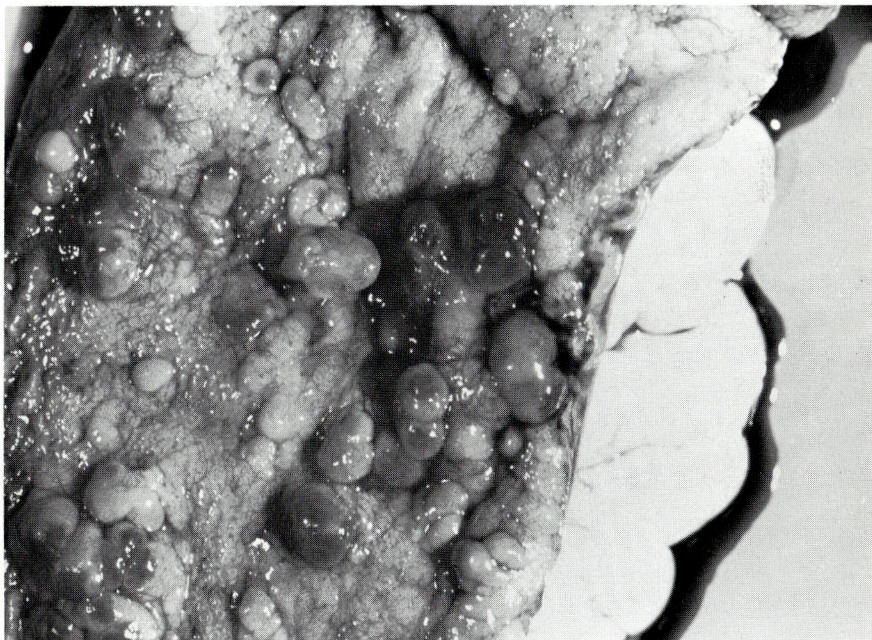

Figure 9-4 Close-up view of the descending colon from the same specimen shown in Figure 9-3. The variability in the appearance of the polyps is shown.

12 of 41 cases had multiple neoplasms, and 5 of 14 cases were reported in another.

Microscopic features of these carcinomas also cover the same spectrum as those of the "ordinary" type (Figs. 9-5 and 9-6). In approximately half the cases, patches of neoplastic atypical glands extending into the submucosa and muscular coat may be seen (Fig. 9-8 A and B). In some they may resemble rather closely the irregular islands of buried epithelial nests that are frequently seen in ulcerative colitis, and the distinction between the two must be made on the basis of the cellular morphologic criteria pertaining to atypical hyperplastic and neoplastic cells. Indeed, whether the neoplasm arises from such epithelial inclusions or not remains an interesting speculation. In the majority of cases there is an intense fibrosis in the mucosa and submucosa extending to the superficial layers of the muscularis with a varying number of chronic inflammatory cells, principally lymphocytes, plasma cells, and monocytes in the stroma of the neoplasm. Often this is sufficiently extensive to give the involved region a linitis plastica-like appearance including some cells with a signet ring shape.

Whether the inflammatory pseudopolyps, frequently identified with ulcerative colitis undergo gradual change into adenomatous polyps that in turn undergo neoplastic change remains moot (Figs. 9-7D, 9-9D, and 9-10B). Some support the concept.[23, 40, 67] The first

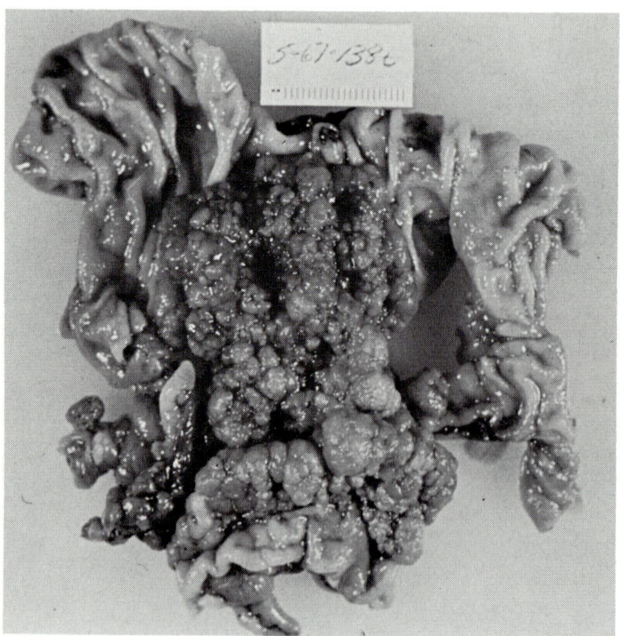

Figure 9–5   Close-up view of a villous (or papillary) adenocarcinoma in the rectum. The sessile growth of the lesion is shown. Also, the neoplastic change has almost extended the total circumference of the mucosa.

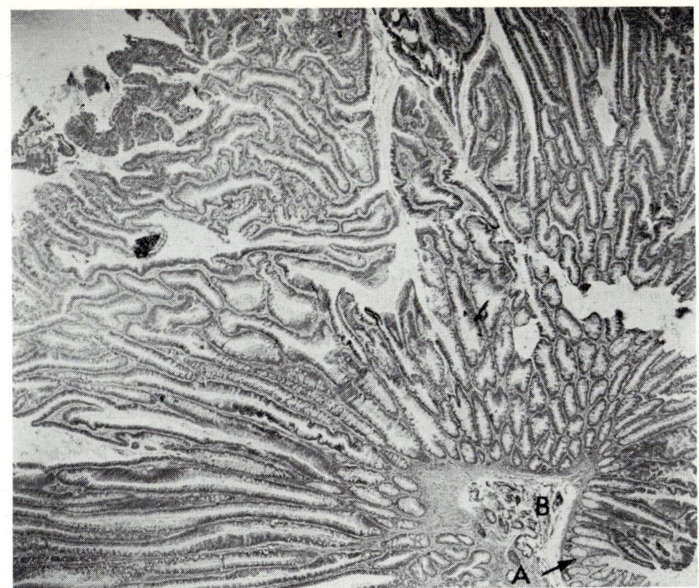

Figure 9–6 Microscopic view of the lesion shown in Figure 9-5. The junction with the colonic mucosa is shown (A). A site of invasion of the subjacent submucosa is also seen (B). The major part of the photomicrograph is composed of elongated papillary mucosal glands. ×10.

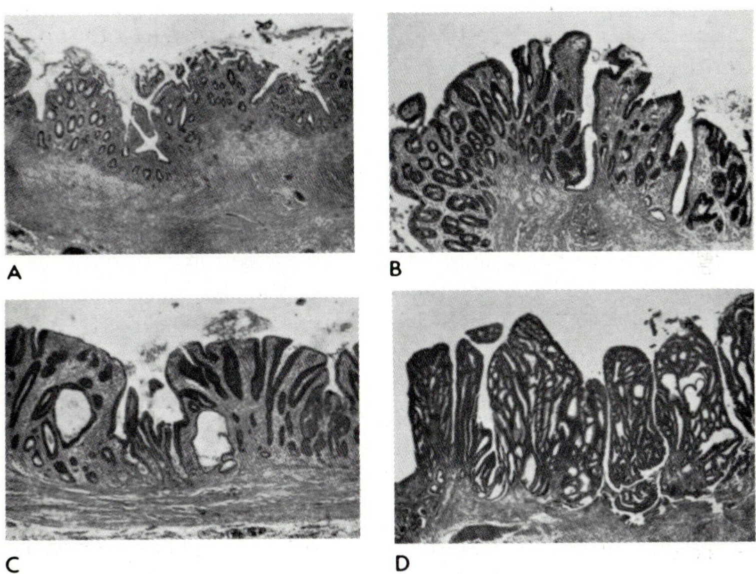

Figure 9–7 *A, B,* and *C.* Various stages of precancerous change in the colon of a 50 year old woman who had total colonic ulcerative colitis for 20 years before the cancerous change. Two areas of invasive carcinoma were found, one in the ascending colon, another in the rectum. Both produced strictures. The patient died of metastases a year after operation. Histologically the tumors were moderately well-differentiated adenocarcinoma. *D,* A characteristic papilloma of the colon from a similar case. For histology of the malignancy in this case see Figure 9–8. ×20. (Courtesy of I. M. P. Dawson and J. Pryse-Davies. Brit. J. Surg. *47*:113–128, 1959, and John Wright & Sons, Ltd. Bristol.)

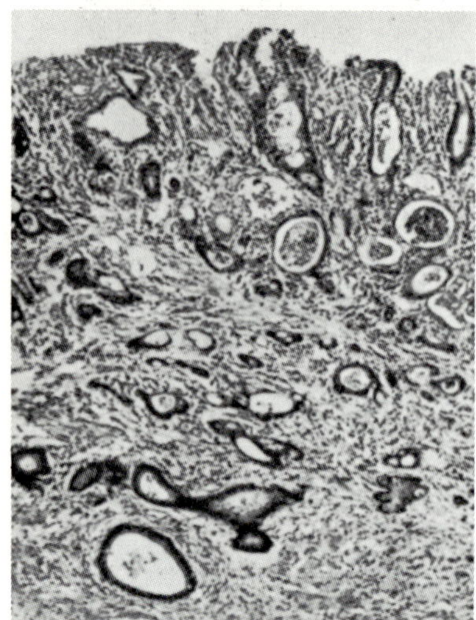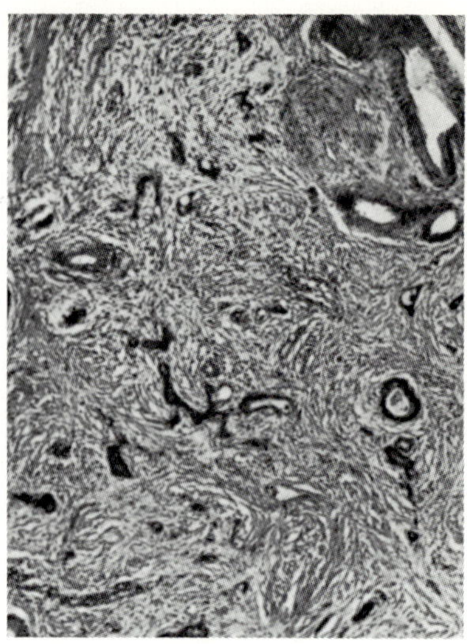

Figure 9–8 Photomicrographs from the two sites of invasive carcinoma described in Figure 9-7. Neoplastic glands are shown infiltrating the subcutaneous and deeper layers. The morphology of these malignant glands contrasts with that seen in colitis cystica profunda (see Figures 5–32 and 5–33.) ×50. (Courtesy of I. M. P. Dawson and J. Pryse-Davies. Brit. J. Surg. *47*:113–128, 1959, and John Wright & Sons, Ltd. Bristol.)

of these authors indicated that they have found polyps that were indistinguishable histologically from true neoplastic adenomas or papillomas and report six cases of transitional lesions between true polyps and pseudopolyps, yet such evidence at best must be regarded as presumptive because of the widespread involvement of the mucosa of the colon and the diffuseness of the atypism of the epithelium observed in long-standing ulcerative colitis (Figs. 9-7, 9-9 to 9-14). The existence of exophytic (polypoid) carcinomas provides no valid evidence for the relationship because whether a neoplasm is exophytic or endophytic depends on the relationship of the neoplasm to the host tissues as a characteristic of the neoplastic cell rather than its histogenesis. Occasionally cancers develop in nonfunctional rectal stumps following subtotal colectomy for ulcerative colitis. Though frequently associated with epithelial nests, distorted morphology, and pseudopolyps and mucosal bridges, occasionally cancers have developed in atrophic mucosa following long-standing quiescent or burned out ulcerative colitis.

Statistical studies by Goldgraber and co-workers compared the colonic cancer risk in ulcerative colitis patients with that in a control series matched for race, sex, and age and found an eightfold increase in frequency of death from colonic cancer in the ulcerative colitis group of patients.[22a, 22b] Slaney and Brooke analyzed 304 cases of carcinoma following ulcerative colitis reported in the literature, and found a five year survival rate of 18.6 per cent. They emphasized that the carcinoma may develop after a quiescent or healing phase or in a

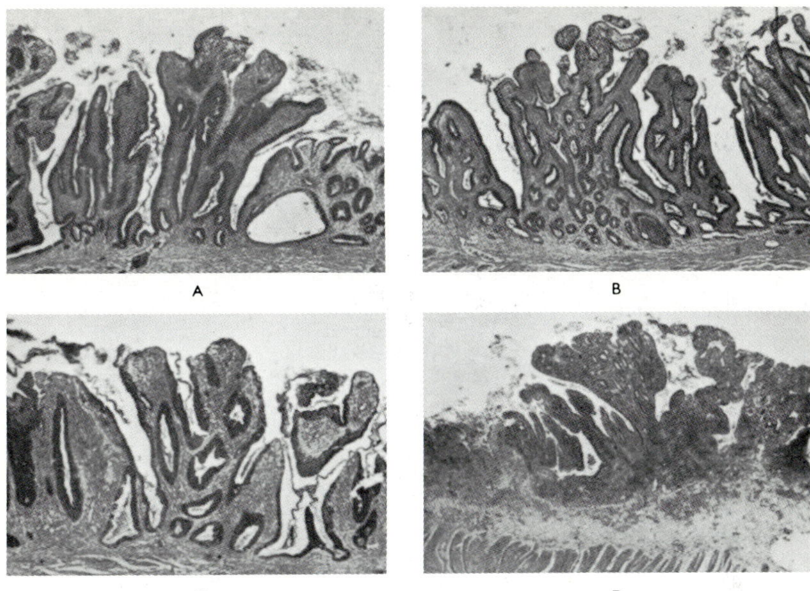

Figure 9–9   Various stages of carcinogenesis are shown in a surgically resected colon from a 57 year old woman who had a total colonic distribution of ulcerative colitis for 18 years prior to neoplastic change. The invasive malignancy occurred in the cecum adjacent to the ileocecal valve and appendix, producing a stricture. *A* to *D*. Four photomicrographs of various types of precancerous change ranging from mild to severe atypism (*A, B, C*) and a pseudopolyp (*D*). The adenocarcinoma was moderately well differentiated. ×20. (Courtesy of I. M. P. Dawson and J. Pryse-Davies, Brit. J. Surg. *47*:113–128, 1959, and John Wright & Sons, Ltd., Bristol.)

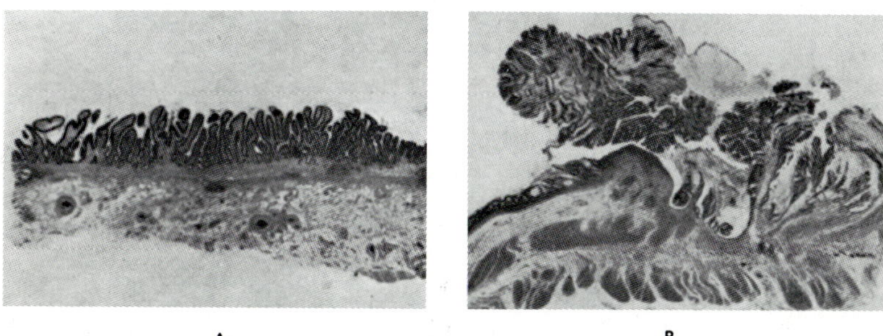

Figure 9–10   Photomicrographs from two sites of precancerous change from patients who had elsewhere developed colonic carcinoma secondary to ulcerative colitis. *A*. Precancerous changes in the epithelial cells in an otherwise atrophic epithelium. *B*. Similar precancerous changes in a papillary polypoid hyperplastic epithelium. ×4. (Courtesy of I. M. P. Dawson and J. Pryse-Davies, Brit. J. Surg. *47*:113–128, 1959, and John Wright & Sons, Ltd., Bristol.)

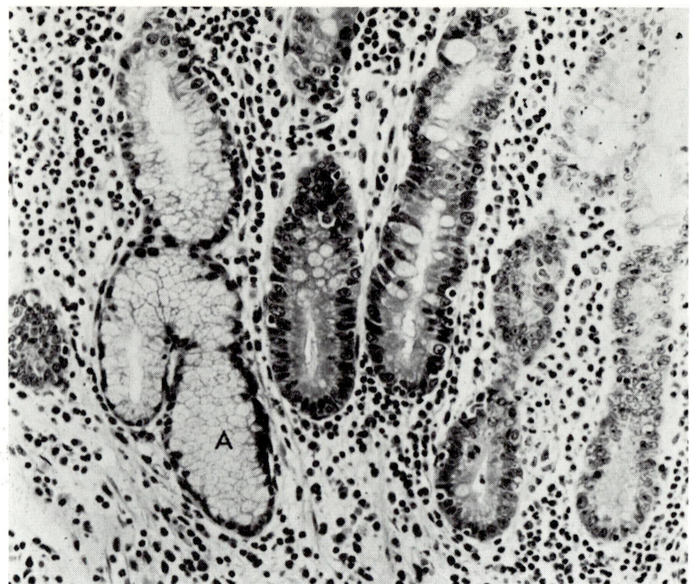

Figure 9–11   Photomicrograph of a region of the mucosa of long-standing ulcerative colitis in which some glands are hypersecretory (A), whereas others have diminished secretion and early precancerous change. ×175.

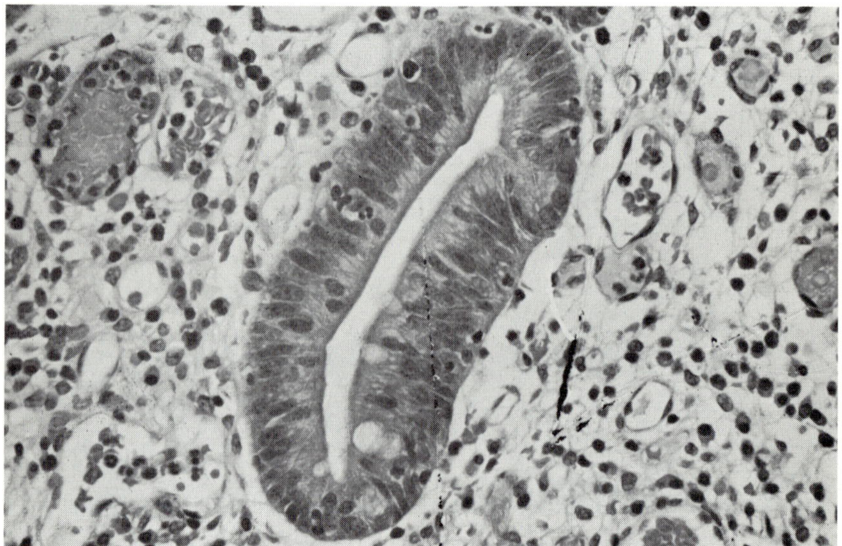

Figure 9–12   Photomicrograph of a gland with diminished secretory activity and hyperplastic changes in the epithelial cells. ×260.

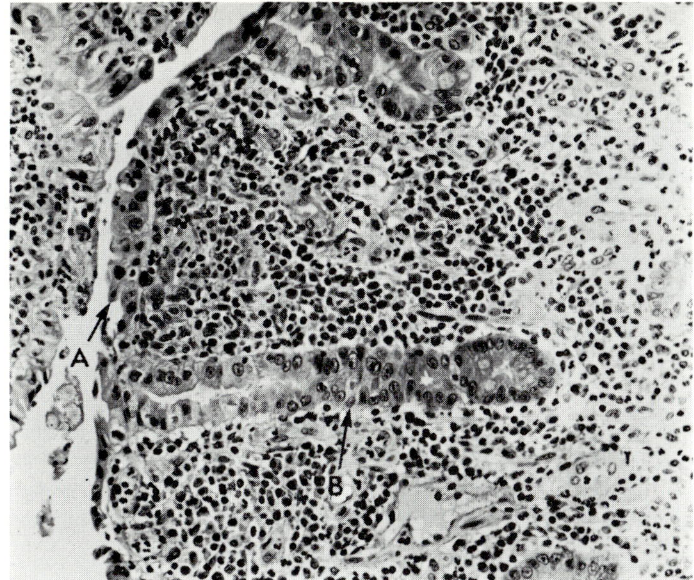

Figure 9–13   Early precancerous change in the colonic epithelium of a patient with long-standing ulcerative colitis. Precancerous changes are seen in both the surface epithelium (A) and the glands (B). Nuclei are frequently central within the cells, enlarged, angular, and irregularly hyperchromatic. Enlarged nucleoli may be seen in some. Mucus secretion is markedly diminished. ×175.

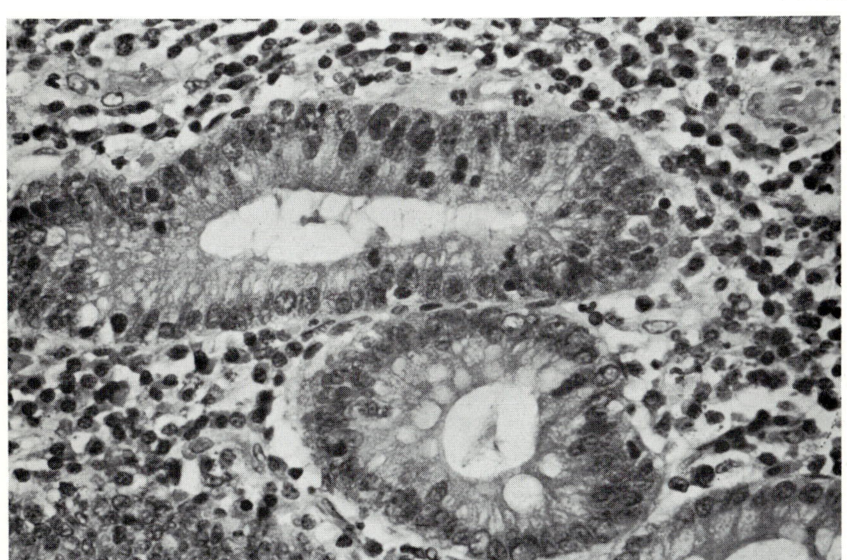

Figure 9–14   Glands from another region of the same specimen shown in Figure 9-13. The changes already described are present, but to a lesser degree. ×260.

segment of the bowel not involved in the ulcerative colitis, adding to the difficulty of detection.[57] Turnbull and Brown reported two cases of carcinoma of the colon in ulcerative colitis in which there was no evidence of inflammatory or adenomatous polyps.[68] Felsen and Wolarsky studied the pseudopolyps of 855 cases of chronic ulcerative colitis and found no malignant change.[69] Otani and Snapper concur that when malignancy develops in the colon it is secondary to pre-existing polyps.[70] Microscopically, the carcinomas range in appearance from highly anaplastic to well-differentiated mucus secreting lesions.

According to Weckesser and Chinn, among patients who have had ulcerative colitis for 10 years or longer, the incidence of malignant disease of the colon was 9 per cent; and according to Rosenquist and co-workers, among patients who have had ulcerative colitis for 10 to 20 years, one in three develop carcinoma.[46, 65] Russell and Hughes reported that the average duration of colitis prior to the development of carcinoma was 13 years and that those patients who have had colitis for 10 or more years have a 25 per cent chance of developing carcinoma.[58] Gazzaniga and Gazzaniga reported the occurrence of chronic ulcerative colitis in two brothers who subsequently developed carcinoma of the colon.[71] Both developed ulcerative colitis before the age of 20 and both died of carcinoma before the age of 35. Hinton reviewed the risk of malignant change in ulcerative colitis in cases from three hospitals in England and added his own experience.[61] He concluded that it was most unlikely that patients with ulcerative proctitis or proctosigmoiditis have any greater risk of developing large bowel cancer than the normal population and that the greatest risk occurred in patients who had total and extensive chronic ulcerative colitis. He also observed, as reported by similar studies already mentioned, that the duration of the colitis is important in the cumulative risk. Those with less than 10 years of colitis had only a 5 per cent risk, but between 10 and 20 years there was a 25 per cent risk. MacDougall demonstrated that those whose colitis began before the age of 25 had twice the cancer incidence of those whose colitis developed after that age.[55] Correlated with this is the fact that in the younger age group the colitis is total and severe in about two thirds of the cases in contrast to that in the older age group.

Exfoliative cytology to identify potential carcinogenesis has been applied to chronic ulcerative colitis patients by Galambos and co-workers and by Boddington and Truelove.[72, 73] The method has not yet proved sufficiently reliable to provide a means of identifying precancerous changes in patients with ulcerative colitis.

Neoplasms of the lymphoma type have also been reported as a sequela of ulcerative colitis, much less frequently, however, than adenocarcinoma. In one review a total of seven cases was presented.[74] More recently another case was added.[75] They have occurred anywhere in the large intestine from the cecum to the rectum, in both sexes, and in an age range of 26 to 64 years. The duration of the ulcerative colitis was 5 to 16 years. The histologic appearance of the lymphomas were also quite variable, covering the entire spectrum of cell types. About half were lymphosarcomatous in type, but reticulum cell and Hodgkin's types have also been reported. The similarity of benign intensely hyperplastic lymphoid tissue commonly associated with ulcerative colitis may at times be confused with a lymphomatous process. In addition to the usual criteria for differentiating between them, one must bear in mind that malignant lymphomas have a propensity not only for invading the muscularis, but also are intensively destructive of it. The muscle necrosis is generally much more extensive than that seen with invasion of adenocarcinoma.

References

1. Bersack, S. R., Howe, J. S., and Rehak, E. M.: A unique case with roentgenologic evidence of regional enteritis of long duration and histologic evidence of diffuse adenocarcinoma. Gastroenterology *34*:703-710, 1958.
2. Hughes, R. K.: Reticulum cell sarcoma: case possibly originating in regional enteritis. Amer. Surg. *21*:770-773, 1955.
3. Wyburn-Mason, R.: Crohn's disease and carcinoma of the colon. Brit. Med. J. *2*:697, 1968.
4. Warren, S., and Sommers, S. C.: Cicatrizing enteritis (regional enteritis) as a pathological entity: analysis of 120 cases. Amer. J. Path. *24*:475-501, 1948.
5. Van Patter, W. N., Bargen, J. A., Dockerty, M. B., Feldman, W. H., Mayo, C. W., and Waugh, J. M.: Regional enteritis. Gastroenterology *26*:347-450, 1954.
6. Ginzburg, L., Schneider, K. M., Dreizin, D. H., and Levinson, C.: Carcinoma of the jejunum occurring in a case of regional enteritis. Surgery *39*:347-351, 1956.
7. Kornfeld, P., Ginzburg, L., and Adlersberg, D.: Adenocarcinoma occurring in regional jejunitis. Amer. J. Med. *23*:493-498, 1957.
8. Crohn, B. B., and Yarnis, H.: Regional Ileitis. 2nd Ed. New York, Grune and Stratton, 1958.
9. Lear, P. E.: The physiologic basis for the surgical management of regional enteritis. Surg. Clin. N. Amer. *38*:545-559, 1958.
10. Buchanan, D. P., Huebner, G. D., Woolvin, S. C., North, R. L., and Novack, T. D.: Carcinoma of the ileum occurring in an area of regional enteritis. Amer. J. Surg. *97*:336-339, 1959.
11. Weingarten, B., and Weiss, J.: Malignant degeneration in chronic inflammatory disease of the colon and small intestine. Amer. J. Gastroent. *33*:203-207, 1960.
12. Steele, D. C., and McNeely, D. T.: Adenocarcinoma arising in a site of chronic regional enteritis. Canad. Med. Ass. J. *83*:379-381, 1960.
13. Zisk, I., Shore, J. M., Rosoff, L., and Friedman, N. B.: Regional ileitis complicated by adenocarcinoma of the ileum: a report of two cases. Surgery *47*:970–974, 1960.
14. Almond, C. H., Neal, M. P., and Moedl, K. R.: Regional ileitis with coincident ileal carcinoma. Missouri Med. *57*:452-454, 1960.
15. Hoffert, P. W., Weingarten, B., Friedman, L. D., and Morecki, R.: Adenocarcinoma of the terminal ileum in a segment of bowel with coexisting active ileitis. New York J. Med. *63*:1567-1571, 1963.
16. Berman, L. G., and Prior, J. T.: Adenocarcinoma of the small intestine occurring in a case of regional enteritis. J. Mount Sinai Hosp. N. Y. *31*:30–37, 1964.
17. Wein, M. A., Spector, N., and Robinson, H. M.: Regional ileitis complicated by adenocarcinoma. Report of a case. Amer. J. Gastroent. *41*:58-63, 1964.
18. Cantwell, J. D., Kettering, R. F., Carney, J. A., and Ludwig, J.: Adenocarcinoma complicating regional enteritis: report of a case and review of the literature. Gastroenterology *54*:599-604, 1968.

19. Sheil, F. O. M., Clark, G. C., and Goligher, J. C.: Adenocarcinoma associated with Crohn's disease. Brit. J. Surg. *55*:53-58, 1968.

20. Tyers, G. F., Steiger, E., and Dudrick, S. J.: Adenocarcinoma of the small intestine and other malignant tumors complicating regional enteritis; case report and review of the literature. Ann. Surg. *169*:510-518, 1969.

21. Bargen, J. A.: Complications and sequelae of chronic ulcerative colitis. Ann. Intern. Med. *3*:335-352, 1929.

22a. Goldgraber, M. B., Humphreys, E. M., Kirsner, J. B., and Palmer, W. L.: Carcinoma and ulcerative colitis, a clinical-pathologic study. I. Cancer deaths. Gastroenterology *34*:809–839, 1958.

22b. Goldgraber, M. B., Humphreys, E. M., Kirsner, J. B., and Palmer, W. L.: Carcinoma and ulcerative colitis, a clinical-pathologic study. II. Statistical analysis. Gastroenterology *34*:840-846, 1958.

23. Dawson, I. M., and Pryse-Davies, J.: The development of carcinoma of the large intestine in ulcerative colitis. Brit. J. Surg. *47*:113-128, 1959.

24. Lynn, D. H.: The relationship of chronic lesions to carcinoma of colon; chronic ulcerative colitis; collective review. Int. Abstr. Surg. *81*:269-276, 1945.

25. Renshaw, R. J. F., and Brownell, T. S.: Carcinoma complicating ulcerative colitis. Cleveland Clin. Quart. *12*:123-127, 1945.

26. Svartz, N.: Le traitement des colites ulcéreuses par la salazopyrine. Acta Med. Scand. *170*:733–741, 1946.

27. Cave, H. W.: Late results on the treatment of ulcerative colitis. Ann. Surg. *124*:716-724, 1946.

28. Ricketts, W. E., and Palmer, W. L.: Complications of chronic nonspecific ulcerative colitis. Gastroenterology *7*:55-66, 1946.

29. Cattell, R. B., and Boehme, E. J.: The importance of malignant degeneration as a complication of chronic ulcerative colitis. Gastroenterology *8*:695–710, 1947.

30. Johnson, T. M., and Orr, T. G.: Carcinoma of the colon, secondary to chronic ulcerative colitis. Amer. J. Dig. Dis. *15*:21-23, 1948.

31. Hayes, M. A.: Chronic ulcerative colitis and associated carcinoma. Amer. J. Surg. *77*:363-370, 1949.

32. Svartz, N., and Ernberg, T.: Cancer coli in cases of colitis ulcerosa. Acta Med. Scand. *135*:444-447, 1949.

33. Kasich, A. M., Weingarten, B., and Brown, M. L.: Malignant degeneration in ulcerative colitis. Med. Clin. N. Amer. *33*:1421-1437, 1949.

34. Sauer, W. G., and Bargen, J. A.: Chronic ulcerative colitis and carcinoma. J.A.M.A. *141*:982-986, 1949.

35. Warren, S., and Sommers, S. C.: Pathogenesis of ulcerative colitis. Amer. J. Path. *25*:657-679, 1949.

36. Strombeck, J. P.: Surgical treatment of ulcerative colitis. Acta Chir. Scand. *98*:414-427, 1949.

37. Lagercrantz, R.: Ulcerative colitis in children. Acta Paediat. (Suppl. 75) *37*:89-151, 1949.

38. Kapel, O.: Medical and modern treatment of chronic ulcerative colitis. Acta Med. Scand. *138*:328-340, 1950.

39. Rice-Oxley, J. M., and Truelove, S.: Complications of ulcerative colitis. Lancet *1*:607-611, 1950.

40. Sloan, W. P., Bergen, J. A., and Gage, R. P.: Life histories of patients with chronic ulcerative colitis: a review of 2000 cases. Gastroenterology *16*:25-38, 1950.

41. Lahey, F. H.: The management of ulcerative colitis. Postgrad. Med. *8*:93-100, 1950.

42. Gleckler, W. J., and Brown, C. H.: Carcinoma of the colon complicating chronic ulcerative colitis. Gastroenterology *14*:455-464, 1950.

43. Lyons, A. S., and Garlock, J. H.: The relationship of chronic ulcerative colitis to carcinoma. Gastroenterology *18*:170-178, 1951.

44. Kiefer, E. D., Eytinge, E. J., and Johnson, A. C.: Malignant degeneration in chronic ulcerative colitis. Gastroenterology *19*:51-57, 1951.

45. Counsell, P. B., and Dukes, C. E.: The association of chronic ulcerative colitis and carcinoma of rectum and colon. Brit. J. Surg. *39*:485-495, 1952.

46. Weckesser, E. C., and Chinn, A. B.: Carcinoma of the colon complicating chronic ulcerative colitis. J.A.M.A. *152*:905-908, 1953.

47. Wheelock, F. C., Jr., and Warren, R.: Ulcerative colitis. New Eng. J. Med. *252*:421-425, 1955.

48. Flood, C. A., Lepore, M. J., Hiatt, R. B., and Karush, A.: A prognosis in ulcerative colitis. J. Chronic Dis. *4:*267-282, 1956.
49. Bacon, H. E., Ouyang, L. M., Carroll, P. T., Cates, B. A., Villalba, G., and McGregor, R. A.: Nonspecific ulcerative colitis with references to mortality, morbidity, complications and long-term survivals following colectomy. Amer. J. Surg. *92:*688-695, 1956.
50. Thorlakson, R. H.: Chronic ulcerative colitis and carcinoma of the colon and rectum. Canad. J. Surg. *1:*218-225, 1958.
51. Maltby, E. J., Dickson, R. C., and O'Sullivan, P. M.: The use of ACTH and cortisone in idiopathic ulcerative colitis. Canada. Med. Ass. J. *74:*4–9, 1956.
52. Colcock, B. P., and Mathiesen, W. L.: Complications of the surgical treatment of chronic ulcerative colitis. A.M.A. Arch. Surg. *72:*399-404, 1956.
53. Hickey, R. C., and Tidrick, P. T.: Cancer in patients with chronic ulcerative colitis. Cancer *11:*35-39, 1958.
54. Dukes, C. E., and Lockhart-Mummery, H. E.: Practical points in the pathology and surgical treatment of ulcerative colitis: a critical review. Brit. J. Surg. *45:*25-36, 1957.
55. MacDougall, I. P. M.: Ulcerative colitis and carcinoma of large intestine. Brit. Med. J. *1:*852-854, 1954.
56. Bargen, J. A., Sauer, W. G., Sloan, W. P., and Gage, R. P.: Development of cancer in chronic ulcerative colitis. Gastroenterology *26:*32-37, 1954.
57. Slaney, G., and Brooke, B. N.: Cancer in ulcerative colitis. Lancet *2:*694-698, 1959.
58. Russell, I. S., and Hughes, S. R.: Carcinoma of the colon complicating ulcerative colitis. Aust. New Zeal. J. Surg. *30:*306-311, 1961.
59. White, M. E. E.: Cancer in ulcerative colitis. Brit. J. Clin. Pract. *16:*719-727, 1962.
60. Goldgraber, M. B., and Kirsner, J. B.: Polyps and carcinoma of the colon. Arch. Intern. Med. *100:*669-674, 1957.
61. Hinton, J. M.: Risk of malignant change in ulcerative colitis. Gut *7:*427-432, 1966.
62. Ascherman, S. W.: Carcinoma of the colon and rectum; review of 461 necropsy cases at Cook County Hospital from 1929 to 1952. A.M.A. Arch. Surg. *66:*208-217, 1953.
63. Tidrick, R. T., and Hickey, R. C.: The catastrophic complications of ulcerative colitis; cancer, perforation and massive bleeding. J. Iowa Med. Soc. *46:*485-492, 1956.
64. Thorlakson, R. H.: Carcinoma of the colon and rectum associated with chronic ulcerative colitis. Surg. Gynec. Obstet. *103:*41-50, 1956.
65. Rosenquist, H., Ohrling, H., Lagercrantz, R., and Edling, N.: Ulcerative colitis and carcinoma coli. Lancet *1:*906-908, 1959.
66. Edling, N. P., and Eklof, O.: Distribution of malignancy in ulcerative colitis. Gastroenterology *41:*465-466, 1961.
67. Yeomans, F. C.: Carcinomatous degeneration of rectal adenomas. Report of seven cases. J.A.M.A. *89:*852-854, 1927.
68. Turnbull, R. B., Jr., and Brown, C. H.: Carcinoma of the colon in chronic ulcerative colitis; report of two five year survivals. Cleveland Clin. Quart. *19:*166-170, 1952.
69. Felsen, J., and Wolarsky, W.: Chronic ulcerative colitis and carcinoma. Arch. Intern. Med. *84:*293-304, 1949.
70. Otani, S., and Snapper, I.: On the incidence of carcinoma in chronic ulcerative colitis. J. Mount Sinai Hosp. N. Y. *19:*275-288, 1952.
71. Gazzaniga, A. B., and Gazzaniga, D. A.: Carcinoma of the colon following chronic ulcerative colitis: report of two unusual cases in brothers. Dis. Colon Rectum *5:*437-443, 1962.
72. Galambos, J. T., Massey, B. W., Klayman, M. I., and Kirsner, J. B.: Exfoliative cytology in chronic ulcerative colitis. Cancer *9:*152–159, 1956.
73. Boddington, M. M., and Truelove, S. C.: Abnormal epithelial cells in ulcerative colitis. Brit. Med. J. *4979:*1318–1321, 1956.
74. Cornes, J. S., Smith, J. C., and Southwood, W. F.: Lymphosarcoma in chronic ulcerative colitis with report of two cases. Brit. J. Surg. *49:*50-53, 1961.
75. Sataline, L. R., Mobley, E. M., and Kirkham, W.: Ulcerative colitis complicated by colonic lymphoma. Gastroenterology *44:*342-347, 1963.
76. Magnes, M., and De Bell, P.: Carcinoma associated with terminal ileitis. J. Med. Soc. N.J. *66:*573-574, 1969.

Chapter Ten

Mixed Forms of Regional Enteritis and Ulcerative Colitis

Two thirds of the cases, approximately, of regional enteritis are limited to the small intestine and have the characteristic microscopic features described in preceding chapters. Similarly, at least three fourths of the cases of ulcerative colitis are limited to the large intestine and also have the characteristic morphologic features (Table 10-1). Their clinical features also have separate and distinct patterns. However, in addition to the majority of characteristic cases for each disease, there is another group that does not exclusively fit into either category. The percentage of patients who are classified in the latter group varies in the several large studies.

To be viewed rationally, the group must be subdivided into at least four categories: (1) the ulcerative colitis type of inflammatory process with "backwash" extending into the ileum, (2) the regional enteritis type of granulomatous inflammation involving the colon with or without small intestinal lesions, (3) coexistent regional enteritis and ulcerative colitis types of inflammatory process in one individual, and (4) inflammations of the small or large intestines with insufficient distinctive features for the diagnosis of either or both diseases.

Descriptions of the first two of these categories have been presented in Chapters Four and Five. Little needs to be added here except to emphasize the existence of the overlap of the anatomic site of the two diseases and the constancy of microscopic features irrespective of organ involvement.[1,2,3] Table 10-2 summarizes in a general way the data on the distribution of the two diseases from several reports. The frequency of involvement of a portion of the bowel is recorded on a scale from 0 to 4 plus.

The ulcerative colitis inflammatory process has lesions that are

236

TABLE 10–1   Regional Enteritis and Ulcerative Colitis Compared

	Regional Enteritis	Ulcerative Colitis
Natural History		
Occurrence in animals	pigs, dogs	none
Occurrence in humans	worldwide	worldwide
Incidence (U.K. & N. Amer. gen. white)	0.8–1.8 cases per 100,000	4.6–6.5 cases per 100,000
(non-white)	? less in Am. negro	? less in non-white
(Jews)	9× higher than general white	2–4× higher than general white
Prevalence	9 cases/100,000	80 cases/100,000
Male to female ratio	1:1	1:1.3–1.5
Familial occurrence	1–2% of cases	1–2% of cases
Age at onset	15–55 equal rate	peaks 20–40 and 65
Annual death rate (U.K. & N. Amer. white)	0.08–0.11 deaths per 100,000	0.05–0.9 deaths per 100,000
Etiology	unknown	unknown
Macroscopic Features		
Distribution of lesions	1. stomach to anus 2. principally terminal ileum and cecum 3. discontinuous lesions	1. ileum to anus 2. principally rectosigmoid 3. continuous lesions
Length of diseased organ	unchanged	decreased
Diameter of diseased organ	decreased	unchanged
Thickness of bowel wall	markedly increased	unchanged
Ulceration	yes	yes
Vascular congestion	yes	yes
Muscular hypertrophy	usually	sometimes
Serosal changes	yes	no
Ileocecal valve	constricted	loose, patulous
Mesentery	short, thick, indurated	unchanged
Adhesions	frequent	rare
Fistulas	common	uncommon
Carcinomatous change	rare	frequent (2–5% of cases)
Microscopic Features		
Inflammation distribution	all layers	mucosa and submucosa
Ulcers	deep clefts	shallow
Mucin production	normal or increased	normal or decreased
Mast cell infiltrate	minimal	increased
Lymphocytosis	extreme	extreme
Histiocytic proliferation	extensive	none
Collagen production	extensive	scanty if any
Crypt abscesses	rare	common
Pseudopolyps	absent	common
Lymphangitis	early obliterative	none
Lymph node hyperplasia	moderate	moderate
Lymph node granulomas	present	absent
Extraintestinal Lesions		
Liver granulomata	present	absent
Sclerosing cholangitis	rare	frequent
Erythema nodosum	occasional	occasional
Arthritis (nonspecific)	3–10% of cases	25% of cases
Spondylitis	2% of cases	2% of cases
Amyloidosis	rare	rare

TABLE 10–2   Distribution of Lesions in the Bowel

	Regional Enteritis	Ulcerative Colitis
Stomach	±	0
Duodenum	1+	0
Jejunum	2+	0
Ileum	4+	1+
Cecum	3+	2+
Ascending colon	2+	3+
Transverse colon	±	4+
Descending colon	±	4+
Rectosigmoid colon	0	4+

continuous, the rectosigmoid region being the location of principal involvement. Only a small proportion of patients have ascending colonic lesions, and even fewer (10 to 25 per cent in various studies) have "backwash" lesions in the terminal ileum. "Skip lesions" are not found in the small intestine. In contrast to this, the granulomatous inflammatory lesions of regional enteritis may be found anywhere in the intestinal tract from the stomach to the anus. The lesions are usually discontinuous. The greatest frequency is in the terminal ileum, with a

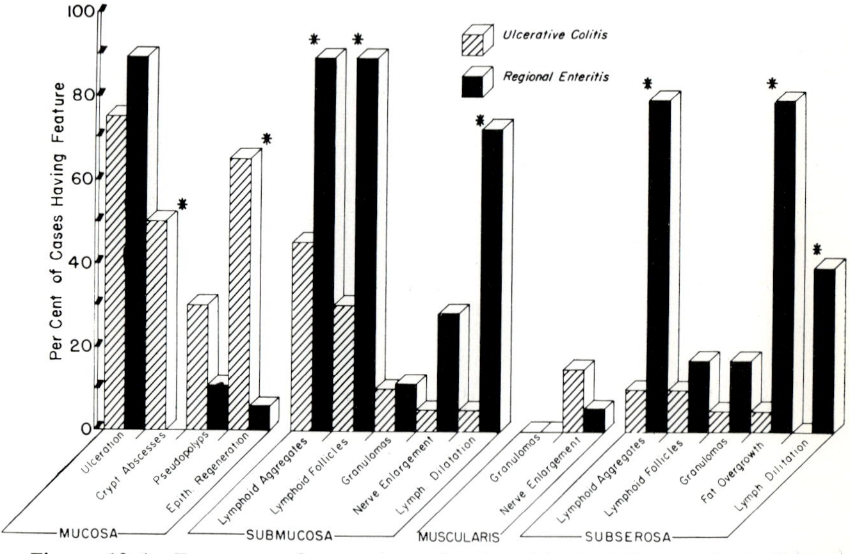

Figure 10–1   Frequency of occurrence of various histologic features in the ileum in ulcerative colitis and in regional enteritis. Note the difference in the pattern of the two diseases, ulcerative colitis resulting primarily in mucosal changes, and regional enteritis in submucosal and subserosal changes. The asterisks indicate statistically significant differences in frequency of occurrence ($\chi^2 > 3.84$; $p < 0.05$; Yates' adjustment[2] for continuity as necessary). (W.U. Ill. #62-8953). (Courtesy of S. L. Saltzstein and B. F. Rosenberg, Amer. J. Clin. Path. *40*:610–623, © 1963, and The Williams & Wilkins Co., Baltimore, Md.)

decreasing incidence as one proceeds proximally and distally from the ileocecal valve.

Figures 10-1 and 10-2 compare the histologic features of regional enteritis and ulcerative colitis in the large and small intestines. It is apparent from these graphs that regional enteritis is transmural in both the ileum and colon (length of dark bars). In contrast, ulcerative colitis inflammatory changes (light bars) are predominantly mucosal. Comparison of individual histologic features such as crypt abscesses, granulomas, and pseudopolyposis reveal extreme discordance as well. Irrespective of the organ involved, the morphologic features of each process remain unchanged.

In addition to the overlap of anatomic site already noted, in a small percentage of patients both diseases definitely exist either simultaneously or in sequence. Yarnis reviewed 654 cases of regional enteritis from his own experience and found 54 cases (8 per cent) had ulcerative colitis also.[4] In 38 instances both diseases were present when the patient was first seen. In 16 cases one of the diseases developed after treatment for the other. The sex distribution of the patients was about

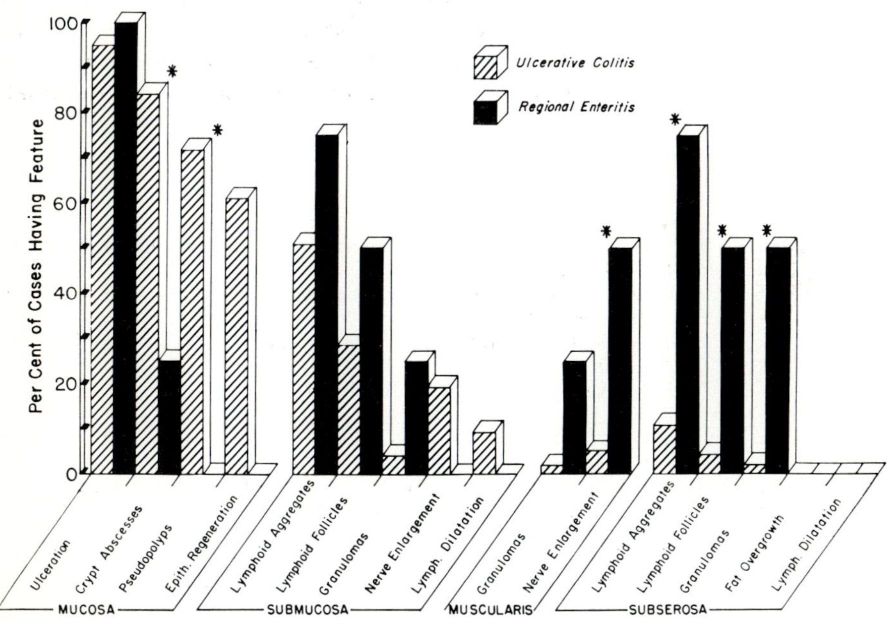

Figure 10–2   Frequency of occurrence of various histologic features in the colon in ulcerative colitis and in regional enteritis. Note the difference in the pattern of the two diseases, ulcerative colitis resulting primarily in mucosal changes, and regional enteritis in submucosal and subserosal changes. The asterisks indicate statistically significant differences in frequency of occurrence ($\chi^2 > 3.84$; $p < 0.05$; Yates' adjustment[2] for continuity as necessary). (W.U. Ill. #62-8953). (Courtesy of S. L. Saltzstein and B. F. Rosenberg, Amer. J. Clin. Path. *40*:610–623, © 1963, and The Williams and Wilkins Co., Baltimore, Md.)

equal, but almost 80 per cent were young (10 to 30 years). The anatomic distribution of the lesions encompassed the same sites commonly involved with either disease. The coexistence of regional enteritis and ulcerative colitis did not occur in the experience of others.[5, 6] In my own experience, I have reviewed several cases that simultaneously had the distinctive features of both diseases. However, in these cases the regional enteritis lesion predominated, whereas the ulcerative colitis changes were minimal.

The last category to be considered comprises the indeterminate cases. Pathologists who are familiar with the morphologic features of intestinal inflammatory diseases generally agree that less than 5 per cent of the cases are indeterminate. Undiagnosed specimens remain either because of (1) superficial observation or insufficient sampling resulting in inadequate assessment of the principal features; (2) examination of the process prior to the development of its characteristic features; (3) insufficient awareness of the features of intestinal diseases, or (4) a combination of these factors. Any one sample of bowel or single microscopic slide may reveal sufficient features to permit definitive diagnosis. More often it will be indeterminate or, worse, misleading. As emphasized in Chapter Three, numerous microscopic slides must be made from appropriate sites of the entire specimen if accurate interpretation is to follow. Inflammatory intestinal disease requires as extensive and thorough a work-up as neoplastic disease. When this is done the number of indeterminate cases will be minimal.

References

1. Warren, S., and Sommers, S. C.: Pathology of regional ileitis and ulcerative colitis. J.A.M.A. *154*:189–193, 1954.
2. Otani, S.: Pathology of regional enteritis and regional enterocolitis. J. Mount Sinai Hosp. N. Y. *22*:147–158, 1955.
3. Reeves, B. F., Carlson, H. C., and Dockerty, M. B.: Segmental ulcerative colitis versus segmental Crohn's disease of the colon. Amer. J. Roentgen. *99*:24–34, 1967.
4. Yarnis, H.: The syndrome of combined ileocolitis. J. Mount Sinai Hosp. N.Y. *22*:159–169, 1955.
5. Lockhart-Mummery, H. E., and Morson, B. C.: Crohn's disease of the large intestine and its distinction from ulcerative colitis. Gut *1*:87–105, 1960.
6. Saltzstein, S. L., and Rosenberg, B. F.: Ulcerative colitis of the ileum, and regional enteritis of the colon. Amer. J. Clin. Path. *40*:610–623, 1963.

INDEX